Psychology Revivals

Experiments in Personality Volume I

Originally published in 1960 these two volumes report a number of experiments in psychogenetics, psychopharmacology, psychodiagnostics, psychometrics and psychodynamics, all of which formed part of the programme of research which had been developing from the late 1940s at the Maudsley Hospital. Presenting the studies together in a book, rather than the more usual route of journal articles, was itself felt to be an experiment at the time, especially given the wide area covered. The decision was deliberate because all the studies reported formed part of a larger whole, which would have been lost if published separately.

Volume I looks at psychogenetics and psychopharmacology.

Experiments in Personality
Volume I

Psychogenetics and psychopharmacology

Edited by
H.J. Eysenck

Routledge
Taylor & Francis Group
LONDON AND NEW YORK

First published in 1960
by Routledge & Kegan Paul Ltd

This edition first published in 2013 by Routledge
27 Church Road, Hove, BN3 2FA

Simultaneously published in the USA and Canada
by Routledge
711 Third Avenue, New York, NY 10017

Routledge is an imprint of the Taylor & Francis Group, an informa business

Publisher's Note
The publisher has gone to great lengths to ensure the quality of this reprint but points out that some imperfections in the original copies may be apparent.

Disclaimer
The publisher has made every effort to trace copyright holders and welcomes correspondence from those they have been unable to contact.

A Library of Congress record exists under LC control no.: 61002085

ISBN: 978-0-415-84243-3 (hbk)
ISBN: 978-0-203-75925-7 (ebk)

EXPERIMENTS IN PERSONALITY

Volume I

PSYCHOGENETICS

AND

PSYCHOPHARMACOLOGY

Contributors

P. L. BROADHURST
Senior Lecturer in Psychology, Institute of Psychiatry

H. J. EYSENCK
Professor of Psychology, Institute of Psychiatry

S. B. G. EYSENCK
Research Associate, Institute of Psychiatry

H. C. HOLLAND
Research Associate, Institute of Psychiatry

IRENE MARTIN
Research Associate, Institute of Psychiatry

EMER TREADWELL
Research Associate, Institute of Psychiatry

R. A. WILLETT
Lecturer in Psychology, Institute of Psychiatry

EXPERIMENTS IN PERSONALITY

Edited by

H. J. EYSENCK, Ph.D.

Professor of Psychology, University of London; Director, Psychological Laboratories, Institute of Psychiatry; Psychologist, Maudsley and Bethlem Royal Hospitals

Volume I

PSYCHOGENETICS AND PSYCHOPHARMACOLOGY

London

ROUTLEDGE & KEGAN PAUL

First published 1960
by Routledge & Kegan Paul Ltd
Broadway House, Carter Lane, E.C.4

Printed in Great Britain
By Butler & Tanner Ltd
Frome and London

It is comfortable to me to find that experiment need not quail before mathematics, but is quite competent to rival it in discovery.

MICHAEL FARADAY

CONTENTS

EDITOR'S INTRODUCTION

IN this book are reported a number of experiments in psychogenetics, psychopharmacology, psychodiagnostics, psychometrics and psychodynamics, all of which form part of the programme of research which has been developing during the past dozen years or so here at the Maudsley Hospital. In itself, such a publication may be regarded as an experiment, written as it is by eleven different people, and covering a very wide area; the more usual method of publication would have been in the appropriate journals of psychology, genetics, psychiatry, statistics, or pharmacology. There are, of course, good reasons why the present course of action was preferred.

In the first place, all the studies reported form part of a larger whole; the programme of research referred to above has a unity which would easily be lost by piecemeal publication in separate journals. This is particularly true when several different disciplines are concerned; geneticists seldom read psychological journals, or pharmacologists statistical ones! Yet our work has touched upon all these varied fields, and no account would do justice to the general theory or set of theories under investigation, which confined itself to only one corner of the evidence. The dividing lines between the biological sciences are arbitrary, but they influence people's reading and thought habits very profoundly; we wished to break down some of these barriers, and publication in this form appeared the best way of achieving this aim.

In the second place, the publication policy of modern journals has become more and more rigid. Articles are required to fit a Procrustes bed—usually a short one!—and anything requiring a somewhat lengthy theoretical introduction, or an extensive discussion, is frowned upon. Few of the studies here reported could have fitted at all easily into the confines of the usual journal article, and consequently we decided on a somewhat novel and unusual form of publication. Monograph publication would of course have been one possible way out, but as the reader can obtain these two volumes for the price of two or three monographs there seemed to be solid economic arguments against this particular solution.

In the third place, it is now ten years since the Institute of Psychiatry was founded as a part of the University of London, and with it the Department of Psychology; some gesture of celebration seemed appropriate, and in view of the concentration of efforts by members of its department on *research*, a kind of *Festschrift* reporting the latest results of such research was thought to be acceptable.

In any case, there is one good precedent for such a venture, namely the publication some twenty years ago of Murray's *Explorations in Personality*; he also, and for not altogether dissimilar reasons to ours, preferred publication in book form to the dissemination of his and his colleagues' work in article form through the journals. The similarity (as well as the difference!) in the title is not accidental; our approach differs in many fundamental ways from Murray's, and a brief discussion of these differences may aid in understanding the lines along which our work has been developing.

It has always been my contention that the study of personality is not in principle different from the scientific investigation of other parts and aspects of nature; John Stuart Mill once put this point very well when he said: 'If there are some subjects on which the results obtained have finally received the unanimous assent of all who have attended to the proof, and others on which mankind have not yet been equally successful; on which the most sagacious minds have occupied themselves from the earliest date, and have never succeeded in establishing any considerable body of truths, so as to be beyond denial or doubt; it is by generalizing the methods successfully followed in the former enquiries, and adapting them to the latter, that we may hope to remove this blot on the face of science.'

Essentially, as I have argued before, this method of choice in the investigation of natural phenomena is the so-called *hypothetico-deductive* method. According to it, the available observations, facts, and experimental data in a given field are combined in the form of a theory which has two functions: it is capable of accounting for all the known facts, and it is capable of pointing to new facts which, while unknown at the time when the theory was formulated, can be discovered by appropriate experiments. Such further experiments support or infirm the theory, which may if necessary be modified, or replaced altogether by a new theory. If possible, the statement of the theory, and the deductions made from it, should be in quantitative form, as this tremendously increases the power of the theory, and also makes it easier to disprove it experimentally. A theory which does not lead to testable deductions cannot be disproved, and is consequently worthless; it 'accounts' for everything and predicts nothing.

All this, of course, is simply a restatement of some of the widely agreed principles of scientific method which can be found discussed in detail in most text-books of logic. I have no hesitation in stating that I believe that these principles apply as much to psychology, and to the study of personality, as they do to physics. I also believe, however, that there is much misunderstanding, particularly among psychologists, of the interpretation of these principles in actual practice; in particular, I believe that many people fail to understand the differences between *strong theories* and *weak theories* in science. As this is a crucial point in research methodology, a brief discussion of it will be given at the end of this book, in an Epilogue entitled: 'The Place of Theory in Psychology' (Vol. II).

In a sense, this book is the sequel to *Dynamics of Anxiety and Hysteria*, just as *The Scientific Study of Personality* was the sequel to *Dimensions of Personality*; in each case the later book has taken up theories elaborated in the earlier one and developed them experimentally in a more decisive fashion than had been possible before. Knowledge of these earlier books, while an advantage in reading the present one, is not essential; brief accounts of previous experiments and the theories underlying them are given wherever necessary. Knowledge of statistical methodology is indispensable for obtaining a full understanding of all the details, but the reader who is willing to take the mathematics on trust will not find it impossible to obtain an idea of the experimental methodology and the main conclusions by means of some judicious skipping.

Acknowledgement is due to the following publishers, authors and editors for permission to quote and reproduce figures from copyrighted works in this part:

American Psychological Association and R. B. Cattell for an excerpt from the *Journal of Abnormal and Social Psychology*.

C. Burt for an excerpt from the *British Journal of Statistical Psychology* (C. Burt, Editor).

Harper Bros. and P. R. David for an excerpt from *Social Psychology at the Crossroads* (1951).

B. I. Hayman for an excerpt and a figure from *Genetics* (C. P. Oliver and W. S. Stone, Editors) and for an excerpt from *Biometrics* (R. A. Bradley, Editor).

J. L. Jinks and J. A. Nelder for excerpts and figures from *Heredity* (K. Mather, Editor).

Methuen and Co. and K. Mather for an excerpt and figures from *Biometrical Genetics* (1949).

Princeton University Press and S. A. Stouffer for an excerpt from *Studies in Social Psychology in World War II*, Vol. IV (1950).

J. P. Scott for an excerpt from *Physiological Zoology* (T. Park, Editor).

In carrying out the experiments here recounted, we were aided by grants from the M.R.C., the Ford Foundation, the Wallace Laboratories, Ciba, the U.S. Army and the Maudsley and Bethlem Royal

Research Fund. Our thanks to these bodies are acknowledged in the appropriate places. Neither they nor the editor, the co-authors, psychiatric colleagues at the Maudsley Hospital, the Board of Control, the Ministry of Health, nor Uncle Tom Cobley are to be held responsible for, or committed by, anything written by any of the authors; such responsibility rests entirely upon the individual contributors!

H. J. EYSENCK

Maudsley Hospital,
1st May 1960

PART ONE

Experiments in Psychogenetics

APPLICATIONS OF BIOMETRICAL GENETICS TO THE INHERITANCE OF BEHAVIOUR

P. L. Broadhurst

1

INTRODUCTION[1]

WHAT follows is an account of a programme of work in the psychogenetics[2] of some aspects of emotional behaviour in the rat, begun in 1954 and still in progress. While the intention has been to make it complete in itself, reference to related investigations published elsewhere will be necessary from time to time. However, the main body of the purely psychogenetical work has not been previously discussed, except in preliminary reports (Broadhurst, 1958d, 1959), and the present account covers the work up to December 1958. It is written

[1] I am deeply grateful to Prof. H. J. Eysenck for infecting me with his enthusiasm for this field of research, and for his unstinting encouragement and assistance.

My thanks are due to Messrs. A. S. C. Ehrenberg, P. Slater, and W. L. B. Nixon for statistical advice and assistance, to Mr. R. G. F. Pretty, and to his successor as animal technician, Mr. K. B. Wraight, for their careful husbandry of the several thousand subjects, and to Miss S. B. Parsons for computational help.

Those familiar with the analytical techniques here employed will at once recognize the extent of my indebtedness to Prof. K. Mather and his colleagues from the Genetics Department at Birmingham University, Drs. J. L. Jinks, E. L. Breese, B. I. Hayman and Mr. R. Morley Jones, who introduced me to the methods of biometrical genetics. I owe an especial debt of gratitude to Dr. Jinks, whose advice and assistance have been generously given on a number of occasions. My understanding of the genetical concepts involved has also benefited from conversations with Prof. C. D. Darlington, Dr. D. S. Falconer, and Prof. H. Grüneberg. None of the abovementioned, however, may be blamed for misunderstandings doubtless still evident.

The financial assistance provided by the Ford Foundation is gratefully acknowledged.

[2] This term, which is a convenient shorthand for 'psychological genetics', is preferred to the term 'behaviour genetics' which appears to be gaining currency, the latter seeming unduly restrictive in its suggestion of emphasis on behavioural responses observed in animals. The analogous term 'psychopharmacology' is now well understood and does not carry this restriction. More preferable than 'psychogenetics', perhaps, would have been the term 'genetical psychology', were it not for the risk of confusion with 'genetic psychology'. The adjective 'genetic', invented by psychologists to mean 'ontogenetic' or 'developmental' only, was taken over by geneticists early in the century (Kalmus, 1955) and its original meaning has become obscured.

for psychologists, so that a knowledge of statistical procedures is assumed, but none of genetics beyond simple Mendelian formulations. Accordingly an attempt will be made, as it becomes necessary, to sketch the main principles of the methods of biometrical genetics which are used. This, however, can be no substitute for the detailed consideration by interested readers of the assumptions, methods and controversies of biometrical genetics, some of which may be sampled in the references given.

SURVEY OF PSYCHOGENETICS

The pioneer work in this field of behaviour study, as in so many others, is due to the genius of Sir Francis Galton. His studies on the inheritance of mental capacities, begun in 1869 and including the significant contribution of the twin-study method, initiated an interest in this field which has rarely lost momentum since. It is not the present intention to dwell on the efforts to assess the size and nature of the genetical influence on human behaviour, but rather to evaluate the contribution that experimental work using animal subjects has made. But in passing it should be noted that progress in the former, real though it has been, still leaves much to be desired. Thus Cattell, whose recent work using multiple variance analysis (1953, 1959a, 1959b; Cattell, Blewett, and Beloff, 1955) represents a methodological advance in this field on the earlier use of the twin study and familial correlation methods independently of each other, writes as follows: 'No argument is necessary to convince the scientific psychologist that personality theory, clinical psychology, and learning theory are bereft of knowledge of about half of the influences at work, in the absence of an understanding of heredity. All learning and adjustment is limited by inherent properties of the organism. Only the unintelligent or the uninformed clinician or educator practices individual guidance without estimating what degree of difficulty a given adjustment or performance offers a particular personality. The general laws of psychology, explaining the genesis of abilities, temperament, and dynamic traits, need also to be more concerned with maturational trends, innate dispositional rigidities, and the effects due to hereditary limits' (Cattell, Stice, and Christy, 1957, p. 143).

But in turning to the animal field, which is an essentially more tractable one for experimental psychogenetics, because of the availability of genetically pure lines, and the control possible over mating, enabling the formation of others, it must be confessed that the situation is only slightly better. Apart from a few significant exceptions in the last decade, it is still possible to agree with Stone when he wrote: 'To many of us who have worked for a long time in the field of comparative psychology it is a matter of shame and regret that only an amateurish beginning has yet been made by psychologists in the utilization of pure lines of animals in fundamental research in the nature-nurture area' (1947, p. 344).

Methods of comparative psychogenetics

Psychological authorities are agreed that there are two main approaches to the study of the inherited determinants of behaviour in animal subjects (Stone, 1947; Hall, 1951; Russell, 1953a). The first is by selection and the second by the analysis of the characteristics displayed by different, preferably pure, strains. In a sense these methods are complementary; the object of the first, selective breeding, is to establish lines which differ in the behavioural characteristics for which they have been selected. The fact that such selection is possible is strong presumptive evidence that the characteristic in question has some hereditary determination. The second method employs established strains, ones selected originally for differences other than those in which a psychologist is interested, such as coat-colour, tumour susceptibility, etc. The criterion for purity of strain in mammals is usually taken as twenty consecutive generations of mating brother with sister (though see Carpenter, Grüneberg, and Russell, 1957; Biggers, McLaren, and Michie, 1958) and can be checked by tissue transplants (Billingham, and Silvers, 1959). Again, the fact of differences between different genetically pure strains is presumptive evidence of the influence of heredity upon behaviour.

The end point reached by the use of both methods is the same—its purpose is, or should be, to arrive at a position from which a genetical analysis can commence using the standard procedures of, for example, cross-breeding with pure strains and the analysis of heritability from selectively bred ones. Both these methods have been employed in the present work.

Strain differences

The use of different strains, particularly of rats and mice, has long been a favourite method of psychogenetics. Bagg was a pioneer in the application of 'the methods of genetics to the study of conduct'. He found strain differences between strains of mice in various learning situations (1916, 1920). The Yerkes, (1913, 1916) and Utsurikawa (1917) compared pure and outbred strains of rats, the latter noting that individual differences exceed strain differences. Sadovnikova-Koltzova crossed albino with wild grey rats and studied the first and second generations of offspring of this cross by means of the Hampton Court maze (1926), publishing further papers later (1928, 1929, 1931, 1933).

The studies on mice of Vicari (1929) and Dawson (1932) show more genetical sophistication but are deficient psychologically. The maze performance measures as used by Vicari are unnecessarily complicated characteristics for study, and it is not surprising that her analyses of three crosses from among four inbred strains did little to clarify the genetics of maze learning, especially since one of her strains, 'waltzer' mutant, is now known to be complex genetically (Grüneberg, 1952). Dawson used as a measure of 'tameness' the speed of unrewarded running in a straight alley, a test which bristles with difficulties to administer and interpret, but for which he claims a reliability of 0·92. He used the standard type of Mendelian analysis with mammals by crossing the parental strains, usually designated P_1 and P_2, to produce a first filial or hybrid generation (F_1), a second filial generation bred from the first (F_2), and then making the backcrosses from F_1 to the P_1 and the P_2–B_1 and B_2 respectively. He does not specify the degree of genetical homogeneity (homozygosity) of the four strains—three tame and one wild—which he used, thus rendering only tentative his conclusions that wildness is determined by a few genes which are dominant and which have no linkage for sex, or for any of the five genes which he knew to be carried by his strains. That this absence of linkage is probably true for one of the genes, 'short ear', has recently been confirmed (Bundy, 1950).

The tendency of young rats to climb up an inclined plane (negative geotropism) has been the subject of a series of studies by Crozier and Pincus (see Munn, 1950, pp. 44 ff., for a review of this work, and the controversy over the nature of the behaviour observed). The main papers of psychogenetic interest are Crozier and Pincus, 1931–2a, 1931–2b, 1931–2c, 1935, 1936. They found that different strains of rats varied in the angle taken up on the inclined plane in response to variations in the angle from the horizontal of the plane itself. Crosses between two of the strains were bred, and backcrosses made to each parental line in turn. The F_1 showed a pattern of geotropic behaviour which was interpreted as hybrid vigour (heterosis) affecting the rear limbs only and giving disproportionate development. The absence of this in the geotropic behaviour of adults of the cross was taken as confirming the hypothesis. Separate consideration is given to each backcross (Crozier and Pincus, 1931–2c, 1936), and despite the very small numbers used it is claimed that the dominance of the genes from one strain can be shown.

Herter (1936) found that strains of mice differed in their preferred floor temperature. By means of F_1's and backcrosses to a wild strain he was able to identify the important determining factor as the density of the belly fur (Herter, 1938; Herter and Sgonina, 1938).

While observations relating to differences between strains of unspecified degrees of genetical purity are still encountered (Schaefer, 1959; Myers, 1959), the post-World War II work on the inheritance of behaviour has concentrated on the use of the inbred strains of rats, and, more especially, mice, which are now available (Staats, 1958). The volume of work on these two species allows a consideration of it topic by topic.

The hereditary determinants of *audiogenic seizures* have been investigated by several workers; their findings are reviewed by Finger (1947) and Bevan (1955). An hypothesis of multifactorial genetical control seems to fit the experimental data rather better than those suggesting one- or two-gene action.

Strain differences in respect of the *hoarding* of food by mice were found by Smith and Powell (1955), and confirmed for rats by Stamm (1954, 1955) who attempted a genetical analysis using three pure-bred lines of different coat-colours. He obtained an F_1 from two of the strains and backcrossed to only one of them (1956). The results did not enable him to specify a genetical mechanism for the hereditary effects disclosed.

The influence of inheritance on *emotional responses* in five strains of rats, which included the three used by Stamm, was confirmed by Broadhurst (1958b), and these findings will be discussed in Chapter 4. Lindzey (1951) had previously shown the same effect with five inbred strains of mice.

Such strains of mice (Carter *et al. mult*., 1952) have been used with good effect in the study of *activity*. Thompson's paper (1953b), employing fifteen of them in three behavioural situations, set a new standard in this field. He went on to confirm the findings on exploratory activity in five strains (1956), two of which had not been used in the previous study. A suggestive parallel exists between Thompson's ordering of these strains in activity and that determined by the thyroid output measured in some of them (Amin, Chai, and Reineke, 1957). The relationship suggests that the higher the output the greater the amount of exploration. The genetical analysis proceeded with the breeding of F_1's (Thompson, 1954), F_2's and backcrosses to the two showing the highest and the lowest activity (Thompson and Fuller, 1957, 1960). This is the most complete analysis of this trait yet reported, and the results are of extreme interest. The heritability, or 'nature/nurture ratio', a measure of the extent to which the character observed is under genetical control, gives a value around 60%, the rest being non-genetical or environmental. An estimate of the number of genes involved is four or more, and there is some suggestion of dominance for those determining higher activity. The use of two somewhat different situations for measuring the activity allows the additional conclusion that the description of a genetical mechanism is in part dependent upon the way it is measured.

McClearn (1959) has also investigated the psychogenetics of exploratory activity in the mouse, on a somewhat broader basis, using four different tests of exploratory behaviour in novel situations, and six mouse strains. Thompson's earlier findings were supported, and an F_1 cross of the two extreme strains, though not, unfortunately, the same strains as in Thompson and Fuller's study, gave results which suggested that the trait as measured is determined multifactorially. The question of exploratory activity in the rat will receive further attention later; that it is subject to hereditary determination has again been confirmed by Carr and Williams (1957), using three strains of rats, one of which has the same origin as the No. 4 in the present studies (see Table 4.4).

Differences in *learning ability* have been surprisingly little investigated. McClearn (1958) found differences in three strains of inbred mice, as did Denenberg (1959) in two sub-lines separated reproductively for some thirty generations. A control for aspects of the post-natal environment did not reveal any important effect attributable to different laboratory conditions. King and Mavromatis (1956) observed differences in the rate of learning an escape-avoidance habit between two inbred strains of mice. Subsequent conflict, induced by electrifying their water supply, modified their relative standing on re-learning. The authors were unable to exclude differences in emotional responsiveness, which seem probable in view of Fredericson's (1953) demonstration of differences in exploration in these strains. King (1958) has studied two sub-species of deer-mice which show innate differences in wildness which is as yet uncomplicated by the selection inseparable from domestication. The reaction to handling in infancy was shown (King and Deshaies, 1959; King and Eleftheriou, 1959) to be different as between the two sub-species and judged to be under genetical control.

Dietary *preferences* in rodents have received renewed attention recently. The work of Williams, Berry, and Beerstecher (1949), Reed (1951) and Mardones, Segovia, and Hederra (1950, 1953) suggested an hereditary influence on inter-strain and even individual differences in the voluntary intake of alcohol. McClearn and Rodgers (1959) surveyed six inbred strains of mice and found one which showed a marked preference for alcohol over water. These were crossed with a strain not displaying this preference and F_1, F_2 and backcross populations bred (Rodgers and McClearn, 1959). Nachman (1959) has investigated the preference of rats for saccharin.

Genetical differences in the *social*, especially *aggressive*, *behaviour* of mice have been extensively reported on by Scott (1940, 1942; Scott and Fredericson, 1951) and others. He showed that three pure-bred strains gave characteristically different patterns of reaction to aggression, and Ginsburg and Allee (1942) confirmed these differences, as did Fredericson, Story, Gurney and Butterworth (1955). Doner, Inman, and Davis (1952) showed that they can be modified by training, and Calhoun (1950) that the differences determined the pattern of social relations of different strains in identical environments, in which the mice were free to range for food. Bauer's (1956) factorial experiment again confirmed the differences and showed that they interact with experiential variables.

The *susceptibility* of different strains of rats to tuberculosis has been linked with behavioural differences by Tobach and Bloch (1955), and

Bendig and Braun (1951) showed, by breeding an F_1 and a backcross, that the retention of a maze habit after electroconvulsive shock is an inherited difference as between an albino and a black-hooded strain. The possibility of investigating differences in sexual potency in the mouse by observing the number of coloured and albino offspring when such males are both mated with albino females has been explored by Levine (1958), who only partly confirmed the previous findings of King (1929) on rats.

Studies using comparable homozygous lines of other species than the rat or mouse for behavioural research are not numerous. Valenstein, Riss, and Young (1954, 1955; Young, 1957) studied the sex drive in inbred and heterogeneous strains of guinea pigs, and found the latter more variable. They suggest that the pattern of mating may be under genetical control, which conclusion receives support from studies on a series of crosses between two inbred strains maintained at the University of Kansas. Filial and backcross generations were bred and the sexual behaviour of both males and spayed females studied. The oestrous behaviour of the latter was observed in response to hormonal injections (Goy and Young, 1957b). These important Kansas studies are among the most complete genetical analyses of a behavioural difference between two strains and present evidence on the mode of inheritance of several components of the behaviour of each sex. Among males (Jakway, 1959) a dominance of the less active strain's behaviour pattern in respect of preliminary sexual behaviour contrasts with some dominance of the more active strain's scores for intromission and ejaculation, but in neither case is the dominance complete. Females (Goy and Jakway, 1959) show a complex pattern of inheritance of mating behaviour, in which some elements are correlated and others operate independently, both of each other and of the environment (Goy and Young, 1957a).

Use of inbred rabbits has shown strain differences in another aspect of reproductive behaviour, maternal care (Sawin and Curran, 1952; Sawin and Crary, 1953; Denenberg, Sawin, Frommer, and Ross, 1958; Denenberg, Petropolus, Sawin, and Ross, 1959), but earlier work appears to have been confined to the study of crosses between wild and domesticated strains (Zimmerman, 1916; Wilson, 1936; Nachtsheim, 1941), and is reviewed by Robinson (1958, pp. 402–6).

Mating behaviour has also been studied in two species of fish (swordtails and platyfish) which share the same habitat (Clark, Aronson and Gordon, 1954). Interspecific crosses were made in aquarium populations and F_1's, F_2's and some backcrosses bred. The analysis of several measures of copulatory behaviour did not reveal any definite pattern, and it was concluded that many different genes were involved in its determination.

Using a very different species, the fruit fly, *Drosophila melanogaster*, Scott (1943) showed that a single gene difference between otherwise homozygous strains of fruit fly could affect behaviour, and Bastock (1956) has shown that the pattern of courtship behaviour (Bastock and Manning, 1955) is radically altered in yellow mutant males, and is attributable to this single gene difference. A multiple (pleitropic) effect of this gene upon behaviour is suggested. Comparable behaviour differences in other insects are probably observable (Von Hörrmann-Heck, 1957) and may sometimes be related to biochemical differences (Gösswald and Schmidt, 1959) analogous to those studied in humans (Harris, 1959). Caspari reviews the effects of gene differences on behaviour in insects (1958, pp. 112–15).

The facility with which the genotype of the fruit fly can be manipulated—by crossing the many well-established homozygous mutant strains—has been put to good account by Hirsch (1959) to construct populations with known chromosomal differences. These have been related to differences between such populations in geotaxis, and the way opened for an analysis of the genetical contribution to individual differences in behaviour.

Observations on the genetical determinants of behaviour in birds have frequently been made in the field, with all the difficulties attendant upon such work. Nevertheless, Leopold (1944) traced the inheritance of wildness in turkeys by following the fate of colonies released to make up the wild population, and studies of sub-species of birds (for example, Blanchard, 1941; Wolfson, 1942; Howell, 1953) have provided evidence on the genetical control, via the endocrine glands, of migration.

Phillips (1912) crossed two species of ducks of varying degrees of wildness and showed heritable effects, and Lorenz (1958) has shown that such hybridization may lead to the suppression of some parental traits in courtship behaviour, or to the exposure of some not seen in either parent. He suggests that 'motor patterns are dependent on comparatively simple constellations of genetic factors' (p. 78). This view is not shared by Hinde, who has discussed the role of the species-specific behaviour in evolution (1959; Hinde and Tinbergen, 1958) and contributed to its experimental study by crosses between three species of finches (1956a, 1956b). He found that the hybrids were generally intermediate in the behaviour studied, whereas Dilger's (1959) study of two species of parrot which differ in the way they carry nesting material showed that the hybrids only successfully employed one method. Metfessel (1940) investigated the inheritance of patterns of song in canaries by rearing them in isolation. The spread across Britain of a new habit among greenfinches of feeding on the fruit of a particular garden shrub (Pettersson, 1956, 1959) may be partly genetically determined, but this is rendered unlikely by the similar spread of a feeding habit among tits (Fisher and Hinde, 1949), this time of opening milk bottles on doorsteps, which is not confined to the one species. Wood-Gush (1959; Wood-Gush and Osborne, 1956) has investigated the mating behaviour of cockerels, but the work on fowl has concentrated on a trait of commercial importance, broodiness in hens (Hutt, 1949). Hurst's (1925) early work suggested a dominant gene mechanism with inhibitors, but more recent workers find two complementary genes, at least in the Rhode Island Red strain (Goodale, Sanborn, and White, 1920; Kaufman, 1948: see Wood-Gush's review (1955)).

Scattered observations on behaviour inheritance in other species can be found, for example, the horse (Estes, 1952), the sheep (England, 1954; Kelley and Shaw, 1943), cattle (Olson and Petersen, 1951; Bane, 1954); the vole (Godfrey, 1959), and the hamster (Lawlor, 1956), but the only body of work comparable in scope to that on the rat and the mouse is that on the dog, and most of this stems from the programme of work at the Roscoe B. Jackson Laboratory at Bar Harbor in Maine. The advantages of working with this species are obvious; the variety of subspecies, the richness of behavioural variation and the availability of well-established laboratory techniques such as conditioning are examples. The disadvantages are expense and, more important from the present point of view, the absence of genetically pure lines formed by brother × sister mating. Most breeds are highly inbred, however, and so this may not be too severe a disadvantage with modern techniques of genetical analysis.

In some early work it was claimed that barking on the trail segregated as a unit linked with short hair (Whitney, 1929), and that the position in which dalmations ran under coaches was genetically determined (Keeler and Trimble, 1940), but neither finding appears to have been confirmed, and it may well be that the optimum time for doing the latter has already passed. Stockard's work at Cornell came to an untimely end with his early death, but not before Anderson (1939, 1941) had completed studies which enabled him to characterize various breeds of dogs by their typical activity measures. His use of F_1 and F_2 crosses sought, though not very successfully, to analyse the genetics of canine activity. Thorne (1944) also worked with Stockard's dogs, and claimed to have traced, by means of pedigree analysis, the influence of one bitch, a 'fear-biter', in the shyness characteristics of the second generation of her descendants. A recent investigator had the excellent idea of tracing the owners of thoroughbred dogs through pedigree records and testing their pets (Mahut, 1958). She suggests that a specific gene difference may exist between the fearless and fearful strains. Krushinski (1944, 1947) studied 'cowardice' in dogs.

The work at Bar Harbor (Scott and Fuller, 1951, 1959a; Fuller and Scott, 1954; Scott, 1954a, 1954b) has concentrated on five breeds of dog only, but representative of the many in existence. Results of profound interest relating to many aspects of canine behaviour and development have emerged in addition to the psychogenetic data, discussed here. Individual differences in the emotional reactivity of dogs were shown to have a physiological basis (Fuller, 1948), which varied reliably from breed to breed (Fuller, 1951; Scott, 1958a). Fuller considers these differences to be the accidental result of selection for other behavioural characteristics, in the development of the strains. Scott and others report further breed differences in ratings of behavioural response to handling (Scott and Charles, 1953, 1954; Scott, 1955; Fuller, 1955; Freedman, 1958), in measures of dominance (Scott, 1952; Pawlowski and Scott, 1956), of avoiding barriers (Scott and Gault, 1953), and in seasonality of mating (Scott and Fuller, 1959b). A programme of psychogenetical research has been initiated with admirable emphasis on the control of environment, and standardization of test procedures, and using standard methods of crossing and backcrossing. The results so far reported are to be found in Scott (1954b) and are discussed in his books (1958b, 1958c). They relate to the crosses between two of the strains, the cocker-spaniels and the basenjis, or African barkless dog. The nine characteristics for which F_1, F_2 and backcross data are presented are a sample from a group of thirty major behavioural tests, which must represent the largest body of experimental data so far collected in psychogenetics. The characteristics range from measures of heart rate and activity to error scores on barrier tests, and ratings of playful fighting. In order to satisfy the assumption that the environmental effects must be purely additive (Scott, 1954a), Scott uses a genetical model which assumes that a threshold of environmental stimulation must exist in order to elicit the response measured (Fuller, 1954). From this he obtains estimates of the number of genetic factors involved which range in size up to two only, though Thompson and Fuller (1960) report a re-calculation for the transformed data on activity which yields a value of four. In general no very clear-cut picture of the genetic mechanisms underlying the traits reported on is forthcoming; it may be that they are too complex genetically, as Scott himself seems inclined to suggest, or that other methods of analysis are required. The data presented enable a number of hypotheses relating to possible genetic mechanisms, especially in relation to the past history of the breeds of dogs concerned, to be discussed.

This, then, concludes our survey of one of the major methods of psychogenetics, the analysis of strain differences. While it is possible to conclude with Hess that: 'Most of the psychological studies of genetic differences have accomplished nothing more than to prove behavioral differences between inbred strains. Only by the grace of our ignorance can these studies be called genetic, since the gene mechanism underlying the behaviour differences have not been found' (1956, p. 311), it is perhaps too much to expect definitive results to have emerged at a time when the nature of the problem has not yet been fully realized (see later), and there is still an undue concentration on the search for major gene effects determining behaviour in straightforward Mendelian fashion. Only the Bar Harbor and Kansas groups may be said to have begun a satisfactory experimental attack on the study of the genetical transmission of behavioural traits in mammals: it is perhaps significant that the former (Fuller, Scott and Thompson) lay some stress on the importance of a multifactorial hypothesis of gene action.

Selection

Selective breeding is the second major method used in psychogenetics. It is a special case of the genetical method of assortative mating in which parents are picked for their possession of some characteristic of interest to the investigator. This may be qualitative, or it may be a quantitative measure. Mating like with like will tend to increase the prevalence of the quality in the strain, or to increase the mean score in subsequent generations, so that the end point may be reached, at which the expression of the character exceeds the level of it shown by any individual in the original, parental generation (Goodale, 1937). It should be noted that it is not necessary to select in more than one direction at once, giving two or more lines, typically 'high' and 'low', as is usually done in psychogenetics. This procedure should also be distinguished from that known as 'reverse selection', which means selection *against* the characteristic of the strain(s) used, and which is usually employed for experimental purposes in selectively bred lines already well established. Thus selection for low scores among a 'high' line, and *vice versa*, would constitute reverse selection. Desirable features of the design of selective breeding experiments are, firstly, the careful constitution of the parental population so that it is as heterogeneous as possible with respect to the character to be studied, and may be reconstituted at will, and, secondly, the maintenance in the experiment of an unselected control group.

Selection has been practised by animal breeders throughout history to improve stock and to establish new varieties of, for example, dogs, and applied experimentally by geneticists to characteristics as diverse as the shape of hen's eggs (Marble, 1943) and the oil content of maize. Falconer (1955, 1957) gives other examples. Selective breeding has been used by students of behaviour in several studies, few of which have reached the stage when genetical analysis was made possible, usually because the experiment was not carried on long enough, or, as we shall see, the method of analysis used was not satisfactory. It should, however, be noted that such was not always the object of the experiments reviewed here. Frequently all that is attempted is a demonstration of the existence of an hereditary influence, not an analysis of its mode of operation.

Thus the work of Coburn (1922), who appears to have been the pioneer in this field, shows that the few generations of selection which he practised added little to his analysis of the inheritance in mice of 'wildness' and 'savageness', which is not surprising since he used somewhat subjective ratings as his measure of these traits. The same considerations apply to Taylor and Reichlin's (1950) study of types of behaviour in a maze situation. On the other hand, Stone and Barker (1940) demonstrated by six generations of selection for early or late onset of mating in the rat that heredity is an important determinant of the behavioural pattern—see also Warren and Bogart (1952)—and Griffiths (1942) showed, also by six generations of breeding, that strains of rats could be selected for their susceptibility to audiogenic seizures. Frings and Frings (1953; Frings, Frings and Hamilton, 1956) confirmed this by selection in mice. Kuppasawny (1947) persisted for ten generations in a study of the effects of selective breeding upon a food-getting habit in the rat, but it is difficult to gather from his published report what the author deems the study to have shown. Dawson (1932) effectively demonstrated the influence of selection by four generations of selecting unidirectionally for slow running speed among his tame strains of mice (see page 6), and for fast speed among the wild one. Rasmussen (1952) used the Columbia obstruction apparatus to select for sex drive in rats. The marked difference achieved after five generations was associated with a decline in fertility in the high line. Two generations only of selection were used in recent studies on rats. Nachman (1959) continued his study of saccharin preference by mating together animals displaying high, or low, preferences, and Sines (1959) selected for the enhanced development of stomach lesions. In neither case do the data do more than suggest hereditary effects.

Selection for body size in the mouse has brought about correlated changes in many characteristics, including temperament, which have been noted by some workers, though without attempts at quantification. Thus, MacArthur (1944a, 1944b, 1949) found his small strain of mice to be more active, excitable, and 'of nervous temperament', compared with his large strain which were sluggish, as well as being obese, as did Lewis and Warwick (1953). Falconer (1953) confirmed the relative inactivity of his large strain, as compared with the higher activity of the small. Others selecting for the same character, body size, do not appear to have observed behavioural differences (Goodale, 1938; Korkman, 1957, though see Waterman and Moore, 1958). A search might reveal further differences in these strains, and in other strains of mice and rats selected for somatic differences.

One experiment in which such selection for somatic characteristics has been deliberately planned with the expectation of correlated behavioural effects is that of Krech and his co-workers at the University of California at Berkeley. It was found that the performance of rats in an apparatus which permitted them to demonstrate the formation of types of response to an insoluble problem depended to some extent on the amount of cholinesterase enzyme in the cerebral cortex; those with low cholinesterase tended to show visual 'hypotheses', those with high cholinesterase, spatial ones (Krech, Rosenzweig, Bennett, and Krueckel, 1954; Krech, Rosenzweig, and Bennett, 1956, though see Peirce, 1959). This finding linking brain chemistry with behaviour is being studied further by selecting strains for high and low cholinesterase (Rosenzweig, Krech, and Bennett, 1958a, 1958b, 1959). This is a particularly laborious undertaking as the brain enzyme can only be determined by sacrificing the rat after the breeding has taken place.

Turning to the few studies, and the repetitions of them, in which selection has been used in connection with a well-defined behavioural characteristic, and which have reached the stage at which some attempt at genetical analysis of it was made, we find that, as in psychogenetical studies on humans, most of them have been concerned with cognitive ability. Tryon's well-known study on the inheritance of maze learning ability—'maze brightness' and 'dullness'—through twenty-two generations (1929, 1932, 1940, 1942) is the classic in this field, and seems to have had its origin in some work by Tolman (Tolman, 1924; Tolman and Jeffress, 1925). Tryon's experiment began in 1927: he used an automatic, seventeen-unit maze (Tolman, Tryon, and Jeffress, 1929), and for the first few generations only maintained an unselected control group. The parental group was heterogeneous with respect to coat-colour, and it was hoped to use coat-colour genes as 'markers'; in the twenty-second generation brights were mostly grey and dulls, black (Searle, 1949). By the eighth generation separation between the strains was virtually complete, and the distributions showed little overlap. Tryon has presented evidence regarding the nature of the difference between his strains (see Tryon, 1942), and Krechevsky (1933) showed that bright rats from the seventh and eighth generations tended to use spatial hypotheses of the type mentioned before, whereas dull ones used visual ones. This finding has not been confirmed in the recent work on brain cholinesterase cited above and using the descendants of these strains, though it has been shown that on some other cognitive measures the brights are superior as well as having lighter brain weights than dulls (Rosenzweig, Krech, Bennett, and Longueil, 1958) and that the strains still differ in sexual behaviour (Whalen, 1959). Meanwhile, however, Searle (1949) had intensively investigated the characteristics of a small sample of the Tryon strains on a variety of tests and concluded that the differences between them were emotional as well as cognitive. Wherry (1941) used the two strains in a study of the changes in the factorial composition of the behaviour as learning progressed. He used large samples, and showed marked differences between the two in the relative importance of the factors.

Heron's study (1935, 1941) of selective breeding through seventeen generations of rats for maze performance broadly confirms that of Tryon. A distinct separation between the groups was achieved by the fourth generation, and by the sixteenth the dulls were operating at chance level only. As with Tryon's strains, other characteristics have been studied. No differences between the strains were found in activity (Rundquist and Heron, 1935), response to food deprivation and shock (Graves, 1936), size of brain (Silverman, Shapiro, and Heron, 1940)—the last in contrast to the descendants of the Tryon strains. There was some evidence of a difference in basal metabolism favouring the brights in the second generation (Heron and Yugend, 1936), and differences in motivation were detectable (Harris, 1940; Kruse, 1941). The dulls showed greater spontaneous recovery from extinction of a bar-pressing habit (Estes, 1942; see also Heron and Skinner, 1940).

Yet a third study of the inheritance of maze ability, originating at McGill University, has used the well-standardized Hebb-Williams test of rat intelligence (Rabinovitch and Rosvold, 1951). Thompson (1954) reports a marked difference in error scores by the sixth generation, though with difficulties regarding fertility. These must have been overcome in view of subsequent reports using animals up to the thirteenth generation, at the University of Manitoba. Thompson (1953a) and his co-workers (Thompson and Bindra, 1952; Thompson and Kahn, 1955) found that maze bright rats show more exploratory drive than dull ones do but no difference in visual curiosity (Thompson and Solomon, 1954), and later studies have shown that the brights benefit more from glutamic acid (Hughes and Zubeck, 1956, 1957; Hughes, Cooper and Zubeck, 1957), and from an enriched early environment (Cooper and Zubeck, 1958).

The conclusion to be drawn from each of these three independent studies of selection is the same: they have demonstrated the existence of an important hereditary effect upon maze brightness, but have not established the size or nature of the genetical transmission of it. In each case there is evidence that the strains differ in ancillary characters for which no selection was deliberately practised.

Selective breeding for a different characteristic, cage activity, was carried on by Rundquist (1933). The record of fifteen days' activity in a revolving drum was used as the measure. Selection was practised on the basis of the size of these records, irrespective of the rats' strain at first, but later taking account of it. Good separation was achieved by the fifth generation, and maintained thereafter. A marked sex difference in the direction of greater female activity occurred. Rundquist found that the active strain was more fertile, and that coat-colour differences occurred. The latter he regarded as fortuitous, however.

Rats from the fifteenth generation were used for studies of basal metabolic rate, which showed a higher BMR for those from the active strain (Rundquist and Bellis, 1933). Selection was practised to the twenty-fifth and thirty-fifth generations for the low and high strains respectively. The strains were not maintained selectively during the years of World War II (Heron, 1940), but ten generations of re-selection established them as before (Brody, 1942, 1950).

The programme for the psychogenetical study of the fruit fly cited earlier (Hirsch, 1958; Hirsch and Tryon, 1956) shows admirable methodological sophistication. The other results reported (Hirsch and Boudreau, 1958) relate to a selection experiment for positive and negative response to light, using a mass screening technique which avoids the laborious individual testing previously necessary (Scott, 1943). The lines had separated well by the seventh generation, and the results at the twenty-eighth and -ninth allowed the calculation of a measure of the heritability of the behaviour, from the decrease in the variances of the selection lines, which showed that at least 57% of the variability is attributable to heredity.

The other major breeding study for a psychological characteristic is that of Hall (1938, 1940, 1941, 1951), who used an open-field test, which he originated, to obtain measures of emotional elimination in the rat. He took the number of successive days on which the rat defecated or urinated during a short period in the open field as the criterion. The parental group was formed from a heterogeneous collection of 145 animals, derived from at least four different university colonies on the Pacific coast of the United States (Hall, 1938), and brother × sister mating was then practised within each strain. The results obtained by twelve generations of selection for high and low response are shown in Fig. 1.1, which is drawn from the data Hall gives (1951). Clearly the selection was having a marked effect. Study of these strains as they were developing showed that the selection, as has been the case in most of the studies cited, had ancillary effects. Thus, it was demonstrated that animals from the high scoring line were more variable in a free choice situation than those from the low (Hall, 1937), and at the sixth and seventh generation the high line was less subject to audiogenic seizures (Martin and Hall, 1941). No difference between the persistence of the two lines at the seventh and eighth generations was found in a paper-tearing test (Hall and Klein, 1941), but animals from the low strain at the eighth and ninth generations showed themselves to be more aggressive than the highs in careful rating studies of aggressivity as seen in response to attack, etc. (Hall and Klein, 1942). Certain differences between the strains in endocrine organs were observed by Yeakel and Rhoades (1941): these will be referred to further in Chapter 2.

Once again it might be concluded that heredity plays an important part in the determination of the character studied, as seen by the divergence of the curves for high and low strains. But Hall's study suffers from a fatal flaw, as, indeed, do most of the studies on mammals reviewed here, but one which is particularly relevant to the inheritance of emotional tendencies. It is the failure to control for the most important environmental factor of maternal influences. In the present case, high emotional reactivity of offspring may be largely learned from the mother; it may be determined during a critical period of development

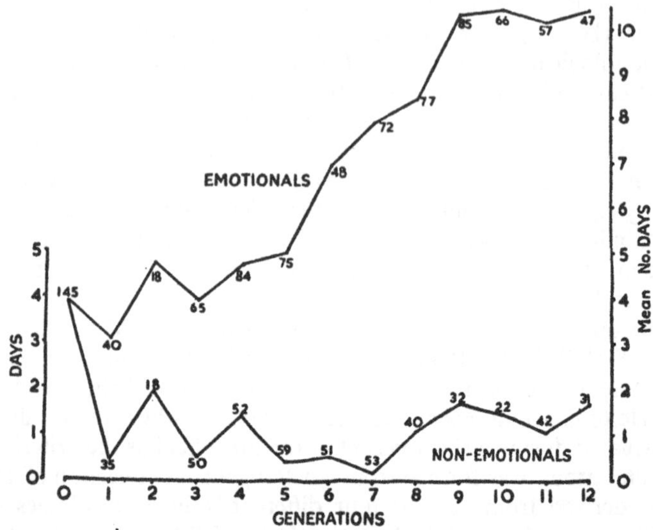

FIG. 1.1. Hall's selective breeding experiment. The graph shows the mean scores of the groups termed 'emotional' and 'non-emotional' in successive generations of selective breeding. Generations, starting with the parental (0), are shown on the abscissa; the ordinates show the mean number of days on which urination and/or defecation occurred. The numbers in the body of the graph indicate the number of subjects on which the adjacent mean is based. (Drawn from data given in Hall, 1951.)

by the experience of being nurtured by, suckled by and caged with, an emotional mother, and *vice versa* for the non-emotional ones. One of the controls for dealing with this problem (which is discussed in detail in the next chapter) is the cross-fostering technique, which, though laborious, has been used in several studies with rats and mice (see, for example, Rasmussen, 1939; Butler and Metrakos, 1950; Fredericson, 1952; Thompson and Sontag, 1956; Thompson, 1957). In the repetition of the Hall study which forms part of the present work it will therefore be found that this and other techniques have been used to control for maternal effects.

Let us conclude this survey of the psychological literature on selective breeding by noting that only three workers have attempted anything approaching a genetical analysis based on crosses from these selectively bred strains. They are Tryon (1940) using his maze bright and dull strains, Brody (1942, 1950) using Rundquist's active and inactive strains, and Hall (1951) using his emotional and non-emotional strains. Tryon crossed his two strains to produce a first filial generation (F_1), and a second filial generation (F_2), and concluded the results supported a multifactorial hypothesis of inheritance of maze brightness, though he was unable to analyse it further. Hall (1951) made three crosses of his strains at the tenth, eleventh, and twelfth generations, obtaining F_1's only from each. He concluded that there was some evidence for dominance of the genes for low emotional elimination. Brody's attempt was the most accomplished genetically. She bred F_1's and F_2's from the twenty-first and twenty-second generations of the inactive and active strains, and also crossed both the F_1's with the original parental lines (P_1 and P_2) to give the backcrosses, B_1 and B_2 respectively. From her results she claimed to have detected the effect of a single major gene pair which, with modifiers, determines spontaneous activity, but was unable to determine the mechanism by which it was transmitted.

In his review of these attempts, Hall (1951) judges them all to have failed, as do Russell (1953a) and Thompson (1953b, 1954). These reviewers are in agreement in assigning the principal cause: it lies, they suggest, in the use of strains of animals which had not yet reached homozygosity, so that the crosses gave wide variability which did not permit the identification of major gene effects. And yet they are all only partly right in these conclusions: more correctly it might be said that the failure of the attempts so far made has been attributable to a failure to adopt appropriate genetical procedures. The emphasis on the purity of line is apposite only in relation to the use of established pure lines for the purpose of the standard type of Mendelian analysis by crossing pure lines to obtain F_1 and F_2, and B_1 and B_2. This is the classical procedure for analysing the effect of one or two genes upon a character in mammals and other dioecious (two sexed) organisms where F_3, F_4's, etc. cannot be obtained by selfing F_2's. While it has been elaborated, as we shall see, to give information about characters which are almost certainly determined by a large number of genes each having a small effect, as in most of the cases discussed above, it is not a method particularly suited to analysing the effects of selection. Therefore the emphasis on inbreeding *combined with selection* is misplaced, and is likely to lead to difficulties in interpreting the results. The point can be best understood at a practical level. The purpose of selection is to create a strain homozygous *for the genes determining the character for which selection is made*. There are usually many genes involved; if there were only a few, the maximum possible advance under selection would be achieved within a few generations by the usual processes of Mendelian segregation.[1] But the aim also is to achieve this homozygosity against a suitably homogeneous background of all other genes determining the other heritable characteristics of the organism. Clearly this can be achieved in two ways; either by seeking to fix all other genetic characteristics as well as the one selected, or to maintain a genetically

[1] The fact that such is not the case in most selection experiments reported is *prima facie* evidence for the multiple factor or polygenic determination of the character under selection. Psychological writers often overlook this point, for example, Hall (1951); though see Brody (1942).

heterogeneous or randomly varying background—and hence, for practical and statistical purposes, homogeneous—with respect to the expression of the selected character. The first will be achieved by practising the maximum possible inbreeding (brother × sister mating with mammals); the second, by avoiding inbreeding as much as possible though inevitably some inbreeding will in time occur in any closed population. The second alternative is to be preferred to the first, for two reasons. Firstly, the genetical models available for analysing the effects of selection (see Lerner, 1950; Lush, 1943; Falconer, 1957) usually assume random mating within the selection line(s); any other assumption tends to complicate the picture beyond the point of usefulness. Secondly, it is virtually impossible in practice to fix all genetical characteristics in a selection experiment without adopting the inconveniently restrictive procedure, from the point of view both of maintaining selection pressure and providing experimental subjects, of breeding from one pair only in each generation in each line. As soon as this is departed from, as, indeed, Hall (1951) notes, sub-lines inevitably arise, and the heritable characteristics not selected for are almost certain to be different as between these sub-lines. Moreover, since these differences are bound to be adventitious, loss of control over the genetic composition of the strain occurs. An example of this involving the coat-colour genes occurred in the experiment to be described in Chapter 3, and referred to shortly. Only Rosenzweig, Krech and Bennett (1958b) have so far avoided this pitfall.

The other methodological failure which has so far dogged psychogenetics, in both studies of selection and of strain differences, has been the effort to apply Mendelian analysis in its simplest form. There are few psychological characteristics which show the all or none, present or absent, appearance typical of simple two- or three-gene determination, such as coat-colour in the rat. The few that do are usually pathological, e.g. phenylketonuria in humans, or of little significance from the broader evolutionary view, e.g. colour blindness, also in humans. David and Snyder (1951) make the point that 'If we pick two unrelated people at random from any human population, we shall probably find that they differ in respect of one or another of the blood antigens, and we may find that one is a taster and the other a non-taster. Beyond this it is highly probable that few, if any, of the observable phenotypic differences between them will be referable to known major genes. Yet we know that the physical characteristics which distinguish individuals are to an appreciable degree determined by genetic differences because of the almost complete physical identity of individuals who are known to have *identical* genotypes, viz., members of monozygotic twin pairs' (p. 63). This striking example might equally be applied to psychological characteristics.

Yet the attempt to cope with the problems of psychogenetics in terms of single gene effects has persisted, especially in the comparative field. The best example is the hypothesis which seeks to relate temperamental characteristics in the rat to the coat-colour gene which in its dominant allele (A) gives rise to agouti or brownish-grey coat-colour, and in its recessive (a) to non-agouti or black coat-colour. Keeler (1942, 1945a, 1945b, 1947, 1948) and Keeler and King (1941, 1942) present evidence to show the effect on the morphological and physiological characters of wild and domesticated rats of the genes controlling coat-colour. They incidentally argue that the process of domestication took place as a result of mutational changes of genes controlling, *inter alia*, coat-colour. The A–a gene is held to be the most important one involved, its recessive allele (a) having, it is suggested, a pleitropic effect on docility or tameness which allowed domestication to occur.

While this hypothesis has been widely (Hall, 1951), and even lyrically (Cook, 1941), acclaimed, it has received little experimental support from workers other than its originators. For example, Thompson (1953b) investigated the emotional and exploratory behaviour in fifteen different pure strains of mice without finding evidence suggestive of a systematic association between behaviour and different types of coat-colour. In preliminary work using five different pure strains of rats, together with a small sample of wild ones, Broadhurst (1958b) similarly did not find any association. It might be argued that such experiments are failing to test the hypothesis adequately, and for two reasons. Firstly, it might quite properly be said that tests of emotionality involving defecation and exploratory activity in strange situations are not measuring behavioural docility as it figures in the domestication process (Richter, 1950, 1952, 1959; Scott, 1954b), especially since the available evidence suggests that wild rats do not defecate more in response to mild stress than domesticated albinos do (Stone, 1932; Broadhurst, 1958b). On the other hand they do show pronounced 'neophobia' or fear and avoidance of novel objects (Barnett, 1956, 1958) which might be expected to reduce their activity in strange and therefore slightly stressful surroundings. But the same argument might equally be applied to the tests used by Keeler (1942), which included emergence tests, and reactions to annoying stimuli such as tickling the rat's nose and blowing cigar smoke at it. It therefore seems that the scores regarded as indicative of emotional responsivity to the mild stress provided by the open-field test may be taken as the most satisfactory available measures for testing the Keeler and King hypothesis.

The second objection is more fundamental. It is that the effect of the differences in the A–a gene can only be properly investigated against a homogeneous background of other genetical characteristics, otherwise there may well be alternative genetical determinants of the behavioural responses studied which will serve to mask or exaggerate the postulated effect of the A–a gene. The obvious and most satisfactory way to meet this objection—which may be held to apply to the original work as well as to the work of Thompson and of Broadhurst referred to above—is to cross two strains known to differ with respect to the A–a gene, breed the F_1 and F_2 generations and observe the effect of the segregating gene among the latter.

This was done in the experiment described below. The genetics of coat-colour will be expounded as we proceed in order to make the rationale of the experiment clear. The two strains of rats in question are a brown-hooded strain whose coat-colour is determined principally by the genes AACChh, and a black-hooded strain, aaCChh. The C–c and H–h genes determine, respectively, the presence or absence of pigmented fur, and its distribution. The former occurs irrespective of other characteristics—an example of epistacy—so that an animal having both alleles cc will always be albino. The distribution of the coloured fur depends on H–h, so that a rat having HH (or Hh, since all the genes here discussed show dominance) will have a self or complete coat-colour, whereas the hh rat will show the piebald or hooded pattern (Castle, 1947) (see Plate II in Chapter 4 for illustrations of these differences: the two strains discussed here are the Brown hooded and Black hooded II, nos. 3 and 4). But since our two strains both have the genotype CChh, we need not consider these genes further, and concentrate attention on the A–a difference. Crossing AA with aa will yield only Aa animals, that is the F_1 will all be of the same genetic composition with respect to coat-colour, and will all be brown hooded, since brown (A) is dominant over black (a). Such was indeed the case for the two litters bred to provide the F_1 in this experiment: one litter came from a brown-hooded mother with a black-hooded father, and the other had the parental sexes reversed (the reciprocal cross) and so had a black-hooded mother with a brown-hooded father. This was done to avoid any possible maternal effects of one strain or the other. These offspring were in turn mated together to provide the F_2, males being randomly chosen for mating with their sisters. Now since each F_1 rat carries both A and a the genes will segregate in such matings as follows, AA, 2Aa, and aa. Since AA and Aa are superficially (phenotypically) identical we shall have the typical Mendelian ratio of dominants to recessives of 3 : 1. A total of sixty-one pups were reared from seven litters; of these forty-three were brown hooded and eighteen black, which is not significantly different by χ^2 test from the expected 3 : 1 ratio.

These subjects were given the standard open-field test to be described in detail in Chapter 2, which yielded the following results. The mean defecation score for the brown animals was 2·1 fecal boluses deposited per trial and for the black ones 2·5; the mean ambulation ('walking around') score for the brown animals was 5·5 metres per trial, and for the black ones 5·1. In neither case did the difference reach statistical significance when the data were subjected to two-way analyses of variance with unequal numbers in sub-groups (Snedecor, 1956). The other variable in these analyses was sex, which was highly significant and in the usual direction in both cases, males having higher defecation and lower ambulation scores (Broadhurst, 1957a). This contrasts with the non-signicant effect of the coat-colour variable, though it may be noted that there was a slight trend in the direction of higher defecation and lower ambulation scores in the contrary direction to that demanded by the hypothesis, that is, the animals carrying the wild type (agouti) gene scored *lower* on the indices of emotional behaviour than those carrying the 'domestication' genes for non-agouti (black). These results, in so far as they go, therefore, fail to support the hypothesis as formulated.

Other evidence from our data can be adduced. In certain crosses from our strain selectively bred for low defecation scores (see Chapters 3 and 4) it became clear that the different sub-lines therein were not homozygous for coat-colour. This had not been suspected, since the coat-colour of the strain is albino (cc), thus masking differences in A–a or H–h. When, at the eighth generation of selection, crosses to the black-hooded lines (aaCChh) were made, it was found that some gave brown hooded offspring (AACChh, probably), and others gave black hooded. This showed that while some albino parents had the expected genotype aacchh, others had A?cchh, probably AAcchh. It was possible, from our records, to show that the sub-lines from which these two coat-colour types came had not diverged until the second generation of selection, and that segregation of the A–a genes took place in the third. A check on the scores of all descendants in subsequent generations which could be unequivocally assigned to one coat-colour type or the other—and this assignment was itself later confirmed by the outcome of appropriate crosses—revealed that, in each generation, animals having the recessive aa gene defecated consistently and usually significantly more in the open-field test than those carrying the A gene, and, contrariwise, they ambulated significantly less. These data confirm the trend of results of the previous test; both, therefore, fail to support the coat-colour hypothesis as stated. While the second is admittedly not such a crucial test as the first, since the results could have been determined by other genetical differences between the strains, and arising from segregation, or from the selection practised (see Chapter 3), these two independent checks agree reasonably well. They reveal a possible effect of a coat-colour gene on behaviour, but not in the expected direction.

It seems probable, therefore, that the hypothesis as stated is too simple, and the experimental digression just indulged in may reinforce this point. It suggests an effect of coat-colour genes upon behaviour, but it is unlikely that it is a major gene effect, operating through pleitropy. It is more likely to be a linkage effect of perhaps several major genes, probably in association with a polygenic system determining behavioural responses. It would clearly be a major undertaking, for which psychogenetics is as yet ill-equipped, to attempt to investigate such an hypothesis. The methods employed in the present studies, however, may be a step in that direction. 'Psychogenetics must imitate biogenetics,' said Hall (1951), but it is important that it should be the biogenetics of today, and not that of forty or fifty years ago.

The multifactorial or polygenic hypothesis

The solution to the problem of the incompatibility between psychological data with its typically continuous distributions and the simple Mendelian method with its emphasis on large discrete differences is fortunately at hand. It lies in the advances in genetics which have come to be called biometrical genetics. The modern school of biometrical genetics has developed from the foundations laid by Fisher (1918) in his reconciliation of the view of the early Biometricians (e.g. Weldon) and those of the Mendelians (e.g. Morgan).[1] 'The original discordance seems to have arisen because neither side understood the full implications of Mendel's fundamental separation of determinant and effect, of genotype and phenotype. The Biometricians seem to have regarded continuous somatic variation as implying continuous genetic variation, and the Mendelians seem to have considered discontinuous genetic variation as incompatible with anything but obviously discontinuous somatic variation. Indeed, de Vries took continuity of variation in the phenotype as a criterion of non-heritability' (Mather, 1949, p. 2). Fisher showed that the familial correlations found by the biometricians could be expected if the hypothesis of multiple genetical factors were adopted. Let Burt take up the narrative, 'At that time, however, Fisher's methods of handling statistical problems were too new and too technical to attract much attention; and it was for long widely supposed that Pearson's results had conclusively shown the "utter inapplicability of any Mendelian hypothesis to continuous variation in man". Thus, for the next fifteen years it was generally agreed by both Mendelians and biometricians that whichever hypothesis came nearer to the truth, the hereditary determination of graded traits was quite incompatible with the segregation of discontinous units postulated by the Mendelian theory. This view still seems to survive in the arguments adduced by many psychological writers. Nevertheless, as the recent advances of genetics have amply shown, on the one point over which the two disputants happened to agree, both, strange to say, were utterly wrong' (Burt and Howard, 1956, p. 96).

It is these recent advances in genetics with which we are concerned

[1] This necessarily condensed account of the origins of the methods to be used ignores the contributions of other workers. The interested reader is referred to the fuller accounts in the sources quoted and in Darlington and Mather (1949) and Wright (1952).

here, and especially those of the biometrical school of genetics of which Mather and his colleagues are prominent members, and whose methods, especially that of analysing the results of diallel crossing (see Chapter 4), have been developed most fully during the past decade. But first it

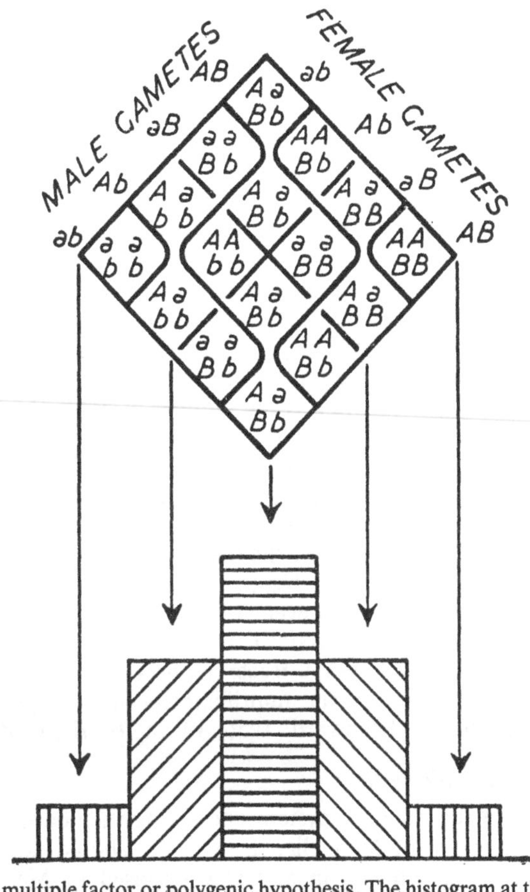

FIG. 1.2. The multiple factor or polygenic hypothesis. The histogram at the bottom of the diagram shows the distribution of phenotypes in an F_2 resulting from the segregation in the F_1 mating—shown at the top—of two genes of equal and additive effect, each having two degrees of expression but without dominance of the one over the other. The phenotypic expression is proportional to the number of capital letters, non-heritable variation being neglected; see text. (From Mather, 1949.)

seems necessary to give some account of the underlying theory, the multiple factor or polygenic theory.

The fact of continuous variation in an observed characteristic is no bar to its being hereditarily determined, as may be seen from Fig. 1.2. Here are shown the results of breeding the F_1 generation derived from two P generations which had the genetic constitution AABB and aabb, that is, they were each homozygous for the two genes involved in this example. Their offspring, the F_1, are also uniform but heterozygous for the two genes, each having the composition AaBb. They in turn will produce the gametes (sperm and ova) as shown at the top of the figure with genes in the four possible combinations indicated, so that their offspring will, in their genotypes, receive the combinations indicated within the body of the diamond as may be seen by reference to the letters at the ends of the appropriate arrays. Now, let it be assumed that the effect of each gene is, firstly, equal, and secondly, additive, and that dominance is absent, so that the usual convention of genetical nomenclature of A for dominant and a for recessive is not operating, the capital and lower case merely indicating two degrees of expression.

Then the distribution of their F_2 phenotypes will be as shown in the histogram at the bottom, and the phenotypic expression is the outcome of the number of capital letters in the genotype. In this way it can be seen that from the action of two genes, five classes will result, from the action of three, seven will result, and so on. In general, the number of classes will be $2n + 1$, where n is the number of genes (Mather, 1949). Other discontinuities caused by non-heritable (environmental) variation will serve on an average to smooth the curve further, so that with a large number of genes the familiar normal distribution for the trait or character in question may be expected.

Comparable demonstration of the theory of the cumulative effects of polygenes has long been available to psychologists in the writings of Tryon (1929, 1940, 1942). However, it is not difficult to see why, in the absence of a method of analysis in these terms, it failed to achieve general acceptance (Hall, 1951). Recently, however, some writers have stressed the importance of the multifactorial view in psychogenetics (Fuller, 1956; Burt and Howard, 1956, 1957a, 1957b; Cattell, 1959a).

Analysis of polygenic systems

The analysis of the genetical system underlying such continuous variation is an extension of Mendelian genetics. It should not be thought that biometrical genetics is in any way opposed to Mendelism; the basic principles of the Mendelian hypothesis of the nature of heredity remain unaltered, it is only an increased complexity of their operational effects which is envisaged. Some principles basic to the polygenic view have already been touched on: they may be stated comprehensively as follows. The variance associated with the phenotypic expression of a continuously distributed character is the outcome of the following determinants: firstly, the non-heritable, which include the effects of environment and errors of measurement of all kinds, and secondly, the heritable or genetically determined which are viewed as the summated effect of a large number of genes each having a small, but additive, effect. This heritable or genetically determined variance can itself be further subdivided into a stable or genetical component expressive of the additivity of the polygenes, and a component which expresses the average dominance of the polygenes and which is consequently unstable and hence non-fixable, since segregation may occur with subsequent breeding. It will thus be seen that some of the concepts familiar from Mendelian genetics, e.g. the emphasis on the interaction of environment and genotype to form the phenotype, and the concept of dominance, are encountered anew, but that the emphasis is always on the cumulative or average effect of large numbers of genes.[1]

A graphical example will perhaps clarify the principles.[2] This is given by Mather (1949), whose work the interested reader is urged to consult for a fuller account of biometrical genetics; see also Darlington and Mather (1949). In Fig. 1.3 we have a representation of the simplest

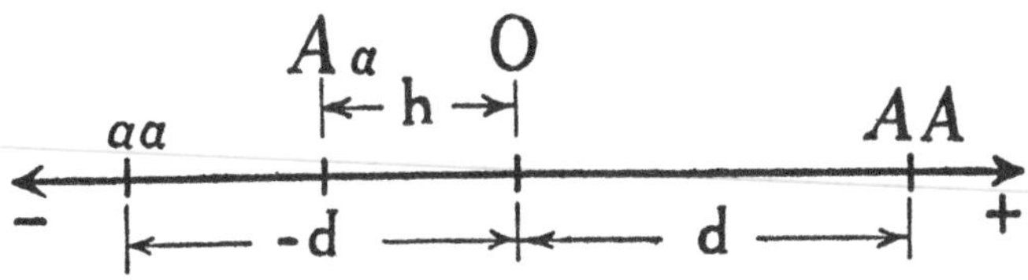

FIG. 1.3. The effect of the three genotypes of the gene A–a. The diagram shows the metric expression of the d and h increments of a gene, the A allelomorph not being dominant over a. Deviations are measured from the point 0, midway between the homozygotes. The heterozygote, Aa, may lie on either side of this point, and the sign of h will vary accordingly. (From Mather, 1949.)

case. The effect of any gene, say, A–a varies over the horizontal scale as indicated, and here again the convention of A for dominant and a

[1] Other familiar concepts such as the linkage of genes, their number, and their interaction in various ways have their place in the polygenic hypothesis, though they are perhaps less generally accepted than the basic tenets and have fewer applications at the moment in psychogenetics. Only some of them will therefore be touched on in the present work.

[2] At this point the reader must share a dilemma in which the writer found himself regarding the conventions of genetical nomenclature to be adopted in the present account. The nomenclature of genetics, and genetical algebra in particular, is a jungle full of pitfalls for the unwary. In addition there are at least two competing systems of notation. This in particular applies to the systems symbolizing the components of variation about to be discussed, one of which has already made its début in the psychological literature (Burt and Howard, 1956, 1957b), and which has certain advantages (Kempthorne, 1957) over that of Mather in ease of recognition. But on balance it was decided to retain Mather's notation, partly because of its historical precedents, and partly because the present writer would have otherwise found himself in the unenviable position of having to invent symbols for certain quantities not yet having a place in the alternative system. In passing this burden on to the reader, the writer is consoled by the thought that geneticists themselves have been sufficiently troubled by it recently to provide comparative tables for translating the different systems (see Lerner, 1958, pp. 55 and 78; Kempthorne, 1957, pp. 373–4).

for recessive is not operative. Leaving aside for the moment consideration of non-heritable effects, and additivity of the gene effects, the cross between the two organisms homozygotic for A–a will yield a value on the scale of 0, the mid-point. Hence the effect of A can be specified by +d, for deviation from 0, and conversely that of a by −d as indicated. But the value for the heterozygote may not fall at 0, it may be nearer to one homozygote or the other by an amount which will reflect the tendency to dominance of the one allelomorph over the other. In the present example therefore, Aa = h, as may be seen in the figure. If we then imagine the effect on the character in question of a large series of genes B–b, C–c, D–d . . . etc., each operating in the manner indicated, it is clear that we can regard their total effect as the outcome of the sum of their individual effects and composed of the sum of the d's, representing the average additive effect of these polygenes, and the sum of the h's, representing the average dominance effect of these polygenes. Thus the magnitude of the sum of the d's will depend on the differences between individuals who are different from each other by being homozygous for the various polygenes, whereas that of the h's will depend on the departure of the heterozygote from the mean of the two comparable homozygotes. These are the primary theoretical components of variation: an example of their application will be given in Chapter 3.

The above is a grossly oversimplified account of the biometrical method. As we shall see in Chapter 4, it is usually the variance of the character under investigation which is analysed into the components corresponding to d and h. The weighted sums of the squares of these quantities are then specified by the capitals D and H respectively, to be read as that part of the observed variance which may theoretically be ascribed to additive gene effects, and that part which may be ascribed to dominance. The genetical algebra by which the partitioning is actually effected into these and other heritable and non-heritable components cannot be entered into here. In general it depends on comparisons of observed generation variances with those theoretically expected on the above scheme. Study of the examples given in Chapter 4, together with the references cited, may clarify the methodology, but perhaps the principle may be grasped by one or two simple examples which must suffice. Thus the theoretical expectation of the variance of any pure line and of that of an F_1 cross is zero, because such strains are regarded as genetically homogeneous, being homozygous for all genes in the first case and uniformly heterozygous in the second. Hence any variance detected is ascribable to non-heritable causation and serves as a measure of environmental effects (E). The variance of the F_2 generation can be shown to be $\frac{1}{2}D + \frac{1}{4}H + E$, hence the variance of F_2–F_1 will give a measure of $\frac{1}{2}D + \frac{1}{4}H$. The variances of other generations and back-crosses to parental lines, as well as certain covariances between them, yield other theoretical expectations, and solution of the requisite equations yields values of the various components together with estimates of their standard error. The method has been applied to partitioning the components of variation of many heritable characters showing continuous variation, for example, growth in mice (Honeyman, 1957), but more especially to those found in plants.

But a word of caution is perhaps in order at this stage. We must not expect too much: we must not expect the precision characteristic of classical genetics when it deals with major gene effects. We have seen what a seductive will-o'-the-wisp such a hope has been in psychogenetics. As Nelder points out, 'The statistical models belonging to the analysis of discontinuous variation in genetics have an elegance and exactness which is rare in applied statistics. . . . The contrast between this state of affairs and that found when continuous variation obtains is indeed striking. The assumption that continuous variation represents the combined effect of polygenic inheritance and a blurring environmental overlay, though necessary as a basic postulate, is too vague to allow analysis to proceed very far. A further difficulty lies in the fact that experimental data on continuous variation, at least as obtained by present methods, do not suggest a detailed hypothetical structure which can be tested in future work. The hypotheses capable of being tested at present are relatively imprecise, and it must be expected, therefore, that the prediction value of analyses of continuous variation will be correspondingly less than that found in discontinuous variation' (1953, p. 111).

Summary

In this introductory chapter, a survey of studies of the inheritance of behaviour in animals (comparative psychogenetics) was made, distinguishing the two main methods used, the study of strain differences, and selective breeding. The differences between strains of mice, rats, and dogs have been most frequently studied; few are adequate both genetically and psychologically. The exceptions relate to the genetical determination of activity in the mouse, of sexual behaviour in the guinea-pig and of many different characteristics in the dog.

Selective breeding has been principally used for the study of cognitive ability in the rat, though other characteristics, including activity and emotional reactivity, and other species, including the fruit-fly, have beeen investigated. Little has so far emerged regarding the genetics of the characters studied.

It was concluded that the use of inappropriate genetical models and methods had frequently occurred, and experimental evidence for this view was given. The greater suitability of the hypothesis of multifactorial or polygenic inheritance in psychology was stressed, and some basic principles of the methods of analysis of biometrical genetics were expounded.

2

METHODS

ON the basis of the conclusions derived from the considerations discussed in the previous chapter, it was decided to institute a programme of research in comparative psychogenetics using the two techniques available to us, selective breeding and the study of pure strains and their crosses. As in any work on the study of inherited capacities, the methods employed in the general maintenance of the subjects, and the control of their environment, are of great importance. Some consideration must therefore be given to the measures taken in the present studies to effect this control.

Several authors give advice to the research worker about to begin experimentation in psychogenetics (e.g. Hall, 1951). That of Scott and Fredericson (1951) is so discouraging as to be worth quoting *in extenso*:

'To begin with, a behavior trait is probably one of the least favorable for the analysis of a precise mode of inheritance, first because the measurement of behavior traits is always time-consuming and may take anywhere from several minutes to even hours on one individual, and, second, because (since all genetic experiments depend upon the analysis of variability) large numbers are always needed. The thorough study of the inheritance of a behavior trait, therefore, becomes an extremely laborious procedure; and, before such studies are made, everything possible should be done to cut down the work, and serious consideration should be given to the question of whether the experiment needs to be done at all.

'One way in which time can be saved is to perfect simple and brief tests of behavior so that each individual can be classified in a short period of time. Great care should also be taken to cut down variability by standardizing the environment and care of the animals as closely as possible. The more the environmentally caused variability can be reduced, the easier it will be to study the genetic variability' (p. 293).

The rest of this chapter will be devoted, therefore, to a description of the 'simple and brief' test of behaviour used in the present studies, to an examination of the available evidence for its reliability and its validity, and to a discussion of the methods employed to reduce environmental variability to a minimum by standardizing the rearing and husbandry of our experimental subjects.

The open-field test

Hall's early work on the open-field test has already been mentioned. What is desired it was felt, in order to achieve the standardization requisite for psychogenetic work, is to adopt the rigorous standards of the psychometric approach and to try to achieve a completely standardized simple and objective test which would be strictly comparable in administration not only from occasion to occasion within our own laboratory, but which would also be readily transferable to others if necessary. In passing it might be noted that such an approach might well benefit other areas of comparative psychology, where it is not so obviously essential as it is in psychogenetics, but which are bedevilled by differences in findings from one laboratory to another being attributable to differences in experimental procedures.

Accordingly, the present studies were begun with a series of experiments designed to investigate some of the parameters affecting behaviour in the test. These have been reported fully elsewhere (Broadhurst, 1956, 1957a, 1958a, 1958b), and it is not proposed to do more here than to sketch the methods and results of these experiments, and to do this only in so far as they affect the ultimate standardization of the test adopted for our present work on emotionality in the rat.

Firstly, an investigation of the situational determinants of the test response was undertaken (Broadhurst, 1957a). Defecation, ambulation, urination, rearing, and preening were observed on five successive days in an experiment designed to establish the optimum conditions for the use of the test. The large ($N = 192$) factorial design permitted simultaneous evaluation of six variables thought to be of importance. They were sex, intensity of noise and light in the test arena, the size of the arena itself, food deprivation, and the administration of a shock to the feet before the test. Each of these variables was at two 'levels' (to speak in analysis of variance terms), sex, of course, necessarily so. Had it been possible, it would have been desirable to have arranged to have more than two levels of variables such as noise and light, so that the relationship of stimulus intensity to response could have been established with greater certainty than was possible with two levels only. The experiment showed that the defecation and ambulation scores were the most satisfactory measures. Analysis of the defecation scores indicated that both higher noise and light stimulated increased emotional elimination and that male rats defecated more than females. It was not possible to exclude definitely the influence of body size on this sex difference, however.

Food deprivation and arena size had no effect on this score. These findings had important implications for the standardization of the test for use in all subsequent work. The ambulation scores, which in general showed the previously reported inverse relation with defecation, were regarded as a less important index of emotional reactivity, probably being related to the intensity of evocation of exploratory drive.

A study of a selection of the many possible antecedent determinants of the defecation and ambulation responses in the standardized open-field test followed. Very few of the variables employed showed any definite effect. Systematic gentling and petting, sexual experience (Broadhurst, 1958a), and a degree of visual deprivation during infancy (Broadhurst, 1956) had no effect on the subjects' defecation, nor was their body build correlated with it (Broadhurst, 1956). Previous experience of the same test decreased the scores of young rats. Ambulation appeared to be even more insensitive, though a somewhat mysterious effect on it of sexual experience was detected (Broadhurst, 1958a). Finally, the analysis of genetical determinants was begun with the study of five different pure strains (Broadhurst, 1958b). The marked differences found between the strains will be discussed more fully in Chapter 4.

Standardization of the open-field test

On the basis of the results referred to above, the open-field test, shown in Plate I (facing page 66), was employed as follows. The smaller arena was used, as the larger size favoured by earlier workers (Hall, 1934) had been shown not to elicit a greater defecation response. This arena is made of plywood on a softwood frame, and is 32¾ in. in diameter. The walls are 12½ in. high and painted flat white. It has no floor, but stands on the granolithic floor of an experimental room. On the floor are marked in chinagraph pencil a series of three concentric circles, divided into segments by lines radiating from the middle. These may be clearly seen in Plate I. These lines are readily renewed as they fade during testing, and they provide the basis for scoring the ambulation of the subjects. The divisions are arranged to give the best approximation to an equal distance across each, no matter in what direction the rat moves, and the number of divisions entered by the animal during the test are recorded on a prepared plan of the arena having the same pattern of lines. An entry of all four feet, excluding the tail, is required before a 'floor unit' of ambulation is counted. The four feet need not all be in the division together—the rat may pass through it. These floor units may later be converted to metres run by multiplying by an appropriate constant (0·216) which relates the best approximation to the distance across the divisions to metres, with some weighting in favour of the distance across the divisions round the circumference of the outermost circle, since they are the ones most frequently entered.

Around and above the arena a light metal structure supports a muslin screen which serves both as a rough one-way screen—the rat being in the brightly lit arena, and the experimenter observing from the darkened room outside—and as a means of diffusing the light to provide a uniform light field over the arena floor. The lights for this purpose are six photographic lamps wired in parallel attached to the metal structure at a height of 44 in. above the floor, which, in the present arrangement, yield an illumination averaging 165 foot-candles at floor level, as measured by an AVO type 2 light meter. Six loudspeakers, 6½ in. in diameter, are also attached to the metal structure at a height of 51 in. To them is fed, via an amplifier, continuous 'white noise', that is, noise of all frequencies together, generated by a small commercial neon lamp. The intensity of this noise at floor level averages 78 db. above the standard reference level of 0·0002 dyne/sq. cm., as measured by a Dawes sound level meter (type 1400 D). These values of stimulus intensity are checked from time to time, and the muslin screen renewed as it gets dirty. In addition to serving as an emotional stimulus, the noise acts as a sound screen to mask distracting noises from outside the experimental room.

The standard procedure adopted is to transport the rat to and from its home cage in the adjoining animal colony room in a white enamelled pail, and expose it in the arena for precisely two minutes to the sound and light fields specified above, this being done at approximately the same time of day on four successive days. The ambulation responses are recorded as described above and the number of fecal boluses deposited in the arena counted. Also noted are the presence or absence of urination, and any rearing, preening, etc., together with any other unusual behaviour. This apparatus and procedure have been in frequent use for more than four years in the form specified[1] and have proved to be reliable and satisfactory. An experienced observer takes an average of four minutes to test one animal, so that some sixty rats may conveniently be tested in one day.

Two main scores are thus obtained, number of fecal boluses deposited —the defecation score—and the number of floor units entered—the ambulation score. Note that each is the sum of four individual days' scores: most of the calculations to be reported in what follows are done on these raw scores: when the results have been averaged over days to yield a score 'per trial', and, in the case of ambulation scores, also converted to metres run, this fact will be noted. None of the other scores from the test have been systematically analysed: some use has been made of the urination score as an ancillary measure of emotional elimination, as will be seen later.

Reliability of the open-field test

The early work on the open-field test indicated reliabilities for fecal

[1] On two occasions departures from this standardization have been made: their purpose and significance will be indicated as they arise in what follows.

counts which never fell below 0·85. However, these were usually derived from split-half correlational techniques, with various corrections applied, and for which tests of significance are consequently not available. One particular difficulty, not unique to this test, is the tendency for scores, especially defecation, to show a marked trend from day to day. While this trend, as we shall see, has important implications relating to validity, it complicates the measurement of reliability and necessitates a further correction to any split-half correlation.

The approach adopted here has therefore been through the analysis of variance. This has the advantage of leading simultaneously to estimates of reliability and tests of their significance. The variance of the defecation and the ambulation scores for the 704 rats comprising the whole of the seventh, eighth, and ninth generations of selective breeding, together with the cross-bred animals from the first two mentioned (see Chapter 3), was analysed with the results to be found in Table 2.1.

It will be seen from the first eight columns of the summary tables of variance in Table 2.1 (those headed 'Combined data') that the variance ratios (F) due to both differences between the mean scores for trials and for those between rats are highly significant for both scores. This, of course, is not surprising, and reflects day-to-day changes in scores, and individual differences between animals, respectively. For the present purpose, attention is directed to the relationship between the estimated variance, s^2 (MS) for rats—($s_R{}^2$)—and for the rats × trials interaction (residual)—$s_I{}^2$, which are combined in the manner indicated to yield the correlation coefficients of 0·82 for defecation scores, and 0·75 for ambulation scores, both reasonably satisfactory figures for this type of work.

It was also thought important to investigate another aspect of test reliability—inter-observer reliability—in view of the number of experimenters[1] who have from time to time assisted in testing animals in the open field. Failing direct observation by two observers simultaneously, which would have been difficult to arrange with our apparatus, the following approach was adopted. The scores of the 704 subjects mentioned above were divided according to whether they had been tested by the same experimenter on all four successive days or whether two or more observers had participated in the testing programme, and analyses of variance performed on the two blocks of data independently. The results are shown in the second part of Table 2.1 in the columns headed 'One observer throughout test' and 'More than one observer'. These yield much the same results as for the combined data, but for the present purpose attention is concentrated on the s^2 for the rats × trials

[1] My thanks are due in this respect to the following members of staff and students of the Animal Psychology Laboratory: Mrs. G. Das, Dr. D. C. Kendrick, Miss S. Parsons, Miss U. Sabbagh, Mr. R. D. Savage, Mr. D. S. Shalman, Prof. S. D. Singh, Mrs. V. K. Singh, Mr. S. N. Sinha, and Mr. K. B. Wraight.

TABLE 2.1

Reliability of defecation and ambulation scores

Source of variance	d.f.	Combined data: Defecation scores MS	Defecation scores F	Defecation scores P	Ambulation scores MS	Ambulation scores F	Ambulation scores P
Between trials	3	23·02	12·70	0·001	6138·33	62·98	0·001
Between rats	703	18·03	9·94	0·001	687·14	7·05	0·001
Rats × trials interaction	2109	1·81			97·46		
Total	2815						
Reliability: $\frac{s_R^2 - s_I^2}{s_R^2 + s_I^2}$		0·82			0·75		

Source of variance	One observer throughout test: d.f.	Defecation scores MS	F	P	Ambulation scores MS	F	P	More than one observer: d.f.	Defecation scores MS	F	P	Ambulation scores MS	F	P
Between trials	3	14·28	4·97	0·001	2035·10	22·11	0·001	3	10·67	7·70	0·001	4154·37	38·39	0·001
Between rats	267	13·91	4·84	0·001	490·91	5·33	0·001	435	13·11	9·48	0·001	739·07	6·83	0·001
Rats × trials interaction	701	2·87			92·03			1305	1·38			108·23		
Total	1071							1743						

interaction, which in the case of multiple observers must contain an additional error term attributable to this source, when compared with that for the single observer. Making these comparisons we have, for defecation scores 1·38/2·87 which gives an *F* less than unity, and for ambulation scores 108·23/92·03 which gives an *F* of 1·18 which, with the given degrees of freedom (701 and 1305), is significant at the 5% level. From this we may conclude that the defecation score from the open-field test is less sensitive to error attributable to differences between observers than is the ambulation score. This is wholly in keeping with the greater objectivity of counting the number of fecal pellets on the floor, as compared with deciding whether a possibly fast-moving rat did or did not enter a floor division.

The logic of the above analyses is not entirely free from question, however. The observant reader will note that the *F*-ratio of error residuals for defecation scores when calculated in reverse yields a highly significant figure which could be taken to mean that two or more observers are *more* reliable than one, and the trend of the reliability coefficients, calculated as before, support this, being 0·66 and 0·68 for defecation and ambulation respectively for one observer, 0·81 and 0·75 for more than one. However, this apparent paradox may have arisen from marked departures from normality of much of the defecation data (see Chapter 3, Fig. 3.3), and the differences between the variances involved in each case is reassuringly small, so that the above caveat need not detract too much from the main conclusion from these analyses, which is that the scores derived from the open-field test appear to be reasonably reliable.

Validity of the open-field test

It is obviously difficult to establish the validity of any test unequivocally, and in animal psychology there are special difficulties to contend with. The most helpful approach to the problem which the writer has encountered is that of Cronbach and Meehl (1955), and the following discussion is concerned with the scores derived from the open-field test, and especially the defecation score, in relation to the different types of validity which they distinguish.

It is clear that the idea, that the defecation score of the rat when placed in a strange situation measures an emotional response, is an example of construct validity, since there is no definite external criterion against which to validate it. Something analogous to Cronbach and Meehl's predictive validity also enters, but only at a later stage. There are several lines of evidence relating to the construct validity of 'emotionality' as here measured. First, there is what may be termed the intuitive-anthropomorphic. Strong emotion, especially fear, is known to induce a tendency to lose control over elimination. This phenomenon is well known in man, and in other species, and its recognition is of considerable antiquity. Thus, Armstrong (1958) records a case of probable emotional defecation plastically recorded in prehistoric times, and Alverez (in Hall, 1938) cites an epic account of a battle in early Persian history in which the flight behaviour of the enemy commanders is described as follows: 'To save their lives they trampled over the bodies of their soldiers, and fled. Like young captured birds they lost courage. With their urine they defiled their chariots and let fall their excrement.' Other historical, anecdotal, and observational evidence could be adduced, but experimental studies are not often found, perhaps because they might be thought to be labouring the obvious. Recourse may therefore be had to questionnaire studies such as those of Stouffer *et al. mult.* (1949, 1950) in which it was reported that in soldiers under battle conditions the need for elimination may become so compelling as to break through cultural restraints. Thus, these authors conclude from a study of the reports of front-line soldiers of their different physiological fear symptoms that 'the symptoms come from a single universe and permit a rank ordering of respondents along a single continuum. There is an intrinsic interdependence among the different fear symptoms which permits them to be ordered from more to less severe. In this case the underlying continuum is probably physiological . . .' (Stouffer *et al. mult.*, 1950, p. 142). Loss of control over elimination is found to be the extreme fear symptom on this continuum, 9% of the men reporting 'urinating in the pants', and 21% reporting loss of control over bowels when under fire, as compared with, for example, 57% feeling sick, and 84% experiencing 'violent pounding of the heart'.

The second line of evidence bearing on the problem of this test's validity relates to the generality of the phenomenon. This is seen not only in the inter-species comparisons alluded to above, but also in the wide variety of situations judged fear-provoking in which it may be observed in rodents. Parker's experiment (1939) in which he intercorrelated the defecation responses of 200 rats to six such situations, ranging from the open-field test itself to dropping or restraining the subject, provides adequate evidence on this point. A factor analysis of the 6 × 6 table of Parker's intercorrelations given by Hall (1941) shows that all tests have very high loading on a first factor which accounts for 66% of the variance among males, and 78% among females, and which is undoubtedly a general factor of responsivity to each of these tests, as seen in the frequency of defecation.

Internal evidence from the open-field test itself has often been taken as supporting the construct validity of defecation. Hall (1934) attempted to validate defecation as an index of emotionality by showing a significant negative correlation with eating in the open field, on the grounds that a frightened animal would not eat in a strange situation. The correlation has been confirmed by some workers (Yoshioka, 1932; Thompson, 1953a), but others have not found it (Evans and Hunt,

1942; Bindra and Thompson, 1953). More convincing, perhaps, since it is a more obvious and direct measure of the idea of habituation which underlies the previous approach, is the simple fact that defecation in the open-field test decreases with successive exposures in it. Hall's original observations on this point have been repeatedly confirmed. A slightly different line of argument provides additional evidence. Evans and Hunt (1942) and Broadhurst (1957a) have shown that increasing the intensity of two of the physical stimuli impinging on the subject under test—noise and light—increases the defecation response. To the extent that these stimuli are accepted as fear-provoking, the validity of defecation as a fear response is supported.

The relationship between defecation in the open field and measures of timidity or fearfulness in other situations provides yet another method of validation—one which has not always met with success. O'Kelly's experiment (1940) leads him to question the validity of an emotionality index which did not correlate with speed of escape and certain learning measures. Similarly, Hunt and Otis (1953) showed that defecation does not correlate with an emergence test of timidity though it does correlate highly with the other component indices of the conditioned emotional response (CER) formed to electric shock in a Skinner box. But since these findings come from tests on two different groups of rats, the relationship between the CER developed in the stressful Skinner box conditions and emotionality as defined by open-field defecation is not established. Experiments which fill this gap will be mentioned later. More convincing however than these findings with unselected groups of animals given one or two tests in addition to the open-field test, are the experiments in which a battery of tests, including the open-field, were used, and the results subjected to factor analysis. Factorial validity has been demonstrated in this way. Billingslea (1942) showed that defecation scores had a high saturation on his factor of 'fearful and inhibited behavior' in rats, and Willingham (1956) showed that in mice an emotional elimination factor exists (incidentally confirming Parker's (1939) observations discussed earlier), but that factors defining other aspects of emotional behaviour must be considered in describing the concept of 'emotionality'. Geier, Levin, and Tolman (1941) also provide evidence of factorial validity, but it should be noted that this study has been criticized on methodological grounds by Royce (1950).

The predictive aspect of the defecation response as a contribution to its validity is perhaps best seen in the series of studies which have used the Maudsley emotionally reactive and non-reactive strains, developed by selective breeding for high and low defecation responses in the open-field test. Without anticipating the details of this experiment, which will be fully discussed in Chapter 3, it may be said that comparison of the performance of rats from the high defecating strain with those from the low in other test situations has shown that the former are consistently more susceptible to fear motivation. This was seen in increased speed of swimming underwater under air deprivation (Broadhurst, 1957b, 1958c), and in the development of CER's in the Skinner box (Singh, 1960), confirmed on two separate occasions (Singh, 1960; Singh and Eysenck, 1960). Savage (1960) has also demonstrated greater susceptibility to frustration (Amsel, 1958), to conflict (Miller, 1944) and to 'freezing' among the high defecators. Studies in which the two strains do not differ (Sinha, Franks, and Broadhurst, 1958; Das and Broadhurst, 1959) employed measures to extinguish fear responses which account well for the lack of differences, and this fact can be taken as supporting the identification of defecation in the open field as a measure of an emotional response with some generality.

The final line of evidence bearing on this problem is one which may be considered to be the most fundamental to the comparative psychologist interested in establishing a sound physiological basis for his observations. The existence of a physiological mechanism underlying emotional elimination has been implied in much of what has preceded. Nervous control of defecation has long been established (Cannon, 1929), and is attributable to the action of the autonomic nervous system (Hess, 1954). Clearly, as a fear response it would be anticipated that the action of endocrine organs, especially the adrenal medulla, would be involved. Evidence on this point is conflicting. Anderson and Anderson (1940) found no evidence of a correlation between the weights of various ductless glands and the defecation and ambulation scores in either male or female rats from a heterogeneous population, whereas Yeakel and Rhoades (1941), on the other hand, did. But they used selectively bred animals from Hall's experiment (1938, 1940, 1941, 1951) and found the results summarized in Table 2.2. They do not record any

TABLE 2.2

Yeakel and Rhoades findings (1941)

	Males		Females	
Gland	High Strain	Low Strain	High Strain	Low Strain
Adrenals	Heavier		No significant difference	
Thyroid	Heavier		Heavier	
Pituitary	No significant difference		Heavier	

differences in body weight between the strains. Broadly speaking, these findings seem congruent with the notion that the high defecators may be considered to be more reactive physiologically. It must however be noted that the size of an endocrine gland is not necessarily a complete indication of its functioning or of the organism's endocrine status. Thus the adrenals may be enlarged by stresses of different types, and it is especially true of the thyroid gland, which may be enlarged in both hypo- and hyperthyroid conditions. Watson (1958, 1960) has analysed some of the biochemical and physiological differences between the Maudsley reactive and non-reactive strains at the fifth and sixth generations. He found weight and other differences between the two strains suggestive of a lowered metabolism among the animals from the high defecating strain. The conclusion was reached that the emotionally reactive strain displays a slight hypothyroidism, and was supported by observations on animals from the low defecating strain which had had their thyroid output reduced by being given methyl-thiouracil. These findings were confirmed and extended by Feuer and Broadhurst (1960). Using rats from the tenth generation, they showed that the high defecating strain has larger but relatively less active thyroids than the low defecating strain. The levels of the thyroid hormones circulating in the blood were within the normal range for the albino rat, however. The evidence suggests that a pituitary mechanism is involved, and it is known that psychological stress can give rise, via the action of the thyrotrophic hormone (TSH), to marked inhibition of the thyroid gland, both acute (Brown-Grant, Harris, and Reichlin, 1954) and prolonged (Carrière and Isler, 1959). Further work on the physiological determinants of emotional defecation is in progress, but it appears certain that our selection for high and low response has involved differences in thyroid output. This is not surprising in view of the evidence that thyroid activity is also genetically determined (Chai, Amin, and Reineke, 1957; Chai, 1958), and that selection for one polygenic characteristic frequently involves correlated responses in others not selected for—see Chapter 1, also Mather and Harrison (1949). Linkage relationships involving the polygenes may be responsible. It is of interest to note that in Hall's selection experiment a similar thyroid difference was detected by Yeakel and Rhoades (see Table 2.2). It would however be improper to place too much weight on this concordance, since the genetical changes correlated with selection for the same characteristic may well be chance determined and hence different in reproductively isolated populations. It is perhaps worth noting in this connection that the difference in audiogenic seizure susceptibility—which may also be an adventitiously correlated response—between the strains selectively bred for high and low defecation by Hall (Martin and Hall, 1941), is shared by rats of the Maudsley strains, the low defecators being the more susceptible.[1]

Despite the problems raised by these findings and which remain to be resolved, it is conceded that the physiological interpretation of the defecation responses of animals in our selected strains is not yet unequivocally established as a valid measure of the construct of emotionality. But it is important for what follows to note that any alternative explanation does not, and as yet seems unlikely to, apply to the defeca-

[1] I am indebted to Mr. R. G. A. Stretch for this observation.

tion responses of our inbred strains, and less still to those of *unselected* populations of rats. It is clear that, in Cronbach and Meehl's terms, there are still several gaps in our nomological net binding this construct.

It will be noted that nothing has been said regarding the validity of the other main score derived from the open-field test—the ambulation score. What is being measured here is probably some aspect of an exploratory drive (Broadhurst, 1957a), since the score tends not to correlate with general cage activity. A negative, though small, correlation between ambulation and defecation has frequently been reported (e.g. Hall, 1936; Biel and O'Kelly, 1940). This suggests that there may well be an emotional component involved (cf. Willingham, 1956; McClearn, 1959), since it is to be expected that an emotional, fearful animal will show decreased activity, representing a partial manifestation, at least, of the freezing pattern characteristic of the rodent response to a fear-provoking stimulus (Nissen, 1946; Riess, 1945, 1946a, 1946b). It has not, however, been found possible to relate the two measures more directly on some continuum representative of intensity of emotional responsiveness. Possible explanatory mechanisms for the decay typically found in ambulation scores during a short period are discussed by Berlyne (1950), Glickman (1958) and re-interpreted by Broadhurst and Eysenck (1960).

Environmental control

The following rigidly standardized procedures relating to animal husbandry were initiated in 1954 for the parental generation of the selection experiment (see Chapter 3), and have been continued ever since, for all rats destined to serve as subjects in the work reported here. They are summarized in Table 2.3. The references to cross-fostering refer only to the selection experiment described in Chapter 3, and their implications will be discussed there.

As soon as possible after birth, the mother and her pups are removed from the cage in which parturition occurs, and the pups counted, sexed, and weighed. All cages are 9 × 9 × 8½ in. high, and have solid metal backs, tops and sides. Nesting material (*c.* 30 gm. of wood wool, Grade 'O') and loose pellets of food (MRC diet No. 41)[1] are now supplied, and the 2-in. gap between the ¼-in.-sq. wire-mesh cage floor and the sanitary tray under the cage is filled with wood wool to exclude draughts. The animals are returned to the cage, thus provided, which is then left undisturbed, except for the addition of food and water as necessary, until the fifth day. A check is then made, without handling the animals, on the number in the litter still surviving. Again the cage is left undisturbed, this time until the twelfth day, when another check on superficial

[1] Diet No. 41B, in which the cod liver oil is replaced by a stabilized vitamin supplement to avoid the destruction of Vitamin E, was used after January 1957, i.e. after the sixth and before the seventh generation.

TABLE 2.3

Summary of schedule of standardized environmental conditions, etc., under which all subjects were reared

Age (in days)	Handling and other procedures	Caging	Diet
(−2 to −5)	(Mother isolated)	(One per cage)	(Loose food pellets and tap water)
0 (birth)	Counted, weighed, sexed (transferred to foster-mother in some cases)	With mother (or foster-mother) and litter-mates	Milk
5	Numbers checked	ditto	ditto
12	Ditto	ditto	Milk, plus (later) loose pellets of MRC diet No. 41, and tap water
21	Weaned; counted, weighed and sexed	Five per cage, same sex; usually litter-mates but always comparable age	Loose pellets of food, and tap water
50	Ears marked under light anaesthesia; weighed	Three per cage, same sex, otherwise as before	Pellets of food in food-hopper, and tap water
100–103 (approx.)	Tested in open field	ditto	ditto
110 (approx.)	Weighed	ditto	ditto

numbers is made. At this time the protective wood wool is removed from under the cage, and daily tray cleaning—removing soiled sawdust and replacing it with fresh—is resumed. This regimen continues, except that from twenty-one days caging is in groups of five pups of like sex, not necessarily, though usually, litter-mates. At fifty days the final cage allocations are made with three rats of like sex in each cage, immediately after punch holes have been made in the ears under light ether anaesthesia. These holes indicate, by means of a simple code, each animal's individual number. The cages are again left undisturbed until the occupants are tested. Throughout the whole period, an automatically controlled lighting system supplements daylight in such a way that the animal colony room is in darkness only during the period from 9.00 p.m. to 3.30 a.m. GMT. It is not possible to ensure that all animals have the same exposure to light and laboratory noises, etc., since each batch of animals occupies two or more batteries of cages, containing five rows of cages at heights varying from about 12 to 65 in. from the floor. An effort is made to equate any possible resultant effect over the two sexes by caging males and females in alternate cages at their final cage allocation.

Summary

This chapter is concerned with the requirements of experimental work in psychogenetics. The standardization of the open-field test of emotional reactivity in the rat, to be used throughout the present work, is described, and consideration given to the evidence relating to the reliability and validity of the test. It is concluded that the reliability is satisfactory, and that the test is probably a valid measure. A description of the detailed control of animal husbandry to ensure uniformity of environment is given.

3

SELECTIVE BREEDING

INTRODUCTION

THE selective breeding experiment was begun in October 1954, and, at the time of writing (April 1959), has reached the twelfth generation of selective breeding (S_{12}).[1] The results to be reported in this part, however, relate to the first ten generations of selection (S_{1-10}) only, which, with the parental generation (P), make a total of eleven.

Subjects

The subjects for the P generation were a group of 222 albino rats (106 males and 116 females) specially bred as subjects for this experiment from a remote Wistar strain originally obtained from a dealer. The strain had been maintained in the laboratory for at least five generations by unsystematic mating, though care was taken in this case to avoid matings of brother with sister, or any other close mating, to ensure as heterogeneous a group as possible with which to commence the selection for emotional defecation.

All of the ten subsequent generations which are reported on here are descendants of this parental group, and were bred from parents in each generation selected by virtue of their defecation scores in the open-field test in the manner described below. The numbers and sexes of the animals constituting these successive generations are shown in Table 3.1. The intention was to have a total population of the order of 200 subjects in each generation. As will be seen from the table, this intention was at first amply met (first and second generations—S_1 and S_2), but not so well achieved in later ones (e.g. S_4), despite an increase

[1] Many psychological writers use the term F_1 (filial generation one), F_2, etc., in designating the successive generations of a selection experiment. This is more correctly reserved in genetics for the progeny of the cross of two distinct lines, usually inbred. The designation adopted here is used by Mather and Harrison (1949).

TABLE 3.1

Numbers and sexes of successive generations during selective breeding

	No. given open--field test			No. selected for breeding next generation					
				Reactive			Non-reactive		
Generation	Total	M.	F.	Total	M.	F.	Total	M.	F.
Parental	222	106	116	32	13	19	31	10	21
First	191	96	95	23	8	15	28	10	18
Second	196	92	104	29	10	19	23	6	17
Third	198	102	96	30	10	20	27	8	19
Fourth	140	70	70	31	9	24	42	14	28
Fifth	176	85	91	35	13	22	33	10	23
Sixth	185	76	109	42	20	22	40	17	23
Seventh	193	99	94	57	23	24	38	18	20
Eighth	166	85	81	42	18	24	38	18	20
Ninth	216	119	97	46	23	23	47	27	20
Tenth	197	103	94	37	16	21	33	17	16

in the number of animals selected for breeding. This reflects a decrease in fertility—or, to be more precise, a decrease in the propensity for, and efficiency of, maternal care, resulting in the loss of many pups before weaning—which has occurred, and about which nothing can be done (see Table 3.10 later). On the whole, however, the breeding programme has been well maintained.

Mating

Immediately after the completion of the testing in the open field, as described in Chapter 2, the individual data sheets are scored and potential parents for the next generation selected. This is done by plotting a histogram of the defecation scores and deciding upon cut-off points which will yield sufficient numbers of high- or low-scoring siblings to serve as parents for the next generation. The actual cut-off scores used in successive generations are given in Table 3.2. It will be noted that the

TABLE 3.2

Cut-off defecation scores for selecting parents

	Emotionally reactive Min. score included		Emotionally non-reactive Max. score included	
	Males	Females	Males	Females
Generation	(Number of fecal boluses deposited per trial)			
Parental*	5·5	4·5	2·0	0·5
First	3·7	3·7	2·0	1·3
Second	3·3	3·5	1·7	0·3
Third	3·3	3·3	0·7	0·3
Fourth	2·3	2·3	0·5	0·3
Fifth	3·0	2·7	0	0
Sixth	3·6	3·6	0	0
Seventh	3·6	3·6	0	0
Eighth	4·3	4·3	0	0
Ninth	3·6	3·6	0	0
Tenth	4·6	4·6	0	0

* The mean scores for this generation are based on the results of testing on *two* successive days only, and are consequently not comparable in absolute size to those of subsequent generations because of the decrease in score from day to day.

criteria have become progressively more rigorous for the non-reactive strain, till a point was reached after the fifth generation when it was not possible to progress further using the defecation scores alone as derived from standard testing conditions. With the sixth generation the following procedure was therefore adopted. At the end of their four days' testing, the animals of the non-reactive strain were given a fifth day under a higher noise level (average sound intensity at floor level of 87·3 db. ref. 0·0002 dynes/sq. cm.). The results were disappointing: very few rats commenced or resumed defecation in the manner anticipated, and consequently the additional data were valueless for the desired purpose of increasing the pressure of selection on this strain. More drastic measures were therefore taken with the next generation (S_7), and the whole group of 193 rats were given their four-day test under the higher noise level. The results were even more disconcerting,[1] since the effect on neither strain was in the expected direction and no additional data of the sort desired were secured. The attempt to increase the selection pressure by manipulating the intensity of the physical stimulation in the open-field test was therefore abandoned, and the routine testing conditions as detailed in Chapter 2 were resumed with S_8 and have been maintained ever since. The alternative of selecting among the non-reactives for urination as well as defecation scores has been used. Breeding animals were required not to have defecated at all and to have urinated in the open-field test on fewer than a certain number of days. For S_7 this was less than two, for S_8 the same, and for S_9 less than one.

No such problems of selection have arisen with the reactive strain, though the rigour of the selection possible has fluctuated somewhat. It will be appreciated that the criteria given in the table are minimal ones, and do not necessarily reflect the mean defecation scores of the parents selected, though the criteria are necessarily determined by the numbers born into any of the sub-groups described.

It was decided to employ mating brother by sister, in order to approach purity of strain as quickly as possible. This decision was unfortunate in view of the considerations discussed in Chapter 1, though their importance was not properly understood at the time the experiment began. But having started by using the closest possible inbreeding, it was decided to continue with it, and brother × sister mating was done throughout, except in the following two cases when it was necessary to depart from it in order to maintain numbers. In the parental non-reactive population eight females were mated with their half-brothers, i.e. males sharing one common parent, and in S_4 one reactive female was mated with a half-brother. The descendants of these parents are no longer represented, however, in the present populations, so that the effect of this necessary relaxation of the closest possible inbreeding probably had little effect.

The actual mating of the subjects, selected by the procedures described above, takes place by bringing the sexes together on a Monday and separating them on a Friday, and repeating this procedure once and sometimes twice in successive weeks. This five-day period of mating ensures, firstly, that few litters are born on a Saturday and even fewer

[1] Having regard to the data showing increased response to increases in physical stimuli, that is. But it may be that the non-reactives were already too far below the threshold of response, and the reactives approaching a physiological limit to defecation.

on a Sunday—since the average gestation period of the rat is twenty-two days, fourteen hours (Farris and Griffith, 1949)—and secondly, that in the usual case in which a female or a group of females is mated with different males during the successive weeks in order to maximize the chances of impregnation, the identity of the father of the litter is preserved. This can be unequivocally ascertained by subtracting the gestation period from the date of parturition and noting which male was running with the female in question at the time. Females judged pregnant on the basis of weight increases revealed by the weekly weighings instituted after open-field testing are removed to individual cages two to five days before the earliest possible date of parturition. No nesting material is provided at this time so that the newborn litters of the next generation may be easily observed for the purposes of weighing, sexing, etc., as described in Chapter 2 (Table 2.3).

Maternal effect

The necessity for controlling for maternal effects in psychogenetic work has been stressed by several writers (Scott and Fuller, 1951; Russell, 1953a) but most explicitly by Hall (1951). The transmission of the character selected for in the present type of experiment may be extra-genetical in that it may result from the operation of pre- and post-natal maternal influences. It is clearly vitally important that the possibility of such artifacts should be ruled out. To control for *post-natal maternal effects*, the technique of cross-fostering of litters at birth was adopted. Essential as this technique is for providing a control for the effects of post-natal maternal influence, it is not to be undertaken lightly. The minimum interference of the mother rat and her newborn litter is desirable to ensure adequate maternal care; removing the mother's own litter completely and substituting another is a procedure calculated to disturb this process. Despite the evidence, therefore (Wiesner and Sheard, 1933), that some albino rats will accept others' pups, or even young of other species, for suckling for extended periods after parturition, the substitutions in this experimental programme were made as soon as possible after birth. In one case only was it necessary to delay for so much as one day. Advantage was taken of the opportunity afforded by the single routine handling of the mothers and their newborn litters at birth to make the substitutions (see Table 2.3). The aim was to cross-foster half the rats of each generation, so that half the rats of emotionally reactive parents are reared by non-reactive mothers, and, conversely, half the rats of emotionally non-reactive parents are reared by reactive mothers, though, for a variety of reasons, it was not possible to achieve this aim precisely. Special care needs to be taken to ensure that the identity of cross-fostered litters is not lost. It is difficult to mark newborn pups physically, and a considerable secretarial problem consequently ensues. The procedure was continued up to and including S_6, when the results so far collected indicated that it could be discontinued.

The necessary control for *pre-natal maternal effects* could not be undertaken until the strains had achieved some degree of separation, since it depends on being able to distinguish the mean scores of parental strains from the (intermediate) ones of their offspring when the two strains are crossed. The genetical considerations underlying the analysis are as follows: if the two strains, high and low, are crossed reciprocally, i.e. high males with low females, and low males with high females, the expectation is that among the two generations thus formed the reciprocal crosses would not differ from each other significantly, because, on an average, they should have inherited the same genetical system controlling defecation from their respective parents, the only difference being that the first had been nurtured pre-natally by a low scoring mother, and the second by a high. A significant association of the scores of the F_1 offspring with those of the mother will thus disturb this equality of the two F_1's, and is *prima facie* evidence of a pre-natal maternal effect. In general terms we may say that the offspring of reciprocal crosses are alike genetically, and any large difference between them suggests a maternal effect.

There are, however, factors which can vitiate this analysis which are discussed by Broadhurst (1960a). Among them are sex linkage and cytoplasmic inheritance. The former may be defined as an association of the expression of a gene with one sex only, and should be easily recognizable. The latter is extra-nuclear, non-chromosomal inheritance, and could result in an effect which might mimic a maternal one. In the case of positive findings it might be necessary to exclude this possibility by distinguishing effects due to maternal uterine conditions, i.e. environmental—the maternal pre-natal effect discussed above—from effects due to the maternal cytoplasm, i.e. genetical. One of the techniques available is the method of transplanting fertilized ova (e.g. Hall, 1947), so that an ovum from, say, a high defecating mother which had been fertilized by a similar father would be removed and transplanted to the uterus of a low defecating mother. In this way the genetical and inter-uterine environmental effects may be disentangled, but the technical difficulties are considerable and, as will be seen below, it was perhaps fortunate that recourse to this method did not seem to be necessary in the present work.

Reciprocal crosses of the sort described were made using the high and low strain at S_6, S_7, and S_8 as parents, and the offspring were reared and tested in the usual manner, except that the offspring of S_7 were tested in the louder sound field. This was done in order to ensure that comparisons with the parental score would not be vitiated by any differences in testing, despite the apparent lack of effect the higher noise had had on the scores returned by S_7.

Results

The results presented here relate to the first ten generations of selective breeding. It is not proposed to stop at this stage, and the experiment continues.

The results are presented diagrammatically in Figs. 3.1 and 3.2 and in tabular form in Table 3.3. It is at once evident from Fig. 3.1 that

TABLE 3.3

Defecation scores for successive generations (units are average number of fecal boluses per trial)

Generation	Males *n*	Males M	Males SD	Females *n*	Females M	Females SD	Both *n*	Both M	Both SD
Parental*	106	3·78	1·62	116	2·40	1·78	222	3·06	1·84
Emotionally reactive									
First	48	3·07	1·46	47	3·10	1·47	95	3·09	1·46
Second	57	3·15	1·16	56	2·68	1·58	113	2·92	1·40
Third	43	3·55	0·76	50	3·23	1·13	93	3·38	0·99
Fourth	27	3·10	1·35	33	3·23	1·54	60	3·17	1·46
Fifth	48	3·21	1·30	37	3·29	1·56	85	3·25	1·42
Sixth	43	3·55	1·42	48	3·81	1·39	91	3·69	1·41
Seventh	45	3·91	1·36	33	3·79	1·13	78	3·86	1·27
Eighth	40	4·56	1·13	43	4·72	1·05	83	4·64	1·09
Ninth	46	3·71	1·15	43	3·76	1·20	89	3·73	1·17
Tenth	52	3·97	0·99	50	4·15	0·84	102	4·06	0·92
Emotionally non-reactive									
First	48	3·26	1·61	48	1·55	1·43	96	2·41	1·75
Second	35	1·70	1·44	48	0·55	0·82	83	1·03	1·26
Third	59	1·48	1·46	46	0·43	0·77	105	1·02	1·32
Fourth	43	0·57	1·09	37	0·18	0·48	80	0·39	0·89
Fifth	37	0·47	0·75	54	0·13	0·30	91	0·27	0·56
Sixth	33	1·61	1·50	61	0·55	1·13	94	0·92	1·37
Seventh	54	0·57	0·84	61	0·10	0·50	115	0·32	0·72
Eighth	45	0·04	0·14	38	0·007	0·04	83	0·03	0·11
Ninth	73	0·31	0·75	54	0·019	0·13	127	0·19	0·60
Tenth	51	0·46	0·94	44	0·86	0·44	95	0·31	0·77

* See footnote to Table 3.2.

selection is having an important effect, and that this effect is asymmetrical. That is to say, it appears to be in the direction of low defecation rather than high, though a trend in the direction of an increase in the scores of the emotionally reactive strain can also be discerned.

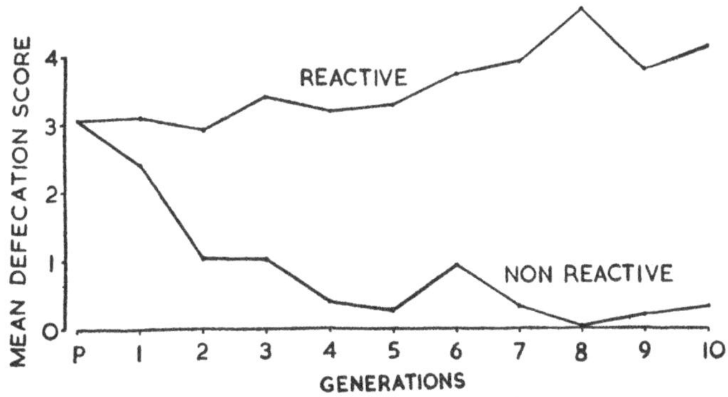

FIG. 3.1. Results of selective breeding for high and low defecation scores. The graph shows the mean scores of the reactive and non-reactive groups in successive generations of selective breeding. Generations are shown on the abscissa; the ordinate shows the mean number of fecal boluses deposited per trial in the test (see text).

Fig. 3.2 demonstrates rather clearly the interaction between sex and strain which results in the marked sex difference, seen in the unselected, parental generation and in other previous work (Broadhurst, 1957a), becoming quickly attenuated in the emotionally reactive strain. It persists, though almost becoming smaller, in the non-reactive strain. The

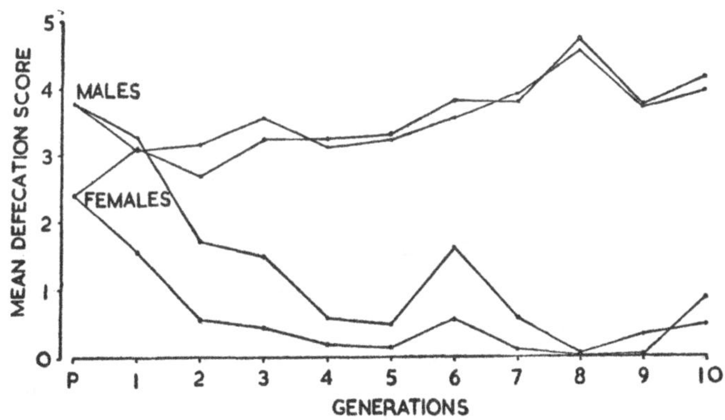

FIG. 3.2. Results of selective breeding for high and low defecation scores: sex difference. The graph shows the mean scores of the reactive and non-reactive groups in successive generations, divided according to sex. Generations are shown on the abscissa; the ordinate shows the mean number of fecal boluses deposited per trial in the test. The higher curves represent the reactive strain, the lower, the non-reactive, males being designated by solid points and females by open ones.

distributions of the scores for the first five generations are shown in Fig. 3.3. The histograms show the nature of the effect of selective breeding, particularly the progressive decrease in the degree of overlap of the scores of the two strains in successive generations. Considered in terms of the percentage of the reactives who have scores higher than any non-reactives, the progression from first to fifth generations is 0%, 0%, 3%, 21%, and 52%. Observe also that after the second

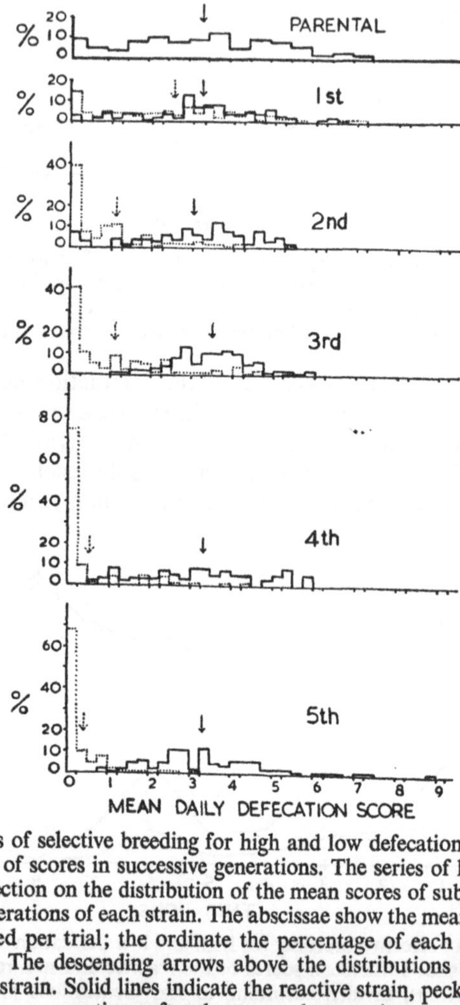

FIG. 3.3. Results of selective breeding for high and low defecation scores: effect on the distribution of scores in successive generations. The series of histograms shows the effect of selection on the distribution of the mean scores of subjects constituting the first five generations of each strain. The abscissae show the mean number of fecal boluses deposited per trial; the ordinate the percentage of each strain having the indicated score. The descending arrows above the distributions show the overall means for each strain. Solid lines indicate the reactive strain, pecked lines the non-reactive—after the parental generation.

generation all of the reactive strain defecate at least once. The distributions for the next five generations, S_{6-10}, are essentially similar and are not shown. An increasing build-up of zero scores among the non-reactive strain occurs, and accentuates the J shape of this distribution. There is some progress towards the separation of the two strains: indeed, in S_8 complete separation was achieved apart from one low-scoring reactive male, but S_9 and S_{10} again show considerable overlap.

Consideration of the standard deviations of the scores shown in Table 3.3 shows a tendency in both strains towards decreased scatter. This doubtless reflects the progress towards homozygosity within the

TABLE 3.4

Ambulation scores for successive generations (units are average number of metres run per trial)

Generation	Males *n*	Males M	Males SD	Females *n*	Females M	Females SD	Both *n*	Both M	Both SD
Parental*	106	3·74	1·91	116	4·41	2·20	222	4·05	2·09
Emotionally reactive									
First	48	5·33	2·33	47	6·75	2·79	95	6·03	2·68
Second	57	7·80	2·06	56	7·66	4·12	113	7·73	3·25
Third	43	7·37	2·25	50	7·73	2·33	93	7·57	2·30
Fourth	27	9·27	2·68	33	9·82	2·22	60	9·57	2·46
Fifth	48	8·77	2·94	37	9·58	2·56	85	9·12	2·81
Sixth	43	7·44	2·78	48	8·84	2·69	91	8·18	2·82
Seventh	45	8·70	2·94	33	10·19	2·20	78	9·33	2·76
Eighth	40	6·79	1·43	43	7·75	1·84	83	7·29	1·82
Ninth	46	6·57	2·22	43	8·37	2·14	89	7·44	2·36
Tenth	52	6·59	2·28	50	8·00	2·45	102	7·28	2·47
Emotionally non-reactive									
First	48	6·61	2·69	48	7·43	2·85	96	7·02	2·80
Second	35	8·30	2·51	48	9·72	2·96	83	9·12	2·86
Third	59	9·03	2·53	46	10·67	2·96	105	9·75	2·85
Fourth	43	10·02	2·84	37	11·16	2·34	80	10·55	2·68
Fifth	37	9·25	2·46	54	10·77	2·11	91	10·15	2·38
Sixth	33	9·16	2·72	61	10·34	3·09	94	9·93	3·12
Seventh	54	10·20	2·34	61	11·54	2·41	115	10·91	2·47
Eighth	45	9·00	2·85	38	10·32	3·08	83	9·61	3·03
Ninth	73	10·45	2·26	54	12·55	2.29	127	11·34	2·50
Tenth	51	10·32	3·15	44	11·28	2·61	95	10·76	2·95

* See footnote to Table 3.2.

strains to be expected from selection and from brother × sister mating.

An effect of selection for extremes of defecation on the ambulation scores is to be expected in view of the correlation between the two measures. Table 3.4 and Fig. 3.4 present the relevant data. It will be observed that there has been an increase in the mean score of both

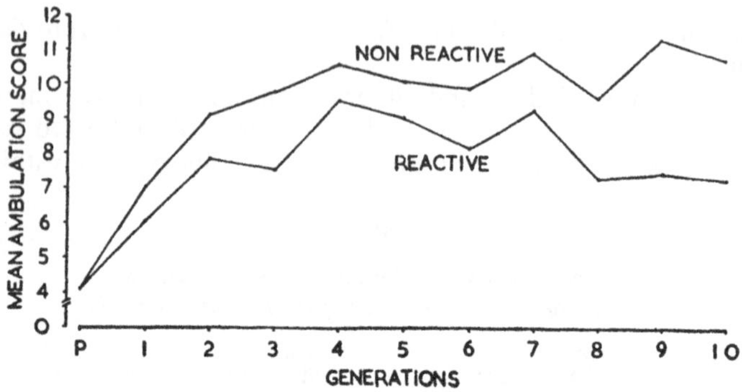

FIG. 3.4. Results of selective breeding for high and low defecation scores: effect on ambulation. The graph shows the effect on the mean ambulation scores of the reactive and non-reactive groups in successive generations of selective breeding. Generations are shown on the abscissa; the ordinate shows the mean number of metres run per trial in the test.

strains, though the increase in that of the non-reactive one is perhaps more marked. The greater overall activity of females in the open-field test is apparent from Fig. 3.5.

The findings suggest that the response to selection for defecation has had a marked effect on a character not selected for; the fact that it is

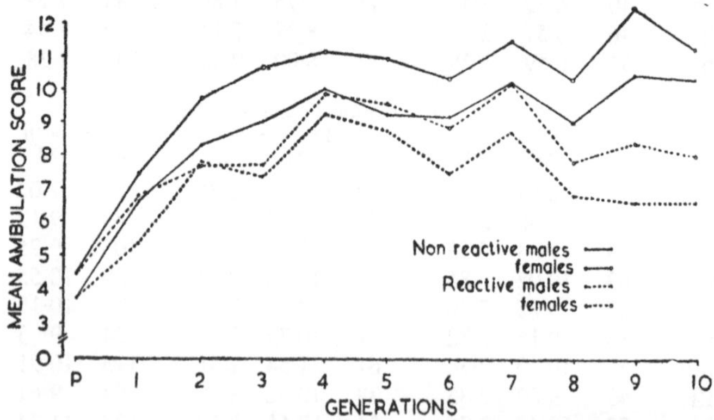

FIG. 3.5. Results of selective breeding for high and low defecation scores: effect on ambulation—sex difference. The graph shows the effect on the mean ambulation scores of the reactive and non-reactive groups in successive generations, divided according to sex. Generations are shown on the abscissa; the ordinate shows the mean number of metres per trial run in the test.

in the same direction in both lines suggests that it may be a response to the other variable operating on both lines equally, that is, inbreeding. The genetical situation is doubtless complicated and may represent a case of genetical correlation (Falconer, 1954). This could be investigated by the technique of selecting separately for the two traits on different populations and observing the correlated response in the other.

Statistical analysis

While the above tables and diagrams demonstrate that changes are taking place, statistical analysis is necessary to confirm the significance of the trends observed. But difficulties which were not foreseen at the start of this experiment have arisen in the analysis of the effect of breeding *per se* in the first ten generations—difficulties which preclude using the analysis of variance in the way that was projected. The principal difficulty lies in the increasing positive skewness shown by the scores of the non-reactive group (see Fig. 3.3). This is doubtless the result of successful selection for a trait in the direction of its own non-occurrence, that is to say, the situational determinants of the defecation response in the open-field test are no longer intense enough to release the response in the non-emotional group despite increases made in the noise stimulus in testing S_6 and especially S_7. Consequently, the assumptions underlying the analysis of variance (McNemar, 1955, p. 249 f.) are grossly violated, and suitable transformations for normalizing the data and rendering their variances homogeneous have not been found. It may well be that an overall analysis involving both strains may not be possible. A further difficulty is the impossibility of ensuring equality among the sub-groups, without extensive over-breeding as was done in the first generation (309 pups were bred, but the total was reduced to 191, principally by random culling). This renders impracticable the application of the analysis of variance to data classified in more than two ways.

Hence the major reliance must be placed for the moment upon the trends of the scores as demonstrated above in the figures discussed. Nevertheless, a more rigorous analysis of certain portions of the data is available and is presented below. Table 3.5 gives in summary form the results of the analyses of variance of both defecation and ambulation scores which were found to be possible in the first six generations. The table needs some explanation. Except in the case of S_1, the number in each sub-group was reduced to that in the smallest by randomly discarding data in order to permit triple classification analyses of variance with equal numbers in each cell. The remaining total is indicated in the fourth column. In each case the random nature of this procedure was checked by running *t*-tests comparing the mean of the scores retained with the mean of those discarded; in no case was a significant difference found. The data were then tested for inhomogeneity of variance of the sub-groups (Pearson and Hartley, 1958), and the results are shown in column 6. It will be noted that the log transformation tried for the S_{2-4} defecation scores was unsuccessful in reducing this inhomogeneity to non-significant levels. Indeed the defecation data for

TABLE 3.5

Summary results of analyses of defecation (D) and ambulation (A) scores of generation $S_{1\text{-}6}$

Generation	Total *N*	*n* in smallest sub-group	Analysis done on eight groups of:	Score	*P* for inhomogeneity of variance	Results of analyses of variance, *P* values for: Main effects: Strain (Reactivity: R)	Main effects: Sex (S)	Main effects: Cross-fostering	Interaction R × S	All other interactions
First	191	23	24 = 192	D	n.s.	n.s.	n.s.	n.s.	0·001	n.s.
				A	n.s.	0·01	0·01	0·01	n.s.	n.s.
Second	196	12	12 = 96	D	0·01					
				log (D + 1)	0·01					
				A	n.s.	n.s.	n.s.	n.s.	0·01	n.s.
Third	198	20	20 = 160	D	0·01					
				log (D + 1)	0·01					
				A	n.s.	0·05	n.s.	n.s.	0·05	n.s.
Fourth	140	7	7 = 56	D	0·001					
				log (D + 1)	0·01					
				A	0·05	n.s.	n.s.	n.s.	n.s.	n.s.
Fifth	176	17	17 = 136	D	0·01					
				A	n.s.	n.s.	n.s.	n.s.	n.s.	n.s.
Sixth	185	16	16 = 128	D	0·01					
				A	n.s.	0·01	0·01	n.s.	n.s.	n.s.

S_1 only permitted an analysis involving both strains. In order to provide the missing score in one of the sub-groups the mean score for the rest of the group was inserted as a further value. Considering these defecation scores first, it is noted that the interaction of sex with strain is highly significant; accordingly it has been used in evaluating the main effects of sex and strain which thereby emerge as non-significant, *F*-ratios being less than unity in each case. Analysis of this interaction by means of *t*-tests of the differences between the means of the appropriate sub-groups gives the results shown in Table 3.6. It is clear that selection

TABLE 3.6

Analysis of the sex × strain interaction in defecation scores of S_1 *(mean number of boluses per trial)*

	Sex		
Strain	Male		Female
Reactive	3·1	n.s.	3·1
	n.s.		$P = 0{\cdot}001$
Non-reactive	3·3	$P = 0{\cdot}001$	1·5

has already operated powerfully upon females, but its effect is not yet evident among males.

The reason for this interaction—the nature of which is best seen in Fig. 3.2—might be thought to be a large number of zero scores (eleven out of the forty-eight) occurring in the group of non-reactive females, rather than a general lowering of all scores in this group. A re-analysis, eliminating all zero scores, gives the altered means shown in Table 3.7.

TABLE 3.7

Further analysis of the sex × strain interaction in defecation scores of S_1

	Males			Females		
	Mean score	No. of 0 scores	Adjusted mean	Mean score	No. of 0 scores	Adjusted mean
Reactive	3·1	1	3·1	3·1	2	3·2
Non-reactive	3·3	2	3·4	3·5	11	2·0

This analysis suggests that, while the large number of zero scores in the non-reactive female group does depress the mean score of that group, the interaction effect is not entirely attributable to this cause. The other females in this group also score low, and the resulting mean is consistent with previous results (Broadhurst, 1957a). The essence of the interaction seems rather to lie in the *high* scores of the group of reactive females, who in fact score higher than do the reactive males. This reversal of the usual sex difference is unparalleled in our previous work with unselected subjects though it occurs again in the subsequent generations of the emotionally reactive strain, as may be seen in Fig. 3.2, and is doubtless an effect of the selection pressure maintained. Turning to the results of the analysis of the ambulation scores, we find in S_1, in addition to the expected differences resulting from the sex and strain variables, a difference due to cross-fostering as such. This is not, however, a significant interaction, such as would be observed if the effect of inactivity of reactive mothers, and the activity of non-reactive mothers (Hall, 1936), were influencing pups reared by them. Instead, it is an overall depression of activity scores among the cross-fostered subjects, mean score (number of metres run per trial) 5·9, as compared with 7·1 for the non-cross-fostered group. The reason for this effect is difficult to see. Since it does not recur in the ambulation scores of generations S_{2-6}, analysed in the same manner, it is perhaps attributable in this case to the operation of unrecognized chance factors.

The fact that analyses of variance of the ambulation data after the first generation were possible will be seen from Table 3.5. The reason lies in the nature of the scores, which tend to give a good distribution, the mean of which does not approach zero as does that of the defecation scores for the non-reactive group. Consequently no markedly significant inhomogeneity of variance[1] is disclosed, and the analyses could proceed in the usual way, after the *n* in each sub-group had been reduced. The results show a significant interaction between strain and sex in S_2 and S_3, which obscures the marked sex and strain differences especially in S_3, and is due to disproportionately high mean scores returned by the non-reactive females (see Table 3.4). Evaluation by *t*-tests of the four mean differences in interaction tables shows this disproportion to be significant in each case. Thereafter the sex and strain differences do not interact, and do not themselves reach significant levels in S_4 and S_5, reappearing as significant at the 1% levels in S_6, principally, it seems, because of the low mean scores of the reactive strain.

Discontinuation of the cross-fostering technique after S_6 simplified the analyses for the remaining generations. The same difficulty as before still precluded an overall analysis of the defecation scores; tests disclosed inhomogeneity of variance significant beyond the 1% level in each case. But the homogeneity of variance of the ambulation scores was in general satisfactory and analyses of variance were carried out using Snedecor's (1956) method for double classification with disproportionate numbers in the sub-groups. Thus it was unnecessary to discard any data to simplify the analyses, the results of which are shown in Table 3.8. It will be seen that the strain difference, which reached significance in S_6, again emerges strongly in S_{8-10}. It is perhaps noteworthy that it was in these generations that the effect of the selection for low urination scores in the open field might be expected to have been shown. The main effect due to sex is uniformly significant in these

[1] Inhomogeneity of variance significant at the 5% level only is ignored.

data, so that after S_5, it has reached significant levels in all the ambulation scores analysed.

It emerges from what has preceded that it has only been possible to demonstrate in statistical terms the effect of selection upon defecation scores in the first generation selected, and even then it was partly obscured by an interaction effect. However, a consideration of Figs. 3.1 and 3.2 and the means and standard deviations given in Table 3.3 should convince even the most sceptical of the reality of the results of selection. But the difficulties which precluded the formal analysis of the effects of selection have unfortunately had the result of preventing rigorous assessment of the effects of the other variables involved. Accordingly the effect of selection was taken as demonstrated, and data divided so that the high and low strains could be considered separately. For generations S_{2-6} inclusive, two-way analyses of variance were carried out wherever the test of homogeneity of variance allowed, and using the reduced data as discussed in connection with the analyses of Table 3.5. The

TABLE 3.8

Summary results of analyses of variance of ambulation scores of generations S_{7-10}

Generation	Total N	P for inhomogeneity of variance	Results of analyses of variance P values for: Main effects Strain	Sex	Interaction
Seventh	193	n.s.	n.s.	0·001	n.s.
Eighth	166	0·05	0·001	0·01	n.s.
Ninth	216	n.s.	0·001	0·001	n.s.
Tenth	197	n.s.	0·001	0·01	n.s.

results are given in Table 3.9, and may be summarized by saying that among the reactive strain the data showed, in general, satisfactory homogeneity of variance permitting the analyses of variance which showed uniformly non-significant results due to sex or cross-fostering differences. The single exception in S_3 is attributable to a significant sex difference at the 5% level occurring among cross-fostered subjects only. The data from the non-reactive strain showed the ubiquitous difficulty relating to inhomogeneity of variance so that analysis was not possible beyond S_2 and S_3. In these two generations, however, the sex difference in the direction of lower scores for females (see Table 3.3) was shown to be very highly significant.

Analysis of the defecation data for S_{7-10} employed t-tests of the differences between the sexes and within the strains, since, it will be remembered, the cross-fostering ceased with S_6. The results may be summarized by saying that they show consistently non-significant differences between the sexes in the reactive strain, whereas in the non-reactive strain the sex difference, still in the direction of lower female scores, reached significance in S_7 and S_{10} at the 0·1% and 5% levels respectively, but did not do so in S_8 and S_9. These analyses therefore support the trends of Figs. 3.2 and 3.5, i.e., an attenuation of the sex difference in defecation in the reactive strain, while it remains fairly evident in the

TABLE 3.9

Summary results of analysis of variance of defecation scores of generations S_{2-6}

Generation	Inhomogeneity of variance	Reactive strain: *P* values for Main effects: Sex	Main effects: Cross-fostering	Interaction
Second	n.s.	n.s.	n.s.	n.s.
Third	n.s.	n.s.	n.s.	0·05
Fourth	n.s.	n.s.	n.s.	n.s.
Fifth	0·05	n.s.	n.s.	n.s.
Sixth	n.s.	n.s.	n.s.	n.s.

Generation	Inhomogeneity of variance	Non-reactive strain: *P* values for Main effects: Sex	Main effects: Cross-fostering	Interaction
Second	n.s.*	0·001	n.s.	n.s.
Third	0·05*	0·001	n.s.	n.s.
Fourth	0·01*			
Fifth	0·01			
Sixth	0·01			

* Using the transformation $D' = \log (D + 1)$.

non-reactive strain. A similar reversal of secondary sex difference under selection is known in the fruit fly (Harrison, 1953).

Maternal effects

The results relating to the cross-fostering and cross-breeding undertaken to check on post- and pre-natal maternal effects respectively are discussed in detail elsewhere (Broadhurst, 1960a). In general, it may be said that they indicate that there is little evidence of any marked effect upon either score. The means of the cross-fostered animals are not systematically different from those of animals in the same strain not cross-fostered, that is, they show no tendency to resemble their foster-parents of the other strain rather than their own. The case of a significant effect of this variable in S_1 has been discussed above, but it does not lend any support to the notion of a post-natal maternal effect.

The results of the cross-breeding for the analysis of pre-natal effects, carried out at S_6, S_7 and S_8 in the selection experiment, are not so clear cut. The defecation scores show no significant differences attributable to the strain of the mother except in one case, the offspring of the S_8 generation, where pups reared by reactive mothers score higher than those from non-reactive ones. However, when the data from the three generations are pooled, there is no overall significant difference. Similarly with the ambulation scores, one group, the offspring of S_7 in this case, show a significant effect in the expected direction, pups nurtured by reactive mothers having a *lower* ambulation score than those born to non-reactive ones. Pooling the data from the three generations of cross-bred litters serves to confirm the significance of the overall trend but at a low level.

OTHER RESULTS

Fertility and maternal care

One of the results which frequently accompanies inbreeding is inbreeding depression. This is seen in decreased fertility, which may indeed endanger the continuance of the strain. A check was therefore kept on this important practical aspect of the present experiment, and in Table 3.10 will be found a summary of the salient features, some of which need explanation.

The third column shows the percentage of females mated which gave birth to litters. While this figure, which serves as a measure of female fertility, shows marked fluctuations from generation to generation, there does not appear to be any systematic effect either over the progress of the experiment, or between the strains. The number of days between the date upon which the sexes were brought together in a fertile mating and the date upon which the female gave birth is shown in column 4 and provides a rough measure of sexual vigour, though not distinguishing between males and females. There seems to be little evidence of any effect here. The number of pups born per litter (columns 5–7) refers to the offspring constituting the next following generation, as does each of the subsequent columns, and suggests a decline in litter size with the progress of the experiment, though this is not accompanied by an increase in the average birth weight of the individual pups (column 8). From S_4 onwards we begin to see the first suggestions of a weight difference between the strains, the non-reactives being lighter. The number of pups born dead (column 9) does not appear to vary systematically with strain or generation, but there is an increase in the number lost before weaning (column 10), which reflects the lack of maternal care, failures of lactation, and cannibalism. As far as these data go, therefore, it seems that the effects found may be attributed to an increase in the failure of maternal care rather than to any major decline in fertility. The weaning weights (columns 11 and 12) do not show as clearly the tendency found in the birth weights, possibly because of the complication of the sex differences in weight.

It was therefore decided to analyse the adult weight of a sample of the animals: the groups chosen were the S_6 and S_7 generations, whose

TABLE 3.10

Effects of selection with inbreeding on fertility, etc., in reactive (R) and non-reactive (N) strains

Generation	Strain	Proportion of females mated giving birth (%)	Time from mating to birth (days)	Mean no. pups born per litter Males	Females	Total	Mean birth weight of live pups (gm.)	Proportion of pups Born dead (%)	Dying before weaning (%)	Mean weight at weaning (gm.) Males	Females
Parental	R	94·7	24·2	5·8	5·8	11·6	5·1	2·9	15·8	33·0	32·7
	N	66·7	24·8	5·6	5·3	11·0	5·3	0·6	9·8	32·9	32·3
First	R	86·7	24·8	5·1	5·3	10·4	5·3	5·9	15·7	31·8	30·6
	N	94·4	24·6	4·5	4·9	9·4	5·4	0·6	12·0	33·2	31·4
Second	R	68·4	24·4	4·8	5·1	9·8	4·8	3·1	24·2	35·7	32·6
	N	76·5	24·5	5·2	4·2	9·4	5·2	1·6	12·5	31·4	30·7
Third	R	65·0	24·8	4·2	4·5	8·7	5·1	7·1	41·0	32·4	33·3
	N	80·0	24·4	4·9	4·5	9·4	5·1	2·7	45·2	31·7	31·4
Fourth	R	79·2	24·4	4·1	3·9	8·0	5·4	6·6	38·0	28·4	27·5
	N	53·6	25·0	3·1	4·1	7·2	5·2	3·7	12·5	28·2	26·9
Fifth	R	86·4	24·3	3·9	4·4	8·3	5·5	1·3	35·3	29·2	29·3
	N	87·0	24·5	2·9	4·4	7·2	5·1	0	25·6	32·0	28·7
Sixth	R	74·1	24·5	4·6	3·8	8·4	5·2	0	52·7	29·3	29·4
	N	80·8	24·9	3·6	4·5	8·1	5·0	1·2	30·9	23·6	27·3
Seventh	R	65·2	24·7	3·5	3·7	7·1	5·5	0·9	26·4	30·6	29·9
	N	65·0	23·8	4·4	4·9	9·3	5·1	1·7	29·4	27·3	27·6
Eighth	R	83·3	24·6	4·0	3·9	7·8	5·6	10·3	31·4	33·3	32·4
	N	89·5	24·5	5·4	5·1	10·5	5·2	3·4	26·0	30·7	28·2
Ninth	R	65·2	25·4	3·9	4·0	7·9	5·8	0·8	12·7	34·4	34·5
	N	85·0	24·2	4·0	3·9	7·9	5·3	2·2	28·0	31·0	30·2
Tenth	R	55·6	24·3	3·7	4·3	7·9	5·7	13·4	20·4	27·2	28·0
	N	75·0	24·5	4·5	4·3	8·8	5·2	0	40·0	29·0	29·1

weaning weights are those shown in Table 3.10 under 'fifth' and 'sixth' generation respectively. The data used were obtained from the routine weighing of the animals after the open-field test (see Chapter 2), at around 110 days of age. Analyses of variance were performed on the two generations separately, and, because of the disparity between the findings with respect to females' mean weights as shown in Table 3.11, with the data for both pooled together also. The levels of significance of the differences between the means are derived from the appropriate two-way analyses of variance, carried out according to Snedecor's (1956) method for dealing with the unequal numbers in the sub-groups. The results show the expected difference in favour of heavier weight for males than for females at a consistently high level of significance. Among the males only there is also a similarly significant effect of strain upon weight; the rats from the reactive strain being heavier than those from the non-reactive one. But among females the effect, present in S_6, is reversed, though at a low level of significance, in S_7. Taking both generations together the trend does not reach significance. We may say, therefore, that there is definite evidence that our reactive strain is heavier than the non-reactive, though this difference may be confined to males. This finding is of interest in view of the observations of the behavioural differences between strains of mice selected for high and low body weight, which led the experimenters to characterize the lighter strains as more active than the heavier: see Chapter 1. In selecting for high and low defecation, we have involved genetical determinants for activity, body size, and probably many other physiological characteristics, e.g. hormonal differences (Chapter 2).[1] As noted above, parallel selective breeding for the various characteristics separately would be needed in order to establish the existence of genetical correlations between the several traits.

Maze brightness and maze dullness

One possible behavioural characteristic which might have been involved in the selection for the defecation response is the one specified by the terms maze brightness and dullness, the genetical contribution to which was brought to the attention of psychologists by the selection experiments of Tryon and of Heron. This eventuality seemed particularly possible in view of the findings relating to the differences in the motivational characteristics of Tryon's maze bright and dull strains found by Searle (1949), and has obvious relevance to other studies in which our selectively bred strains might be used, and which involved

[1] In this connection it may be mentioned that a few determinations of the cholinesterase content of the brains of rats from the two strains do not point to the existence of any large difference between them in this respect. This observation, for which I am indebted to Dr. R. H. J. Watson, is of interest in view of the known possibility of selectively breeding rats for different levels of brain cholinesterase (Rosenzweig, Krech, and Bennett, 1958b).

TABLE 3.11

Differences between mean adult weights of rats according to sex and strain (units are grams)

	Generation								
	Sixth			Seventh			Both combined		
	Reactive		Non-reactive	Reactive		Non-reactive	Reactive		Non-reactive
Males	279·3	$P = 0{\cdot}001$	241·7	260·0	$P = 0{\cdot}001$	239·3	269·4	$P = 0{\cdot}001$	240·2
	$P = 0{\cdot}001$		$P = 0{\cdot}001$	$P = 0{\cdot}001$		$P = 0{\cdot}001$	$P = 0{\cdot}001$		$P = 0{\cdot}001$
Females	182·9	$P = 0{\cdot}001$	161·7	153·1	$P = 0{\cdot}05$	170·0	171·7	n.s.	165·7

learning. It was therefore decided to investigate this possibility using the most satisfactory measure of animal 'intelligence' available, the Hebb-Williams closed field test (Rabinovitch and Rosvold, 1951).

Forty-eight rats from S_7 and including the extremes of high and low defecation response were therefore given the Hebb-Williams test under standardized conditions. The results are given in detail elsewhere (Das and Broadhurst, 1959), but are easily summarized since no significant trends relating error scores to emotional defecation could be detected. It was concluded that emotional reactivity is orthogonal to intelligence in the rat as measured in this experiment, and support for this view was derived from the results of the Thompson and Bindra (1952) study of the McGill maze bright and dull strains. Their subjects, selectively bred on the basis of their scores in the Hebb-Williams test, showed no difference in the measures of emotionality which they used.

Genetical considerations

The main purpose of the selective breeding experiment was to provide homogeneous populations of subjects of known degrees of expression of the emotionality variable for use in other experimental work in which it was required. This work has been summarized in the discussion of validity of the defecation measure in Chapter 2 and it is not proposed to review it here beyond saying that the strains have fulfilled their purpose well, and that the results have in general supported the original interpretation of the nature of the characteristic for which they have been selected.

Secondary to this main purpose, but of major interest in the present connection, are the psychogenetical aspects. One of the strains, the non-reactive, was incorporated in the experiment in biometrical genetics to be described in the next chapter, and its contribution to our understanding of the genetical system affecting the expression of defecation and ambulation in the open-field test may be assessed there. But consideration of the results of the present experiment are also informative, though in a less precise way. Firstly, it is clear that, having excluded the possibility of major environmental effects, a profound influence of heredity upon tendency to emotional defecation has been demonstrated by the differences brought about by selection.

Our work in this respect closely parallels that of Hall (1951) (cf. Figs. 1.1 and 3.1), whose findings are thus shown to be repeatable, despite his omission of any control for maternal effects.

It will have been noted that Hall used as his measure the number of days upon which emotional elimination—urination as well as defecation—occurred. While such an elimination frequency score is in some ways an unsatisfactory measure, as has been discussed elsewhere (Broadhurst, 1957a), it is clearly adequate to reveal changes brought about by selective breeding. A re-calculation of the scores of the present non-reactive groups in S_{1-5} in terms of Hall's frequency measure shows a systematic decrease over the five generations which parallels closely the results given by the defecation score and shown in Fig. 3.1. This re-analysis was confined to the non-reactive strain because the reactives reached the possible maximum of four days almost at once.

The second finding of interest is that the selection was asymmetrical, that is, progress has not been equally rapid in both groups. This is frequently found in experiments in which selection is practised simultaneously in more than one direction (Falconer, 1955). The asymmetry is so marked in the present experiment as to suggest, on the scale used, a selection operating mainly in the direction of low defecation only. Thus ten generations of selection have resulted in a mean increase of one unit in the high line whereas the decrease in the low line reaches the value of 2·29 by S_{10}. Hall's data, while resembling ours closely if attention is confined to the first five generations only, later shows an increasing tendency in the high selection line, which is not paralleled in our own. It may be that this delayed selection effect in Hall's experiment—a phenomenon not infrequently encountered in selective breeding (Mather and Harrison, 1949)—has been even more delayed in our strains and is yet to appear. However, the inadmissibility of detailed comparisons of this nature between strains selected differently from different parental stocks, despite the many tempting similarities, must again be stressed.

The third item of psychogenetical interest is the possibility the production of these strains allow us of estimating the genetical parameters contributing to the expression of the defecation and ambulation scores. As has been noted earlier, the practice of inbreeding along with selection for high and low expression of the defecation character has meant that without making entirely unreasonable assumptions it has not been possible to apply the usual genetical analyses applicable in selective breeding experiments, of which Falconer's work on body size in mice (1953) is such an excellent example (see also Lerner, 1958, p. 132 f.). The use of a control group, maintained from the same parental stock as the selected lines, but differing from them only by the absence of selection practised upon them, would have permitted a partial solution of the difficulties into which the use of inbreeding has led us. Indeed, the use of this control is frequently advocated by those discussing selective breeding (Chapman, 1951) but appears to be equally infrequently practised. Not least among the advantages accruing from the use of such a control group, combined with the two selected groups, is that three groups, each differing from the others in the selected characteristic, can then be used instead of two for predictive purposes in experiments of the kind noted in Chapter 2.

There is, however, a way in which the use of inbreeding can be turned to good account, and that is if we make the assumption that the selectively bred lines are homozygous in respect of the characteristics under investigation. Then a simple biometrical analysis of the weighted sums of the components of variation of the generation means can be applied (Jinks and Jones, 1958). Now it is unlikely that such an assumption can be rigorously met in our data. We know that the non-reactive strain is heterogeneous in respect of coat-colour (see Chapter 1), though this does not necessarily imply heterozygosity in the genetical system determining defecation responses. Moreover, eight to ten generations of inbreeding by brother × sister mating may be expected to have reduced the original heterozygosity of the system by an appreciable amount (Wright, 1921). Finally it may be said that the effect of the failure to meet this assumption may be expected to result in inflated values for the variances obtained, hence lowering the significance of the components calculated. In particular, the estimate of E, the component resulting from non-heritable, especially environmental, variation, may be larger than would otherwise be the case. It is calculated in this case from the average of the variances of the parental, filial, and backcross generations so that genetical variation between individuals due to the absence of homozygosity, e.g. segregation, will be confounded with the non-heritable variation thus obtained.

The method requires the data for P_1, P_2, F_1, F_2, and the backcrosses B_1 and B_2. The selectively bred strains at S_8 served as parental generations, high and low being P_1 and P_2 respectively, and the reciprocal cross of them made for the purpose of ascertaining pre-natal maternal influence served as F_1. From the 106 animals of two sorts of F_1 thus available, sufficient were randomly selected for mating in the four possible combinations of sexes and reciprocals to provide an F_2 of 240 subjects, a B_1 of 150 subjects, and a B_2 of 270 subjects. These rats were reared and tested in the precisely standardized manner specified in Chapter 2. In what follows the defecation and ambulation scores thus obtained were pooled over the reciprocals in each generation.

The means and standard errors for the six generations are given in Table 3.12 both separately for the two sexes and combined. In Table 3.13 will be found the equalities derived from Jinks and Jones (1958) and Mather (1949), and upon which the estimates of the components given in Table 3.14 are based. They represent a summation of the genetical parameters d (additivity), h (dominance) (see Fig. 1.3 and the discussion in Chapter 1), and the three components expressive of non-allelic interaction, i, j, l (Hayman and Mather, 1955). The latter may best be thought of as representing genic interaction within and between the additive and dominance components of the general form d,d, d,h, and h,h respectively.

The results for defecation suggest that only the values for the component relating to additivity, (d), is significantly different from zero, being more than three times their standard error in each case. These

TABLE 3.12

Generation means and standard errors of defecation and ambulation scores for crosses and backcrosses of reactive (P_1) and non-reactive (P_2) selectively bred strains

	P_1	P_2	F_1	F_2	B_1	B_2
			Defecation scores (boluses per trial)			
Males	4·6 ± 0·2	0·04 ± 0·02	2·5 ± 0·2	2·8 ± 0·15	3·7 ± 0·15	1·4 ± 0·2
Females	4·7 ± 0·2	0·01 ± 0·01	1·1 ± 0·2	1·1 ± 0·1	2·8 ± 0·2	0·5 ± 0·1
Both	4·6 ± 0·1	0·03 ± 0·01	1·75 ± 0·15	1·9 ± 0·1	3·2 ± 0·1	1·0 ± 0·1
			Ambulation scores (metres per trial)			
Males	6·8 ± 0·3	9·0 ± 0·4	8·6 ± 0·3	7·6 ± 0·2	6·6 ± 0·3	7·3 ± 0·3
Females	7·7 ± 0·3	10·3 ± 0·5	10·1 ± 0·3	9·3 ± 0·2	7·7 ± 0·3	8·9 ± 0·4
Both	7·3 ± 0·2	9·6 ± 0·3	9·4 ± 0·2	8·5 ± 0·2	7·2 ± 0·2	8·1 ± 0·3

findings are reasonably consistent over the two sexes. The significance of (d) allows us to determine an estimate of heritability for the character. This is done using a linear estimate of E, the non-heritable component, derived from the average of the variances of the means of the P_1, P_2,

TABLE 3.13

Equations for estimating certain genetical parameters and their variances from generation means

$$(d) = \bar{B}_1 - \bar{B}_2 \qquad V_{(d)} = V_{\bar{B}_1} + V_{\bar{B}_2}$$

$$(h) = \bar{F}_1 - 4\bar{F}_2 - \tfrac{1}{2}\bar{P}_1 - \tfrac{1}{2}\bar{P}_2 + 2\bar{B}_1 + 2\bar{B}_2 \qquad V_{(h)} = V_{\bar{F}_1} + 16V_{\bar{F}_2} + \tfrac{1}{4}V_{\bar{P}_1} + \tfrac{1}{4}V_{\bar{P}_2} + 4V_{\bar{B}_1} + 4V_{\bar{B}_2}$$

$$(i) = 2\bar{B}_1 + 2\bar{B}_2 - 4\bar{F}_2 \qquad V_{(i)} = 4V_{\bar{B}_1} + 4V_{\bar{B}_2} + 16V_{\bar{F}_2}$$

$$(j) = 2\bar{B}_1 - \bar{P}_1 - 2\bar{B}_2 + \bar{P}_2 \qquad V_{(j)} = 4V_{\bar{B}_1} + V_{\bar{P}_1} + 4V_{\bar{B}_2} + V_{\bar{P}_2}$$

$$(l) = \bar{P}_1 + \bar{P}_2 + 2\bar{F}_1 + 4\bar{F}_2 - 4\bar{B}_1 - 4\bar{B}_2 \qquad V_{(l)} = V_{\bar{P}_1} + V_{\bar{P}_2} + 4V_{\bar{F}_1} + 16V_{\bar{F}_2} + 16V_{\bar{B}_1} + 16V_{\bar{B}_2}$$

F_1, F_2 and backcross populations. Then heritability is calculated as (d)/((d) + e). An advantage may be claimed for this formulation as a measure of heritability over those usually employed, as it is independent of the non-fixable genetical components relating to dominance, (h) here.

TABLE 3.14

Summated genetical parameters

	(d)	(h)	(i)	(j)	(l)
	Defecation scores (boluses per trial)				
Males	2·3 ± 0·3	−1·0 ± 0·9	−1·2 ± 0·8	0 ± 0·6	0·7 ± 1·4
Females	2·3 ± 0·3	0·8 ± 0·7	2·1 ± 0·7	0·2 ± 0·5	−1·8 ± 1·2
Both	2·3 ± 0·2	0·01 ± 0·6	0·6 ± 0·6	0·1 ± 0·4	−0·7 ± 0·9
	Ambulation scores (metres per trial)				
Males	0·7 ± 0·4	−1·8 ± 1·3	−2·5 ± 1·3	0·8 ± 1·0	7·6 ± 2·2
Females	1·2 ± 0·5	−2·9 ± 1·3	−4·0 ± 1·2	0·3 ± 1·1	9·0 ± 2·1
Both	0·9 ± 0·3	−2·5 ± 1·1	−3·5 ± 1·1	0·4 ± 0·7	8·5 ± 1·7

The values obtained are 92·9 for males, 93·8 for females and 95·0 for both combined.

Examination of the results for ambulation scores shows a somewhat different picture, the pooled dominance component, (h), being significant, but negative, suggesting a preponderance of dominants among the genes for low ambulation.[1] A rough measure of the mean dominance is

[1] It should be noted that the effect of dominant genes is not necessarily to increase the phenotypic expression of the character, nor recessives to decrease it, and that in

available in the ratio (h)/(d) (Mather, 1949) which here takes a value of −2·78. The interaction components (i) and (l) are significant for the data for both sexes, which points to multigenic determination, since there must be a mutiplicity of genes involved for interaction to occur. Heritability is estimated as before and gives values of 69·1 for males, 77·7 for females, and 79·8 for both combined.

Further calculations could be carried out using the present data and proceeding along similar lines, especially with reference to estimating and interpreting the components of variation (D, H, etc.) derived from the second degree statistics (Mather, 1949). But no attempt is made to do so here, firstly because of the not entirely satisfactory nature of the data available for such an analysis, and secondly because of the more extensive analysis of the same characteristics available using the data and methods to be presented in the next chapter. Examples of the complete biometrical analysis of psychological data from parental, filial and backcross populations will be found in Broadhurst and Jinks' (1960) re-analysis of suitable experiments reported in the literature, which have been drawn from among those reviewed in Chapter 1.

Summary

This chapter describes the progress of the selective breeding experiment for high and low defecation responses of rats in the open-field test up to and including the tenth generation. The methods of selecting the subjects for mating and the techniques for investigating the pre- and post-natal maternal effects are described. The results show a profound effect of selection upon the level of defecation and upon sex differences in it, with an ancillary effect upon ambulation, and also upon body size. A decline in maternal fitness may be due to the inbreeding unfortunately practised. A biometrical analysis of the genetical components of certain generation means suggests a high heritability for defecation, and a moderate one for ambulation.

a polygenic system the resemblance of an F_1 to a parental population does not necessarily imply the presence of dominants in that population, as it does in simple Mendelian genetics.

4

ANALYSIS OF A DIALLEL CROSS

THE concepts of biometrical genetics have been introduced (Chapter 1) and a simple application of some of them made to data from our selectively bred strains (Chapter 3).

In the present chapter use will be made of the alternative approach to the investigation of hereditary characteristics in animals, the analysis of the properties of pure-bred strains and their crosses. An experiment will be described which is more ambitious in scope, and which, being expressly designed to use the methods of biometrical genetics, may serve to show decisively their application in psychogenetics.

Scaling

There is one important aspect of the biometrical method, discussion of which has been postponed till now, since it can most conveniently be expounded in describing the present experiment. It is the problem of scaling. This problem is a familiar one in psychology where statistical procedures, especially the analysis of variance, have certain assumptions relating to normality of distribution, homogeneity of variance, and the like which must be fulfilled in the data before they can properly be applied. But it has been shown that the consequences of violating the assumptions are not particularly serious (Lindquist, 1953), so long as these violations are not too gross, and in practice failure to meet assumptions is frequently ignored, as may be seen in several examples in the present work. Serious failures can sometimes be countered by re-scaling the data, when it may be found that the assumptions are then met. It is not often that these difficulties are sufficiently great to demand recourse to fractionating the data or to the use of non-parametric statistics.

In biometrical genetics similar considerations apply, but for somewhat different reasons; and it must be stressed at once that the assumptions involved are fundamental to the biometrical models and must be taken seriously. In biometrical genetics we are not partitioning observed variances into component parts, as in the analysis of variance, in order to apply statistical tests of significance to estimate if certain components are larger than others. Instead we are seeking to use observed variances to calculate certain parameters based on theoretical models derived from Mendelian theory. These models have two most important assumptions, firstly, that gene effects are additive, over the range of variation encountered, and secondly, that no environmental-genotype interaction is present. The second case shows itself in various ways, and is easy to detect in the diallel cross method to be used here. It is seen most obviously as a significant inhomogeneity of variance indicating that some strains or crosses (genotypes) are more sensitive to the effect of the experimental environment and possible small undetected changes in it. It can sometimes be dealt with by re-scaling; an example of such a case will be given later.

It is the first assumption that concerns us now—that of additivity. To test this, Mather (1949) and his colleagues (Jinks and Jones, 1958) have devised and used certain *scaling tests*, and the reader is referred to the first reference cited for a full exposition of them. Briefly, they relate to the assumption that if all genes have additive effects, then mean scores for the backcrosses (B_1 and B_2) between the F_1, itself derived from a cross between two homozygous parental lines (P_1 and P_2), and those parental lines themselves, must fall midway between the F_1 and P_1 or P_2 values respectively. That is:

$$\bar{B}_1 = \tfrac{1}{2}(\bar{P}_1 + \bar{F}_1),$$

and

$$\bar{B}_2 = \tfrac{1}{2}(\bar{P}_2 + \bar{F}_1).$$

From these relationships scaling tests A and B are derived; similar considerations relating to F_2 and F_3 give rise to tests C and D respectively, though the last is irrelevant to work with mammals and is omitted here. The tests are given in Table 4.1. It will be seen that the tests are devised so that, if the scale is adequate, the result is zero in each case. Also given in the table are the variances of the means which

TABLE 4.1

Mather's scaling tests

Test	Variances
$A = \bar{P}_1 + \bar{F}_1 - 2\bar{B}_1 = 0$	$V_A = V_{\bar{P}_1} + V_{\bar{F}_1} + 4V_{\bar{B}_1}$
$B = \bar{P}_2 + \bar{F}_1 - 2\bar{B}_2 = 0$	$V_B = V_{\bar{P}_2} + V_{\bar{F}_1} + 4V_{\bar{B}_2}$
$C = \bar{P}_1 + \bar{P}_2 + 2\bar{F}_1 - 4\bar{F}_2 = 0$	$V_C = V_{\bar{P}_1} + V_{\bar{P}_2} + 4V_{\bar{F}_1} + 16V_{\bar{F}_2}$

are derived as indicated from the variances of the component means. In this way a standard error may be computed for each, and any difference from the zero expectation assessed for significance.

A high degree of overdominance is one of the factors which will necessarily give rise to a failure of the tests, and indeed the effect known as overdominance or hybrid vigour (heterosis) occurs when the mean value for F_1 falls outside the range defined by P_1 and P_2. Analysis of this phenomenon in plants by means of these and other tests (Cavalli, 1952) has shown that heterosis can often be attributed to a failure of additivity (Jinks and Jones, 1958). This is detected by the presence of non-allelic interaction, so that, for example, the effect of two genes acting together is greater than the sum of the two acting separately. Dominance itself may be regarded as allelic interaction, one allelomorph of the *same* gene having a different effect from the other, and it is held that disturbance of additivity from this source is less serious, especially since its effect can be assessed on the scale selected (Mather, 1949). It should also be noted that it may not always be possible to remove from the scale, by transformation of the data, the non-additive effects of non-allelic interaction.

Application of the scaling tests

Before commencing on the main experiment to be discussed in this part it was decided to investigate the adequacy with respect to the assumption of additivity of the scales for ambulation and defecation scores which have been used throughout. The scaling tests were therefore applied to two sets of data, firstly, to the P_1, P_2, F_1, F_2, and backcrosses bred from the reactive and non-reactive strains as described in Chapter 3, and secondly to the P_1, P_2, F_1, and F_2 bred from the brown- and black-hooded strains bred for the purpose of segregating the coat-colour as described in Chapter 1, reciprocal crosses being pooled in each case. The results are given in Table 4.2, from which it will be noted that scaling tests A and B, which use the backcrosses B_1 and B_2 respectively, could not be applied to crosses using the brown- and black-hooded strains, since these were not bred. The values, together with their standard errors, are given separately for males and for females in each case, as well as being combined. The results are in general satisfactory and compare well with similar analyses in the genetical literature (see Mather and Vines, 1952; Butler, 1952; Honeyman, 1957). There is apparently no sex difference and significant non-additivity is confined to the crosses from the selectively bred strains, and hardly appears in the defecation scale, but is detected more frequently in the ambulation scale. In two of the four cases of its occurrence, however, it is absent in scaling test C, which is held to be the most sensitive to departures from additivity, since it involves scores from more phenotypes than the others (see Table 4.1). But, as we shall see, only one of the two selectively bred strains was used in the experiment to be described, whereas both the hooded strains were. Mather cautions against the application of scales derived from one set of data to another set, so perhaps greater weight should in this case be placed upon the values derived from data from the

TABLE 4.2

Results of scaling tests

Cross		Defecation scaling test A	Defecation scaling test B	Defecation scaling test C	Ambulation scaling test A	Ambulation scaling test B	Ambulation scaling test C
Reactive × non-reactive	Males	−0·2 ± 0·4	−0·2 ± 0·5	−1·6 ± 0·8	+2·1 ± 0·7	+2·9 ± 0·9	+2·5 ± 1·2
	Females	+0·3 ± 0·5	+0·03 ± 0·3	+2·6 ± 0·6	+2·4 ± 0·7	+2·6 ± 0·9	+1·0 ± 1·1
	Both	0 ± 0·3	−0·1 ± 0·3	+0·5 ± 0·5	+2·3 ± 0·5	+2·7 ± 0·7	+1·5 ± 1·0
Brown hooded × black hooded	Males			−1·2 ± 1·7			−1·2 ± 1·7
	Females			−0·1 ± 1·9			−0·03 ± 2·7
	Both			−0·5 ± 1·4			−0·02 ± 1·8

hooded strains. In each case scaling test C is non-significant, and so it may be concluded that the defecation and ambulation scores meet the first criterion of a satisfactory scale, that of additivity. The methods employed to test for the second criterion, absence of environmental-genotype interaction, will be discussed later in connection with the results obtained. Meanwhile, we must turn to a consideration of the method employed.

The diallel cross method

The diallel cross method appears to have been devised by Schmidt (1919). He gave it the alternative title of 'the method of complete intercrossing', which is perhaps more self-explanatory than the term 'diallel', though the latter has become firmly fixed. It is derived from the Greek, and from the same root as the prefix of 'allelomorph', frequently contracted to 'allele' and meaning 'the same'. In 'diallel' therefore we have a term meaning 'twice the same', and referring to the fact that from each pair of lines involved *two* crosses are made—the cross A × B, and its reciprocal B × A, for example. But, as the alternative name implies, each line is crossed with every other in this reciprocal fashion, so that if there are n lines in the experiment, there will be $n(n-1)$ crosses, counting reciprocal crosses separately. In addition there will be matings within the parental lines themselves, and there will be only n of these since reciprocals are not possible. Altogether, therefore, there will be n^2 matings. Thus, 'a *diallel cross* is the set of all possible matings between several genotypes. A *diallel table* is an arrangement in a square of n^2 measurements corresponding one to one to the mating combinations of a diallel cross, each row and column of the square corresponding to the offspring with a common parental genotype' (Hayman, 1954a, p. 789). The diagrammatic illustration of a 4 × 4 diallel table, given in Table 4.3, will clarify the method.

TABLE 4.3

An illustration of a diallel table showing the genetical constitution of the offspring used in the analysis

		Strain of male parent			
		A	B	C	D
Strain of female parent	A	AA	AB	AC	AD
	B	BA	BB	BC	BD
	C	CA	CB	CC	CD
	D	DA	DB	DC	DD

Taking an analysis of four strains as an example we see that there will be sixteen possible matings, six crosses and six reciprocals, making a total of twelve, together with the four kinds of offspring from the four parental strains. Observe that these are included in the table along the leading diagonal. They need not, of course, contain the actual parents of all the crosses, but need merely be contemporary representatives of the parental lines from which those crosses are derived. Further examples of diallel tables may be found in Tables 4.8, 4.12, and 4.14. Schmidt used a form of the method to investigate the value for breeding purposes of boars, but the most convincing example of its usefulness which he provides was done using fish to investigate the genetical determinants of length and number of vertebrae. Kudrjawzew (1934) later used the method, also with swine, and apparently erroneously attributing it to Nachtsheim (1925).

Mather (1949) discussed the possibilities of the method, but it is only in the past few years that a series of papers from Birmingham have shown the full extent of its potentialities (Hayman, 1954a, 1957, 1958; Jinks, 1954, 1955, 1956; Dickinson and Jinks, 1956). Critics appear to have shown increasing acceptance of it recently (Kempthorne, 1956, 1957).

The diallel cross method appears to be ideal for psychogeneticists, especially for those working with mammals. As we shall see, it reveals much information about the nature of the polygenic system determining the continuously variable characters selected for study, and it does this all in a single generation, the F_1, so that we do not need to wait for the results of breeding the F_2, backcrosses, and even the double backcrosses necessary for the complete biometrical analysis as formerly advocated. To be sure, breeding further generations of the sort mentioned within the diallel cross design can yield further useful information as has been shown (Jinks, 1956; Hayman, 1958), but given the present imperfections of our behavioural measures, it is perhaps questionable whether the comparatively small additional information in the way of refinement of the genetical picture is worth the additional labour involved. The method compares even more favourably with that of selective breeding, both in respect of the temporal aspect and of the information it yields, though, of course, selection has its value in other ways, as we have seen. Diallel crossing can perhaps best be thought of an extensive analytical method, rather than an intensive one, since it surveys the genetical basis of behaviour in a sizeable number of strains at once, rather than concentrating on a perhaps more exhaustive analysis of that to be found in two or three. It is believed that at the present stage of development of the field, the former is preferable to the latter. It is nevertheless one of what Russell has called 'the exacting procedures of biometrical genetics' (1953b), and while the experimental and computational labour involved is probably not more than that expended in prosecuting a large-scale factor analytical study, it should not be undertaken lightly and without an acquaintance with the general principles underlying it. It is hoped that the account of the present experiment may serve to introduce the methodology to psychologists. In doing so it must be stressed that it has not been considered possible, or even neces-

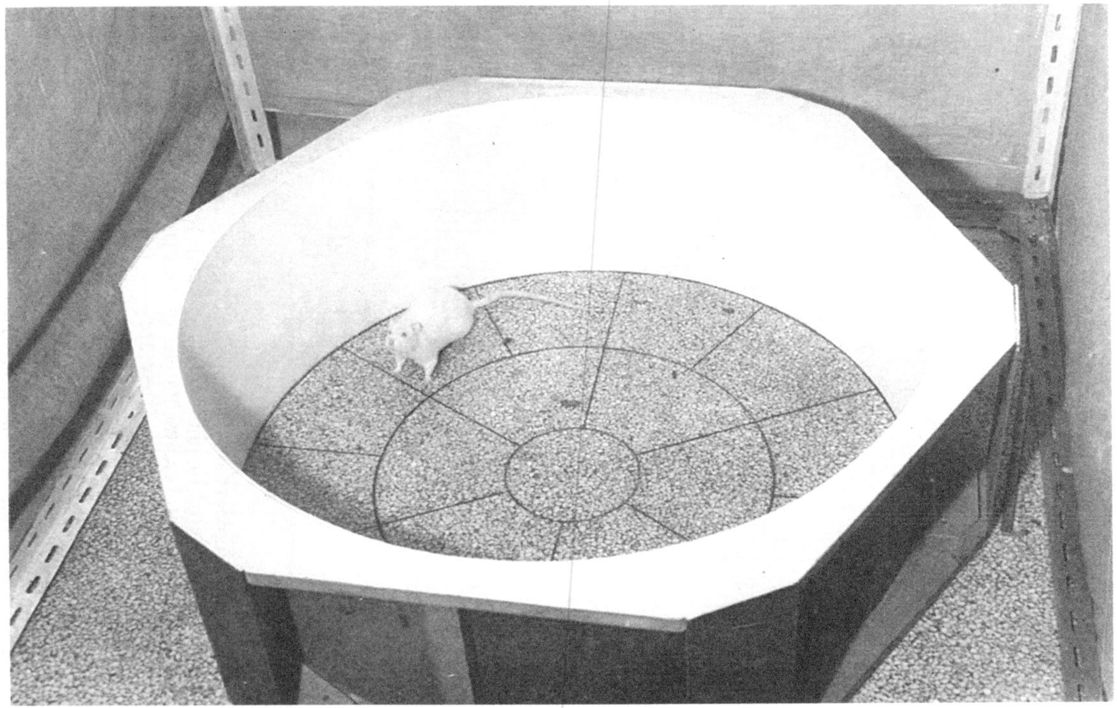

PLATE I. Standardised open-field test. The photograph shows the open-field test as finally standardised for use in the studies described here; see text. The albino subject shown under test has already deposited four fecal boluses.

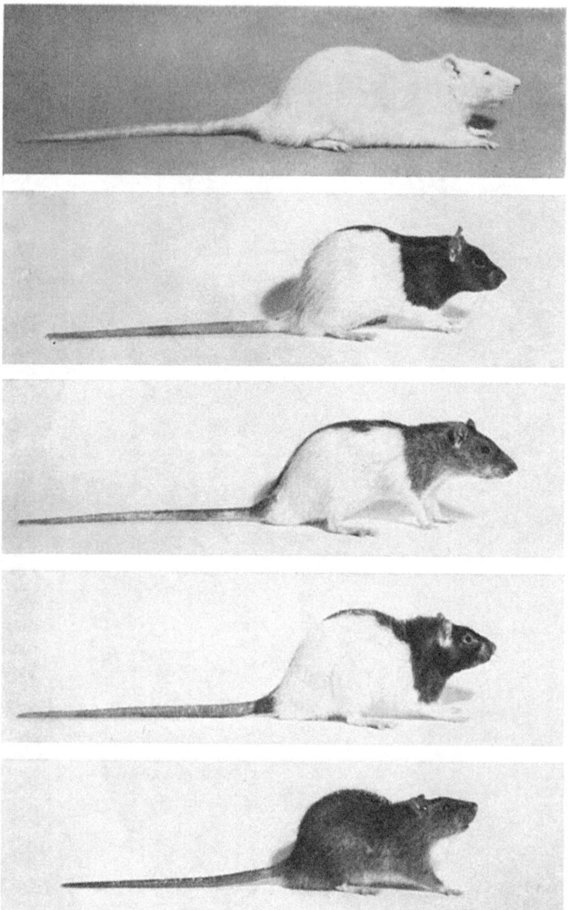

PLATE II. Coat colours of the pure-bred strains of rats used. The strains are illustrated by photographs of adult male animals which were chosen as typical representatives of their strains, though minor individual variations occur. They are arranged in the order 1-5, reading from the top downwards, as in Table 21 (no. 6 not shown). 1 is the *Albino*, devoid of pigmentation, and having pink eyes. Genotype: AAcchh. 2 is the *Black-hooded I*, with the typical piebald distribution of black fur over the head and shoulders with a more-or-less continuous stripe of the same colour down the back, and sometimes a few spots on the belly. The tail is patchily pigmented. Genotype: aaCChh. 3 is the *Brown-hooded*, having the same piebald distribution of coloured fur as no. 2 but agouti in colour. Genotype: AACChh. 4 is the *Black-hooded II*, with coat colour identical with that of no. 2. Genotype: aaCChh. 6 is the *Brown*, having a completely agouti coat, except for the belly, which is gray with white patches. The tail is usually completely pigmented. Genotype: AACCHH.

sary, to attempt exposition of the genetical considerations underlying the procedures used. They will be referred to as they arise, but the interested reader must follow the references given to find the necessary justifications in terms of the genetical model used.

Subjects

The subjects for the experiment were 595 rats from six strains; 94 of them came from the six parental lines, and the rest were bred to complete the diallel table. Five of these strains comprise a collection of pure-bred strains of rats, assembled and maintained in the Animal Psychology Laboratory of the Institute of Psychiatry, and their emotional characteristics as shown by open-field test scores have already been reported (Broadhurst, 1958b).

The previous work had shown that the strains had mean defecation scores ranging from 0·9 to 2·2 fecal boluses per trial, and mean ambulation scores ranging from 2·3 to 7·6 metres run per trial, though with some variations in the order of magnitude between the sexes in the latter case. A sixth strain was added to the diallel table in order to increase the range of scores under investigation. As mentioned previously, this was the non-reactive strain at S_8, which, as may be seen from Tables 3.3 and 3.4, had overall scores of 0·03 for defecation and 9·6 for ambulation. The genetical characteristics and other information regarding these six strains is presented in Table 4.4 which is modified from that given previously (Broadhurst, 1958b),[1] and the coat-colour characteristics of the five pure-bred strains illustrated in Plate II (facing page 77). A representative of the No. 6 (non-reactive) strain is not shown here; it is typical albino and not distinguishable from No. 1 (albino). The table also shows the number of animals used as parents to breed the various cross- and pure-bred litters. The experiment was replicated by breeding two litters of each. In order that these two litters should represent as great a possible genetical diversity, even within the pure-bred lines which constitute the bulk of the experiment, it was stipulated that the parents of the two litters representing each entry should be as unrelated as possible. Thus, in no case was the mother the same, and in only two cases out of the thirty-six pairs of litters were they sisters. For practical reasons relating to animal supply it was not possible to maintain a similar rigour with respect to the fathers: in sixteen pairs of litters the fathers were the same, and in another one they were brothers.

[1] It will be observed that the non-reactive strain is not pure-bred in the sense that the other five strains are, that is, over twenty consecutive generations of brother × sister mating. Though a diallel cross analysis has been developed making no assumptions about the homozygosity of the strains used (Dickinson and Jinks, 1956) the analysis to be used here does so. This departure from the strict requirements of the method was nevertheless accepted in view of the increased information to be expected; its effect was anticipated as an increase in the imprecision of the estimates of genetical parameters.

TABLE 4.4

Designation in this experiment	Name of strain		Description		Subjects obtained from	Original source	No. of generations inbreeding of parents of subjects in diallel table	No. of parents used	
	Short	Full	Coat-colour	Eyes				Male	Female
1	Albino	WAG/C (Wistar albino, sub-lines Glaxo Compton) (LAC No. 163a)*	White	Pink	Agricultural Research Council	Wistar Institute in 1924	68–70	7	11
2	Black hooded I	PVG/C (Piebald, sub-lines Virol, Glaxo Compton) (LAC No. 163b)	White with black non-agouti hood	Black	ditto		40–43	4	10
3	Brown hooded	August Line 990 (LAC No. 163c)	White with black agouti hood	Black	University of Miami, Florida, U.S.A.		56–58	4	9
4	Black hooded II	August Line 35322 (LAC No. 163d)	White with black non-agouti hood	Black	ditto	27th generation of August 990 line (at Miami)	22 & 23	4	8
5	Brown	A × C 9935 (Irish) (LAC No. 163e)	Black agouti	Black	ditto		45–47	5	11
6	Non-reactive	Maudsley emotionally non-reactive (LAC No. 163g)	White	Pink	Selectively bred in laboratory (see Chapter 3)	Wistar strain from dealer, 1951	8	6	12

* Numbers refer to the listing in the *Uniform Strains Catalogue* (Laboratory Animals Centre, 1958).

A further restriction in the choice of subjects was that each litter assigned to the experiment should contain at least two males and at least two females: in four cases out of the seventy-two, however, this condition could not be met, despite the extensive overbreeding that was practised for the purpose, and there was either only one male or one female. The two litters representing the non-reactive parental line were obtained by taking the first two litters born in the S_9 generation of the selective breeding experiment and which met the above criteria. The diallel tables therefore finally contained seventy-two litters with a mean size of 8·3 (4·2 males and 4·1 females), the smallest having two males and one female and the largest, six males and eight females.

All the subjects were bred, reared and tested in the open field in the standardized manner described in detail in Chapter 2. The mean age of the litters at the time of testing was 100·8 days, with a range 94–114 and with an SD of 3·2 days. The data available therefore consist of the behavioural measures of ambulation and defecation, measures of growth as defined by the records of increases in weight, and, in addition, a rating of their degree of pigmentation in the case of the self-coloured and hooded animals (strains 2–5), made with the aid of Castle's scale (1930). The present report is concerned with the behavioural measures only; the investigation of the genetics of growth is to be undertaken (Broadhurst, 1960b), and, as regards the investigation of coat-colour, it may be summed up by saying that no striking anomalies in coat-colour inheritance were detected, though some information regarding the genes carried epistatically by the two albino strains was obtained. As noted in Chapter 1, it was shown that the non-reactive strain (No. 6) was heterozygous with respect to the agouti–non-agouti gene (A–a), while it became obvious from the uniformly agouti coat-colour of crosses with strains 2 and 4 that the albino (No. 1) strain was homozygous for it, but in its dominant form (AA), contrary to the expectation of recessive homozygosity (Castle, 1947; Little, 1958).

RESULTS

Parental lines

Before proceeding to a presentation and a consideration of the results of the biometrical analyses of the defecation and ambulation scores for the whole replicated diallel table, it seems worth while devoting some attention to the results of the ninety-four subjects derived from the parental lines 1–6 alone. In effect the results from strains 1–5 duplicate those of an experiment reported earlier, and, since they were obtained on subjects from the same five inbred strains, up to three generations later but under the same standardized conditions, these results represent a replication of that experiment (Broadhurst, 1958b). They have accordingly been analysed, together with the data from strain 6, by the same methods previously used, that is, analysis of variance for two-way classification with disproportionate numbers in the sub-groups (Snedecor, 1956). A square root transformation reduced the highly significant inhomogeneity of variance in the defecation data to around the 5% level, and the results are given in Table 4.5.

TABLE 4.5

Summary of results of analyses of variance of open-field test scores: parental lines only

Source	d.f.	Score: Defecation *F*-ratio	Score: Ambulation *F*-ratio
Strain	5	10·2*	
Sex	1	2·1	
Interaction	1	2·0	8·0*
Individuals	86		
Total	93		

* Significant beyond the 1% level.

The analysis of variance of defecation scores shows a significant strain difference and the significance of the differences between the strain means was therefore calculated by means of *t*-tests and is shown in Table 4.6. These significance levels suggest a grouping of strains 3, 5, 4,

TABLE 4.6

Significance of differences between strains: defecation scores

Strain no. (descending order of size)	Mean no. boluses per trial	*P* value for comparison with 5	4	1	2	6
3	3·0	n.s.	0·01	0·05	0·001	0·001
5	2·0		n.s.	n.s.	0·01	0·001
4	1·7			n.s.	0·05	0·01
1	1·5				0·01	0·001
2	0·3					0·05
6	0·1					

and 1 as relatively high defecators, and 2, and, of course, 6, as low. This is somewhat different from the findings previously reported, from which 1 and 4 emerged as relatively high defecators as opposed to 2, 5, and 3 which formed a group of low defecators. There is some concordance in the rank order of the means, however, the correlation being + 0·51, though not significant with so few cases.

The analysis of variance of the ambulation scores shows a significant interaction between strain and sex, and so was not continued beyond this point. Instead the significance of the differences between the mean scores for strains was again calculated, but within sexes separately. As

TABLE 4.7

Significance of differences between strains: ambulation scores

Males							Females						
Strain no. (ascending order of size)	Mean no. of metres run per trial	*P* value for comparison with					Strain no. (ascending order of size)	Mean no. of metres run per trial	*P* value for comparison with				
		4	3	5	1	6			3	4	1	5	6
2	2·5	n.s.	0·05	0·05	0·001	0·001	2	2·4	0·05	0·05	0·001	0·01	0·001
4	3·6		n.s.	n.s.	0·001	0·001	3	6·0		n.s.	0·05	0·05	0·001
3	4·9			n.s.	0·01	0·001	4	6·6			n.s.	n.s.	0·001
5	4·9				0·05	0·001	1	9·3				n.s.	0·001
1	8·0					0·05	5	9·7					0·05
6	11·1						6	14·0					

may be seen from Table 4·7 these results suggest rather clearly a grouping of 3 and 4 as forming the nucleus of an intermediately scoring group in both sexes, which includes 5 in males but not in females, and is opposed to a higher scoring group represented by 1 in males, and 5 and 1 in females. No. 2 is lowest in both sexes, though not completely differentiated among males, and 6 is uniformly highest. These groupings correspond very closely to those found in the previous experiment, and the correlations between the mean orders of +1·0 for males and +0·95 for females reflect this fact.

This preliminary analysis suggests, therefore, that the ambulation response in the open-field test is a more stable characteristic of our inbred strains of rats than is the defecation response. A replication on a fresh sample less than half the size of that previously used (75 from lines 1–5, as opposed to 199 previously) has yielded remarkably consistent results in the case of ambulation scores, even in the nature of the interaction of strain with sex, whereas no more than a general congruence was found in the case of defecation. It may be that the genetical determinants of the defecation response are more subject to fluctuation, perhaps as a result of environmental interaction.

This further demonstration of the significant differences between the strains, now including the non-reactive one (No. 6), in both the characteristics under investigation, confirms the suitability of the animal material selected for study, in that it gives a wide range in both scores. One of the assumptions of the diallel cross analysis is that the strains studied are a random sample of a general population of such strains (Griffing, 1956). While it seems unlikely that such a condition can ever be fulfilled exactly, and indeed has not been met in the investigations in plant genetics upon which the present study is modelled, the broader the range available, the more nearly we may expect to approach this ideal.

Diallel cross analysis of ambulation scores

The ambulation scores will be dealt with first, since the analysis presents fewer technical difficulties. In Table 4.8 will be found the mean ambulation scores for the two litters comprising each cross and pure line (the latter forming the leading diagonal; compare Table 4.3). Note that each score was divided by 10, and the value rounded off to one place of decimals for convenience, after calculations had been completed. The analysis then closely follows the example given by Hayman (1954a, 1954b). The first step was to test for the second criterion of scaling, that of the absence of genotype-environment interaction as manifested by inhomogeneity of variance between the sub-groups in the two diallel tables. The ratio s^2 max./s^2 min. yielded a χ^2 value of 38·9, which with 71 degrees of freedom is not significant. We may therefore assume for the moment that the ambulation scores represent a scale which is adequate for biometrical analysis.

TABLE 4.8

Results of diallel cross: ambulation scores (mean ambulation score in floor units × 10^{-1} per litter of the progeny of six strains of rats)

	Strain of father								
Strain of mother	1	2	3	4	5	6	V_r	W_r	$W_r - V_r$
LITTER 1									
1	13·0	10·8	13·8	13·1	19·1	14·0	9·5	16·8	7·3
2	6·0	3·7	9·4	10·5	7·7	12·3	6·4	12·6	6·3
3	16·5	10·4	8·7	11·1	11·4	16·5	9·9	17·5	7·6
4	9·9	6·5	9·1	9·3	10·1	19·0	19·1	28·2	9·1
5	11·1	11·3	11·9	15·5	15·5	13·4	4·1	6·7	2·6
6	19·1	9·5	16·3	21·3	11·6	23·7	23·5	23·4	−0·1
LITTER 2									
1	18·1	6·7	15·3	15·9	10·9	17·3	14·4	21·1	6·7
2	9·1	5·7	10·2	6·3	10·3	8·5	3·8	7·5	3·7
3	11·2	10·5	11·1	8·7	8·8	19·4	6·8	14·3	7·5
4	11·5	7·9	6·4	7·9	7·4	18·6	19·6	28·1	8·4
5	12·9	9·2	14·1	12·6	9·8	14·6	3·0	10·4	7·4
6	17·2	12·9	11·7	16·8	12·4	22·9	13·8	22·9	9·1

The next step is to calculate the quantities V_r and W_r, which are also shown in Table 4.8. V_r is the variance of the *r*th array, and W_r the covariance of that array with the leading diagonal, that is, the covariance of the means of the offspring of one parent with those for the non-recurrent parent, but including the value for the common parents. Therefore, the sums of squares for obtaining W_r are run up as follows, adopting a notation similar to that shown in Table 4.3: $AA^2 + (AB \times BB) + (AC \times CC) + (AD \times DD)$, etc., for the first array, and for the third, for example, $(CA \times AA) + (CB \times BB) + CC^2 + (CD \times DD)$, etc. . . . It should be noted that the values of V_r and W_r shown in the table are calculated using data for the reciprocal crosses pooled (not shown), and not the separate values as given in the body of Table 4·8, since we are not at this point concerned with reciprocal differences which will be analysed later. We are then in a position to calculate the quantities $W_r - V_r$. The genetical hypotheses underlying the analysis require that the quantity $W_r - V_r$ should be homogeneous over arrays.

The following test employs an analysis of variance to investigate the strain (array) and litter (block) differences, and the results are shown in Table 4.9. Both *F*-ratios are less than unity, and we may therefore

TABLE 4.9

Analysis of variance of $W_r - V_r$

Source	d.f.	Mean squares	*F*-ratio
Arrays	5	5·5	0·5
Blocks	1	7·9	0·8
Residual	5	10·0	
Total	11		

conclude that the values in the present experiment do not show significant lack of homogeneity either over arrays or over the two litters used. and proceed to plot the variance-covariance diagram.

The variance-covariance diagram has important properties in the diallel analysis especially with respect to the estimation of dominance. If the values of W_r and V_r from a diallel table are plotted it may be shown that, firstly, they should define a line of unit slope if dominance is present in the genetical system, and secondly, that the intersection of the line with the W_r axis will indicate the degree of dominance. If dominance is absent, the points cluster as shown in Fig. 4.1, and a line of unit slope ($b = 1$) through the cluster gives an intersection point estimating the value of one-quarter of D, the weighted sum of d^2, the component of variation defining the additive genetical effect (see Fig. 1.3). If dominance is complete, on the other hand, the line passes through the origin, and H_1, the component defining the average dominance, is equal to D. Between these two extremes, incomplete or partial dominance may occur, in which case the relationship takes the form shown in

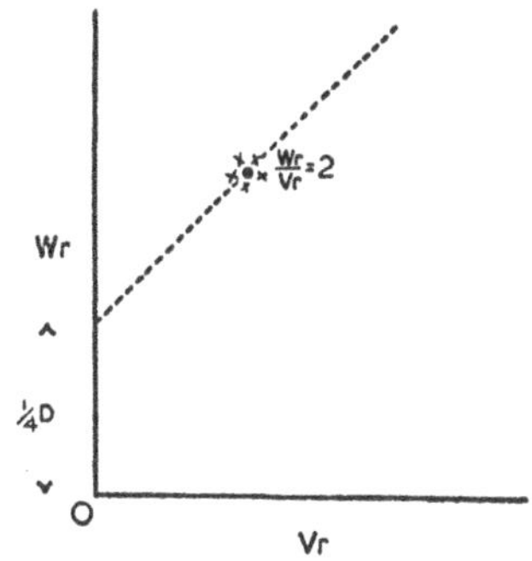

FIG. 4.1. The variance-covariance diagram, illustrating the absence of dominance. In the absence of dominance there is no regression of W_r (array covariance: see text) on V_r (array variance), and all W_r and V_r in the diallel table are estimates of a single point where $W_r/V_r = 2$. A line of unit slope through the points cuts the W_r axis at a value estimating $\frac{1}{4}D$: see text. (From Jinks, 1955.)

Fig. 4.2. Here the intersection of the line defines the quantity $\frac{1}{4}(D - H_1)$. Overdominance (heterosis) is seen when the line intersects the ordinate below the origin, H_1 being greater than D, and $\frac{1}{4}(D - H_1)$ consequently

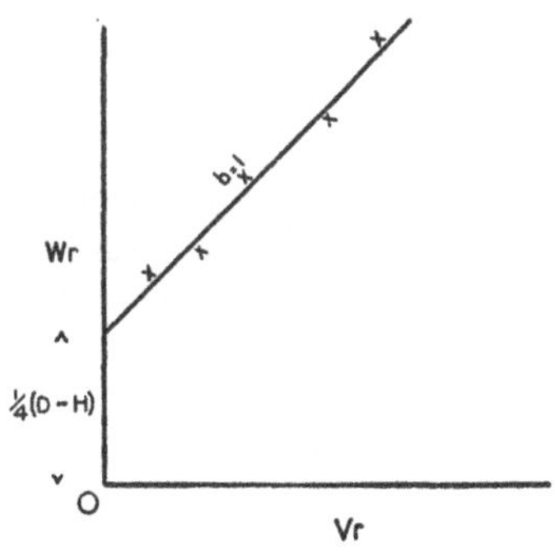

FIG. 4.2. The variance-covariance diagram, illustrating incomplete dominance. If partial dominance is present the regression of W_r on V_r defines a line of unit slope ($b = 1$), which cuts the W_r axis above the origin at a value which estimates $\frac{1}{4}(D - H_1)$: see text. (From Jinks, 1955.)

negative, as seen in Fig. 4.3. Fig. 4.4 illustrates these various possibilities, the point $H_1 = 0$ corresponding to Fig. 4.1, the line $H_1 = \frac{1}{2}D$ to Fig. 4.2, $H_1 = D$ to complete dominance (not illustrated), and $H_1 = 2D$, 3D, and 4D to various degrees of overdominance (compare Fig. 4.3). In addition the figure discloses other properties of the variance-covariance diagram. It can be shown that all points on the diagram must lie within a parabola defined by $W_r^2 = V_r . V_1$, where V_1 is the variance of the parental array on the leading diagonal, and that the points of intersection of this parabola with a line of unit slope define the values at which the percentage proportion of dominant to recessive genes in the polygenic system is extreme (0 : 100 respectively at the top, and 100 : 0 respectively at the bottom). Consequently subdivision of the line into four equal parts gives the other proportions, 25 : 75, 50 : 50, and 75 : 25 as indicated. It thus becomes possible to estimate graphically this proportion

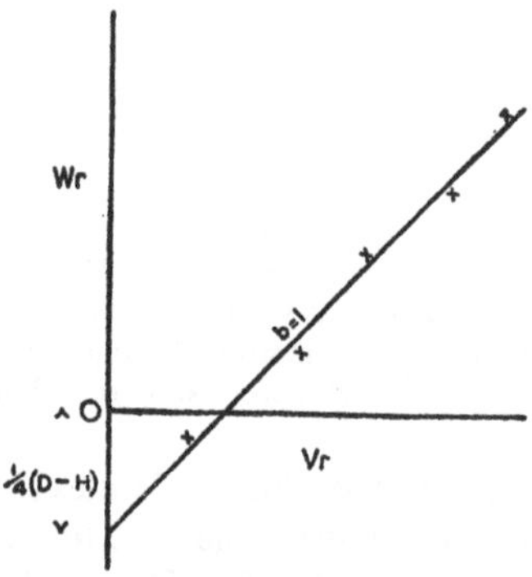

FIG. 4.3. The variance-covariance diagram, illustrating overdominance. If overdominance is present the regression of W_r on V_r defines a line of unit slope ($b = 1$) which cuts the W_r axis below the origin at a value which estimates $\frac{1}{4}(D - H_1)$. (From Jinks, 1955.)

for the various strains in a diallel experiment. The value of AB/OB defines the quantity H_1/D, which is a measure of the mean degree of dominance, and in Fig. 4.4 is taken as $H_1/D = 4$, as an illustration. The failure of the points on the variance-covariance diagram to define a line of unit slope can take several forms. One possibility is shown in Fig. 4.5. This is a case of spurious overdominance seen arising from the presence of non-allelic interaction combined with complete dominance. The deviations can take other forms, many of which can be recognized as implying particular genetical characteristics in the heritable determination of the character. However, in all such cases the failure of some of the genetical hypotheses is implied, with the consequence that the genetical analysis is complicated. In some cases where the failure is due to the action of certain crosses only, it may be possible to remove the offending arrays from the diallel or to estimate new values. In other cases re-scaling may be necessary, and in yet others it may not be possible to proceed with the full analysis. Hayman (1954a) gives examples of the methods employed to overcome some of these difficulties. But such considerations make it imperative to test whether or not the points do in fact define a line of unit slope. In the variance-covariance diagram for the ambulation scores in the present experiment,

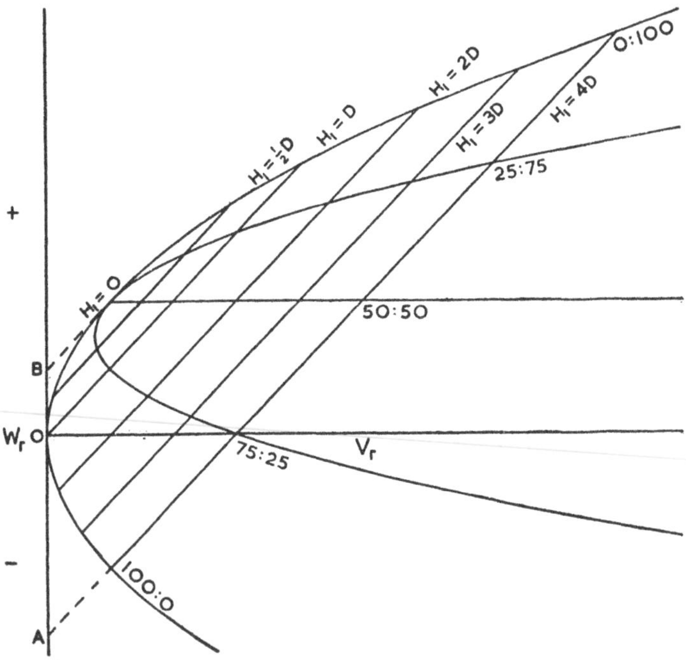

FIG. 4.4. The variance-covariance diagram, illustrating the various relationships. The limiting parabola, $W_r^2 = V_r . V_1$, where V_1 is the variance of the parental array (see text), encloses the points which cluster at $H_1 = 0$, or define one of the parallel lines of unit slope, depending on the dominance relationships in the diallel cross, and indicated by the size of H_1 in relation to D. Note the progression of lines across the diagram, from incomplete dominance, through complete dominance ($H_1 = D$), to overdominance of various degrees, when a continuation of the line may cut the W_r axis below the origin, at a point A, for example. If the parallel line at a tangent to the parabola cuts it at B, then AB/OB defines H_1/D, the mean dominance (= 4 in the example shown). The position of any point W_r, V_r gives the relative proportions of dominants to recessives in the parental strain, the value of this proportion being indicated by the intersections with the lines labelled 100 : 0, 75 : 25, 50 : 50, 25 : 75, and 0 : 100. That is, parents with a *larger* proportion of dominants give points *lower* on the graph, and *vice versa*. (From Hayman, 1954a.)

shown in Fig. 4.6, the *t*-test devised by Hayman for this purpose[1] yields a value of 0·24, which is non-significant. Taken in conjunction with the results of the analysis of variance of $W_r - V_r$, it can be concluded that

1 $$t_{n-2} = \left[\frac{n-2}{4} . \frac{(\text{Var. } V_r - \text{Var. } W_r)^2}{\text{Var. } V_r . \text{Var. } W_r - \text{Cov.}^2 (V_r . W_r)}\right]^{\frac{1}{2}},$$

which is equivalent to rotating the axes of the diagram through 45°, and testing the significance of the regression in the new axes.

these two tests, neither of which is statistically perfect, together confirm the absence of significant deviation from unit slope, and we may finally be assured of the adequacy of our scale.

The variance-covariance diagram shows immediately that we are dealing here with a case of incomplete dominance, since the line of unit slope drawn through the points intersects the W_r axis above the origin. The agreement between the points representing the two litters is also good, so that the order upwards along the line which as we have seen represents the proportion of dominants to recessives is well defined. It is clear that strain 5 is highest in this respect, and strain 4 lowest. In no

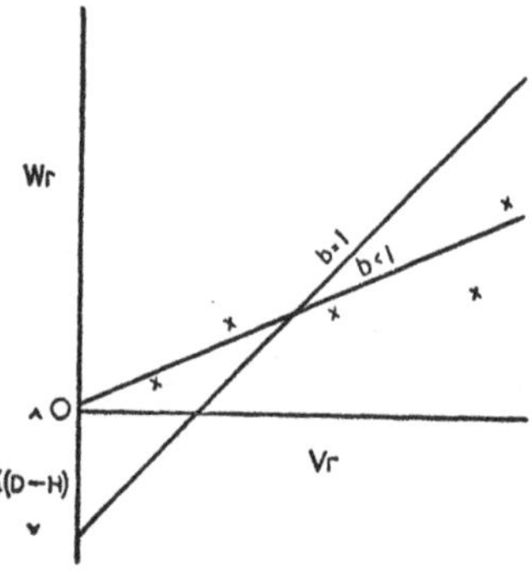

FIG. 4.5. Variance-covariance diagram, illustrating failure of assumptions. If non-allelic interaction is present, a line of unit slope ($b = 1$) might spuriously suggest overdominance, when in fact complete dominance exists, but $b < 1$, due to the interaction. In this case re-scaling might achieve unit slope. (From Jinks, 1955.)

case is the proportion of the occurrence of dominants to recessives as low as 25 : 75. The dominance order, as determined by eye or by the average of $W_r + V_r$ is 523164. Now the ambulation scores as determined by the array means is 234516, which accords well with that previously given for the parental lines alone (Table 4.7), though it should be noted that these latter are of course included in the array means. The correlation between this order of ascending ambulation score and the dominance order is 0·37. This is non-significant, and probably too small to allow any statement about the more usual direction of effect of the dominant genes: probably equal proportions of them are positive and negative in their effect on ambulation.

Other qualitative information of this nature can be derived from the diagram, and it would be possible to cease the analysis at this stage. It is, however, proposed to pursue the various possibilities of the diallel analysis as far as they have been taken by biometrical geneticists, and thereby provide an illustration of the method. The two main tasks that therefore follow are, firstly, to estimate the components of variation as previously defined, especially E—the effect of non-heritable and particularly environmental variation—together with some others which have not yet been encountered, and, secondly, to provide estimates of significance of these components.

A contribution to both these tasks is to be found in the analysis of

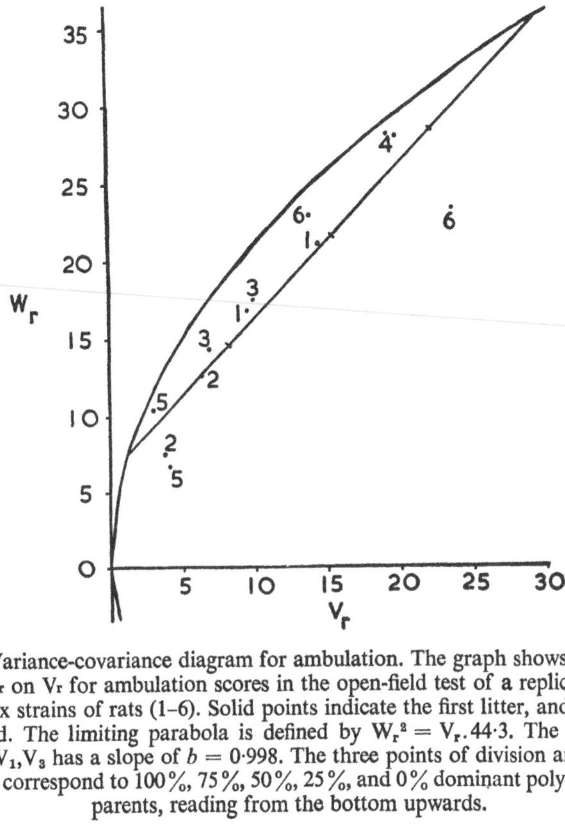

FIG. 4.6. Variance-covariance diagram for ambulation. The graph shows the regression of W_r on V_r for ambulation scores in the open-field test of a replicated diallel cross of six strains of rats (1–6). Solid points indicate the first litter, and open ones the second. The limiting parabola is defined by $W_r^2 = V_r.44{\cdot}3$. The line drawn through W_1,V_3 has a slope of $b = 0{\cdot}998$. The three points of division and the ends of the line correspond to 100%, 75%, 50%, 25%, and 0% dominant polygenes in the parents, reading from the bottom upwards.

variance of the diallel table, constructed by Hayman (1954b) and following an earlier analysis proposed by Yates (1947). This provides, together with an estimate of E, statistically adequate tests of some of the components of variation to be calculated, a further test of the effects of different litters, and a test of reciprocal differences (maternal effects). It is consequently performed on the mean scores as given in the body of Table 4.8 and not on the pooled reciprocals, used for computing all the other statistics given. The results shown in Table 4.10, together with, for convenience, those for defecation scores which will be considered later.

TABLE 4.10

Analyses of variance of diallel cross: ambulation and defecation scores

Quantity	Source	d.f.	Ambulation Mean square	Ambulation F	Defecation Mean square	Defecation F
a	$D - F + H_1 - H_2$	5	165·3	33·7***	1·8740	5·1*
b_1	h^2	1	0·05	0·01	0·0239	1·0
b_2	$H_1 - H_2$	5	7·7	1·6	0·0706	1·1
b_3	See text	9	16·6	3·4**	0·1219	0·6
b	H_2	15	12·5	2·5*	0·0982	
c	Reciprocal differences	5	9·7	2·0	0·1401	1·1
d	Reciprocal differences	10	4·7	1·0	0·0780	0·8
Total		35	31·7		0·3521	
B	Overall block (litter) differences	1	5·2	1·1	0·0793	0·5
Ba	Interaction with block differences	5	3·4		0·3651	
Bb_1	Interaction with block differences	1	4·7		0·0238	
Bb_2	Interaction with block differences	5	2·7		0·0662	
Bb_3	Interaction with block differences	9	2·7		0·1975	
Bc	Interaction with block differences	5	2·7		0·1236	
Bd	Interaction with block differences	10	9·3		0·1008	
Bt	Interaction with block differences	35	4·9		0·1596	
Total		71				

* Significant at the 5%, ** the 1%, and *** the 0·1% levels.

This analysis of variance of the diallel table provides estimates of the significance of the components of variation as indicated in Table 4.10. The quantity (*a*) measures the variation between the mean effects of each parental line (V_2 later), and estimates, in terms of the biometrical model, the quantity $D - F + H_1 - H_2$. D represents the weighted sum of d^2 and H_1 that for h^2, the additive and dominance components respectively (see Fig. 1.3 and discussion in Chapter 1). F indicates whether dominant or recessive alleles occur more frequently in the parental lines, and is positive if dominants are in excess, and negative if recessives predominate. The component H_2 also relates to dominance and is measured directly by the mean square (*b*) in the analysis of variance, the variation in reciprocal sums not ascribable to (*a*). This mean square may be subdivided as indicated, (b_1) estimating h^2, the square of the mean dominance, and (b_2), the difference between H_1 and H_2. This latter quantity relates to the symmetry of the distribution of alleles, so that, if some loci show dominance, $H_1 - H_2 = 0$ means that the positive and negative alleles are in equal proportions in the parents. If insignificant, it implies that (*a*) detects only additive variation. 'The mean square (b_3) also estimates dominance but has no simple interpretation, though, when the gene frequencies satisfy the symmetry relation, (b_1) and (b_3) together provide a test of dominance equivalent to (*b*)' (Hayman, 1954b, p. 239). The mean square (*c*) measures the average maternal effects of each parental line, and (*d*) the variation in the reciprocal differences not ascribable to (*c*), that is, both of these terms measure reciprocal differences. The block (litter) difference in the estimates of the above components are computed, and form the lower part of the variance table and provide error variances against which to test the significance of the corresponding mean effect. In the present case, however, a test of the heterogeneity of these variances having given a non-significant value, they were pooled and (B_t), the between blocks total variance estimate, used to test the significance of the others.

It is important to note that this between blocks total (B_t) estimate of variance also serves as a direct estimate of the size of E.

TABLE 4.11

Components of variation: ambulation

$$D = V_1 - E = 39{\cdot}4 \pm 0{\cdot}7$$
$$F = 2V_1 - 4W_1 - 2(n-2)E/n = 12{\cdot}2 \pm 2{\cdot}1$$
$$H_1 = V_1 - 4W_1 + 4V_3 - (3n-2)E/n = 6{\cdot}0 \pm 2{\cdot}2$$
$$H_2 = 4V_3 - 4V_2 - 2E = 6{\cdot}0 \pm 1{\cdot}9$$
$$h^2 = 4(M_0 - M_p)^2 - 4(n-1)E/n^2 = 1{\cdot}6 \pm 1{\cdot}3$$

Estimates of the following other components of variation are obtained as shown in Table 4.11 from the statistics calculated from the diallel tables, where V_2 = variance of the means of the arrays, V_3 = the mean of the array variances (V_r), W_1 = the mean of the array covariances with the non-recurrent parent (W_r), M_o = the overall mean of offspring (reciprocal crosses), and M_p the overall mean of parents (the leading diagonal). The values shown in the table represent the mean of both blocks (litters), the statistics having been similarly obtained. The standard errors shown are derived from a least squares procedure. There are several possible ways of obtaining them (Mather, 1949; Hayman, 1954a), but the method used here is a simplification of that given by Hayman. The differences between the two observed values, one from each block of each of the five statistics computed, is used to estimate the error variation of the five components shown in Table 4.11, with, in this case, five degrees of freedom. This s^2 is then multiplied by the appropriate values from the matrix given by Hayman, which is a covariance matrix and the inverse of the matrix of the coefficients in the least squares equations. The square roots of these variances give the standard errors shown in Table 4.11. As may be seen, all except h^2 may be judged to be significantly greater than zero.

The concordance between the various analyses of the genetical determinants of ambulation so far presented will be immediately apparent from a comparison of Tables 4.10 and 4.11. Both the analysis of variance and the standard error agree in assigning no significance to h^2. The dominance components H_1 and H_2 may be judged significant from their standard errors; the latter is confirmed from the analysis of variance. The additive component D is significant, and in the absence of significance of (b_2) in the analysis of variance—indicating symmetry of distribution of alleles—the highly significant value of (a) therein confirms this. The absence of significant litter differences in the analysis accords well with the analysis of $W_r - V_r$ (Table 4.9) and the impressions from the variance-covariance diagram.

These findings make it possible to evaluate D/(D + E), which we have previously encountered as a measure of heritability, and which gives the value of 88·9%—of a similar order to the value of 79·8% derived from the analysis using data from backcrosses (Chapter 3). It seems probable that the present value is the more reliable, not only because of the defects in the previous analysis which were pointed out, but also because of the greater range both of parental scores and types of crosses used in the present experiment.

The quantity $(H_1/D)^{\frac{1}{2}}$ = 0·23 and is a measure of the mean degree of dominance over all loci. Another estimate of the same quantity can be derived from the variance-covariance diagram shown in Fig. 4.6, in the manner illustrated in Fig. 4.4, using the distances there defined as AB and OB in the ratio AB/OB, which here gives 4·8/11·1 = 0·43, the square root of which is 0·66. Since this is not free from the effects of E, the earlier estimate must be regarded as the more precise. Nevertheless there is good general agreement between the two. These estimates

TABLE 4.12

Results of diallel cross: ambulation scores
(Mean ambulation scores in floors units × 10^{-1} for the two sexes in the progeny of six strains of rats)

Strain of mother	Strain of father 1	2	3	4	5	6	(From values above diagonal, repeated below) V_r	W_r	$W_r - V_r$	$W_r + V_r$	(From values below diagonal, repeated above; reciprocal crosses) V_r	W_r	$W_r - V_r$	$W_r + V_r$
MALES														
1	14·9	6·0	13·1	10·1	13·0	14·4	11·3	15·3	4·1	26·6	18·6	24·2	5·6	42·8
2	5·7	4·7	6·9	5·8	8·7	8·9	2·9	6·3	3·4	9·1	4·4	8·5	4·2	12·9
3	12·1	8·7	9·1	8·1	8·9	18·4	18·5	25·2	6·7	43·7	5·6	9·9	4·3	15·5
4	7·9	5·7	5·6	6·7	7·8	17·5	18·0	24·1	6·1	42·1	16·6	20·2	3·6	36·9
5	11·6	6·5	10·7	10·1	9·1	11·0	3·6	8·5	4·9	12·2	3·0	4·0	1·0	7·0
6	17·3	10·1	11·4	16·3	9·2	20·6	20·5	16·1	−4·4	36·6	20·9	21·1	−0·2	42·0
FEMALES														
1	17·2	11·9	15·7	17·9	17·5	17·2	5·1	11·9	6·8	17·0	15·1	22·6	7·6	37·7
2	9·0	4·5	12·0	10·5	8·2	11·5	6·6	12·7	6·0	19·3	9·7	17·9	8·2	27·6
3	16·0	11·0	11·0	11·8	12·1	18·5	8·5	16·9	8·4	25·4	8·0	16·3	8·3	24·3
4	12·5	8·3	10·2	12·2	9·7	20·2	18·5	22·7	4·2	41·2	24·8	34·1	9·3	58·8
5	12·4	12·9	15·9	17·5	17·9	18·3	20·3	29·0	−8·7	49·4	5·3	5·0	−0·3	10·3
6	19·7	12·3	15·7	21·7	16·0	25·8	21·4	28·9	−7·6	50·3	23·5	28·4	−4·8	51·9

should be considered in relation to the position of the line through the points W_r, V_r in Fig. 4.6, which supports their suggestion of a low degree of dominance.

The quantity $H_2/4H_1$ measures the distribution of alleles, and provides an estimate of the product of the proportion of alleles having positive or negative effect at loci exhibiting dominance. It can be shown to have a maximum value of $\frac{1}{4}$, when the two are equal. In this case

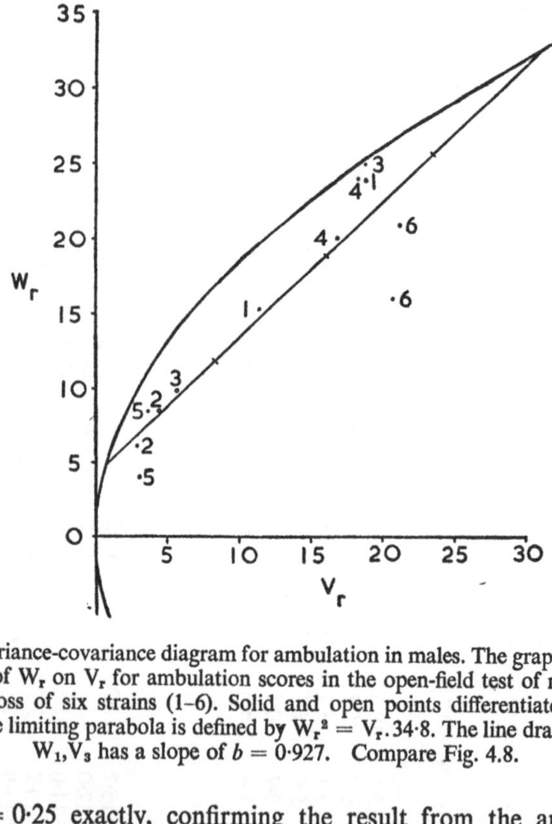

FIG. 4.7. Variance-covariance diagram for ambulation in males. The graph shows the regression of W_r on V_r for ambulation scores in the open-field test of male rats in a diallel cross of six strains (1–6). Solid and open points differentiate reciprocal crosses. The limiting parabola is defined by $W_r^2 = V_r.34{\cdot}8$. The line drawn through W_1,V_3 has a slope of $b = 0{\cdot}927$. Compare Fig. 4.8.

$H_2/4H_1 = 0{\cdot}25$ exactly, confirming the result from the analysis of variance (b_2) that H_1 and H_2 do not differ significantly. The quantity $[(4DH_1)^{\frac{1}{2}} + F]/[(4DH_1)^{\frac{1}{2}} - F]$ measures the ratio of the total number of dominants to recessive genes in all parents, and here equals 2·3.

In view of the persistent finding of sex differences between the ambulation scores of the strains used, and which indicated not merely an overall difference in level for the two sexes—as with the defecation scores—but one which modified the relative standing of the strains, it was decided to repeat part of the analysis for the two sexes separately. Accordingly the data were subdivided so that the scores of the 301 males formed one diallel table, and those of the 294 females another. Because of the absence of litter differences in the previous analyses, the scores from both litters were pooled in each table. The test of the heterogeneity of the new variances thus generated did not reach significance in either case. Values of V_r and W_r were calculated as before, but not using the pooled reciprocals as the previous results had provided no evidence of a significant effect due to reciprocals. Instead two diallels were analysed

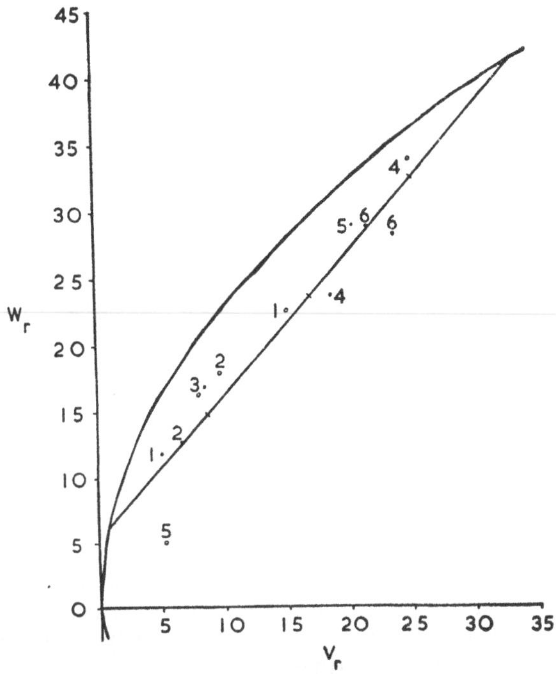

FIG. 4.8. Variance-covariance diagram for ambulation in females. The graph shows the regression of W_r on V_r for ambulation scores in the open-field test of female rats in a diallel cross of six strains (1–6). Solid and open points differentiate the reciprocal crosses. The limiting parabola is defined by $W_r^2 = V_r . 52{\cdot}7$. The line drawn through V_1,W_3 has a slope of $b = 1{\cdot}094$. Compare Fig. 4.7.

for each sex; they were formed by repeating the values above the leading diagonal below it in one table, and the values below the (same) leading diagonal above it in the other. The data are given in Table 4.12, for males and females, but the working tables described above and from which the two sets of values of V_r, W_r, etc. shown were derived are not given. The resulting variance-covariance diagrams are given as Figs. 4.7 and 4.8.

The two tests for homogeneity of $W_r - V_r$, the analysis of variance of strain and block—in this case, reciprocal—differences, and the test of departure from unit slope of the line through the points, both gave non-significant results. This incidentally confirms that the previous findings on these tests could not have been due to a balanced failure of the assumptions, operating in different directions in the two sexes. Inspection of the diagrams shows good agreement in the placement of the V_r, W_r line, indicating partial dominance, the graphical estimate of $(H_1/D)^{\frac{1}{2}}$, using AB/OB, being 0·73 for males and 0·75 for females, but some departures from consistency in the degree of dominance of some of the strains, as indicated by their relative positions, may be seen. In order to test whether or not these and other differences reach significance, an analysis of variance was performed on the most suitable measure for this purpose, the quantity $W_r + V_r$, as given in Table 4.12. The results are given in Table 4.13, and confirm the reality of the strain differences,

TABLE 4.13

Analysis of variance of $W_r + V_r$

Source	d.f.	Mean squares	*F*-ratio
Strain	5	577·2	4·0*
Sex	1	307·2	2·1
Reciprocals	1	1·1	
Residual	16	145·4	
Total	23		

* Significant at the 5% level.

as well as the absence of differences due to sex or to reciprocal crosses. The similar absence of any significant first or second order interactions, which allowed their pooling in the analysis, shows that there is no reason to suppose that differences between the positioning of the points in, or between, the diagrams is other than chance determined. It was therefore decided not to pursue these analyses of the separated male and female data any further.

From the above findings it may be concluded that the polygenic system determining rats' ambulation in the open-field test at 100 days of age does not differ as between the sexes, and that the conclusions regarding the genetical nature of the system reached on the basis of the combined analysis may be taken to hold for both sexes within the limits of the present experiment. This conclusion is not surprising when the nature of the polygenic hypothesis is recalled: any association of a large number of genes with sex differences is an improbable event. Most of the examples of sex linkage or sex limitation in genetics are due to the effects of single genes.

Except, therefore, in a few minor particulars, the interpretation of the findings relating to the genetical system determining the ambulation scores of six strains of rats in the open-field test is unequivocal. The picture emerges of an additive polygenic system with a low degree of dominance, and a relatively high heritability. It is interesting to note that, to the extent that dominance exists, the order of the six strains in respect of it, 523164, has some suggestion of a correlation with coat-colour, in that the albino strains 1 and 6 are low, and the list is headed by the brown coat-colour, which is nearest to that of the wild Norway rat. The finding of greater dominance in the wild type is a commonplace of genetics; the finding of more recessives in No. 6, the Maudsley non-reactive strain, accords well with the suggestion from the analysis of the two selectively bred strains given in Chapter 3, and invites speculation regarding the part natural selection might play in determining optimum ambulation behaviour in a strange situation. Perhaps 'Curiosity killed the cat' is valid for species other than the feline!

Diallel cross analysis of defecation scores

The analysis of the defecation data follows closely the steps taken in the ambulation analysis. However, in the first stage, the test of the second criterion of scaling, a different finding emerged. Application of Pearson and Hartley's exact test for inhomogeneity of variance (1958) gave the significant value of 258·1, with 65 degrees of freedom. There were six fewer degrees of freedom than the $N - 1$ of 71 for both litters, because of the occurrence of zero scores. These were ignored in this connection. Investigation showed an association between the size of means and variances, which was diminished, but not abolished, if strain No. 6 which was contributing most of the very low mean scores in the diallel was omitted. It was clear, therefore, that re-scaling of the data was called for. This was done by transforming each score as follows, $D' = (D/4)^{\frac{1}{2}}$, the factor of 4 being introduced to reduce the total score to the average per trial. This square root transformation was successful, the s^2 max./s^2 min. ratio now being reduced to 22·7, and non-significant. The diallel tables of the transformed scores are presented as Table 4.14. The quantities V_r, W_r, etc. were again calculated using the scores for reciprocal crosses pooled. In this case this procedure had the additional advantage that it eliminated all the zero mean scores, except one, the score for the second pure-bred litter from strain No. 6, for which there is, of course, no reciprocal cross. The same tests as before were applied to $W_r - V_r$, and disclosed no significant heterogeneity or departure from unit slope of the points plotted in the variance-covariance diagram, shown in Fig. 4·9, thus resolving any doubts about the adequacy of the scale. The overall picture suggests another case of partial dominance, though somewhat more complete than in the case of ambulation, $(H_1/D)^{\frac{1}{2}}$ being 0·83. There are some difficulties associated with this interpretation, as we shall see.

We next proceed to the analysis of variance of the diallel tables as given in Table 4.14. In the present case, the six error variances were significantly inhomogeneous, and so each mean effect was tested against

TABLE 4.14

Results of diallel cross: defecation scores

(Mean defecation scores in boluses per trial, square root transformation, of the progeny of six strains of rats)

Litter 1 Strain of mother	Strain of father 1	2	3	4	5	6	V_r	W_r	$W_r - V_r$	$W_r + V_r$
1	0·9821	0·5294	0·6449	1·0109	0·7892	0·4725	0·0798	0·1243	0·0445	0·2041
2	0·6998	0·5841	0·5858	0·6937	0·8738	0	0·0653	0·0900	0·0247	0·1553
3	1·3855	0·9896	1·7358	0·6469	1·7569	1·0095	0·2662	0·3194	0·0532	0·5856
4	0·9265	1·1100	0·5753	0·3384	1·0417	0	0·1344	0·1326	−0·0018	0·2670
5	1·1476	0·7633	1·1034	0·6899	1·4303	0·2845	0·1689	0·2395	0·0706	0·4084
6	0·2845	0·3268	0·0962	0·0643	0·5646	0·1756	0·0235	0·0862	0·0627	0·1097
Litter 2										
1	1·0838	1·1196	1·2553	0·9445	1·4822	1·1130	0·0604	0·0638	0·0034	0·1242
2	0·4163	0·1010	0·2666	0·8154	0·7887	0·1179	0·1047	0·1365	0·0318	0·2412
3	1·6044	0	1·4236	1·6869	0·5590	0·5428	0·3868	0·3915	0·0047	0·7783
4	0·8191	0·3347	1·5959	1·5672	1·8466	0·6315	0·2925	0·3423	0·0498	0·6348
5	1·0540	0·5351	1·2012	0·6722	1·1797	0·3961	0·1963	0·2648	0·0685	0·4611
6	1·1359	0	0·2338	0	0·1798	0	0·1614	0·1368	−0·0246	0·2982

its own interaction. The results were shown in Table 4.10. It will be seen at once that none of the sources of variance is significant except the quantity (*a*) representing the additive heritable contribution (since (b_2) is also non-significant). Observe that there is no significant effect of litter differences (B).

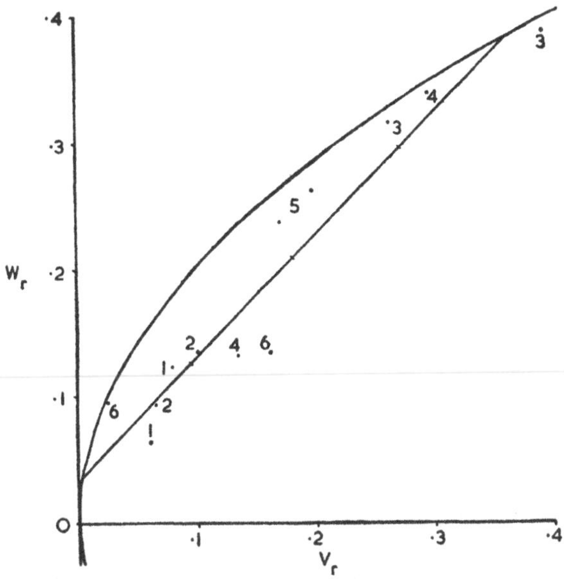

FIG. 4.9. Variance-covariance diagram for defecation. The graph shows the regression of W_r on V_r for defecation scores in the open-field test of a replicated diallel cross of six strains of rats (1–6). Solid points indicate the first litters, and open ones the second. The limiting parabola is defined by $W_r^2 = V_r.0{\cdot}42$. The line drawn through V_1, W_3 has a slope of $b = 0{\cdot}994$.

The components of variation were calculated as before and gave the following values:

$$D = 0{\cdot}2606 \pm 0{\cdot}0265$$
$$F = -0{\cdot}1484 \pm 0{\cdot}0748$$
$$H_1 = -0{\cdot}1346 \pm 0{\cdot}0775$$
$$H_2 = 0{\cdot}0740 \pm 0{\cdot}0693$$
$$h^2 = -0{\cdot}0868 \pm 0{\cdot}0469$$

The additive component (D) is clearly significant, being many times its standard error. The sign of F suggests a preponderance of recessives in the parents but in the absence of satisfactory significance may not be interpreted. The weighted mean square dominance component, H_1, gives a meaningless result, being negative, but need not trouble us on that account as it is not significantly different from zero. Neither H_2

nor h^2 are significant, as judged by their standard errors, though the latter gives another meaningless negative result. On the basis of the analysis of variance, moreover, all these quantities, except D, are confirmed as being statistically insignificant. It is clear that most of the difficulty stems from the large value for E derived from this analysis, and which enters into the calculation of these components, as was shown in Table 4.11. Leaving this consideration aside for the moment the question can be asked whether or not there is any real evidence of strain differences in dominance order as seen in the variance-covariance diagram. An analysis of variance of $W_r + V_r$ was performed with the results shown in Table 4.15. It is apparent that, while the analysis confirms the absence of litter differences, the differences in dominance order

TABLE 4.15

Analysis of variance of $W_r + V_r$: defecation scores

Source	d.f.	Mean squares	F
Strains	5	0·0826	7·1*
Blocks (litters)	1	0·0540	4·7
Residual	5	0·0116	
Total	11		

* Significant at the 5% level.

of the six strains can be regarded as doubtfully significant. This order, as determined by the average of $W_r + V_r$, is 126543: the descending order of size for array means is 351426, which is the same as that given for the pure lines only in Table 4.6. The two correlate + 0·49, but not enough to suggest other than equal proportions of positive and negative contributors to defecation scores among the dominant genes.

Heritability may properly be calculated using the same formula as before. In this case $D/(D+E)$ gives 62·0%, a value which agrees poorly with that of 95·0% derived from the previous analysis. The present value for heritability seems to be more appropriate in view of the extent of the actual progress made in the selective breeding.

Beyond this it is not possible to go in the absence of assurance of the significance of the components. The phenotypic measurement of the defecation response clearly has a large amount of error associated with it, which makes the analysis of the genetical system indeterminate, despite the demonstrated adequacy of the scale used. The instability of the rank order of the parental means commented upon earlier gives some confirmation of this. The effect does not seem to be particularly associated with error of measurement: the reasonably high reliability of the open-field test measure, the absence of inter-litter differences in the diallel analysis, and the progress made in selection all attest to this. It may be that the defecation response is particularly environmentally sensitive. The findings, therefore, may be interpreted with a lower degree of confidence than those for the ambulation measure. They indicate that the genetical system determining the defecation scores of six strains of rats in the open-field test is an additive polygenic system with some degree of dominance and a moderate heritability.

Conclusions and outlook

The tentative conclusions reached regarding the nature of the hereditary determinants of two small segments of behaviour in the rat may seem disproportionate in relation to the experimental effort expended. While it would have been possible to make estimates of other items of interest relating to linkage, number of genetic units in the systems, and the prediction of the outcome of selection, the assumptions necessary are even more complex than those already implied, and even less likely to be completely fulfilled. It was therefore deemed that a somewhat conservative attitude to the method used is the proper one at the present time. The future will doubtless see both corrections and elaborations.

One such elaboration which is already beginning to take sufficient shape to suggest a useful role in psychogenetics is the more rigorous formulation of the effects of environment on polygenic systems. Falconer's experiment (Falconer and Latyszewski, 1952, 1952–3) on the response of mice selected for different body size to high and low planes of nutrition is an example of the sort of technique which might be used with variables of psychological interest. Careful choice of them may help to resolve the sorts of difficulties encountered in our analysis of the defecation response. The ways in which problems involved in the analysis of the interaction of genetical parameters with such environmental variables may be overcome has already received considerable attention (Haldane, 1946; Falconer, 1952; Allard, 1956; Mather and Jones, 1958; Jones and Mather, 1958; van der Veen, 1959).

In sum, therefore, it is suggested that the experiment described in this chapter has demonstrated the feasibility of applying the diallel cross method of biometrical genetics to the analysis of behavioural characteristics in mammalian subjects. The method in its contemporary form has hitherto only been applied to two species of mammals, to cattle (Dickinson, 1954) and to sheep (Dickinson, personal communication, 1959), in small diallels for the investigation of characteristics related to physical growth. The transition to psychological characteristics has not been accompanied by any insuperable scaling problems, and the placing of the points on the variance-covariance diagrams has fulfilled the criterion of linearity at least as well as many of the published diallels in plant genetics. While this is a cause for satisfaction, it need not be a cause for wonderment. On the one hand, psychological characteristics are by the nature of their multidetermination quantitative variables *par excellence*; on the other hand, biometrical genetics has been developed as the method of choice for analysing the heredity of such characteristics. It may be that we are fortunate enough to have been provided with a method well suited to the type of material to be encountered and the type of problem to be attacked in psychogenetics. If the present work has provided a step in this direction, however faltering it may seem in the light of future developments in both psychology and genetics, the writer will be well rewarded.

Summary

In this chapter an experiment in biometrical psychogenetics is reported using the diallel cross method on six strains of rats and their F_1 reciprocal crosses. The method is discussed and the results from the pure lines related to previous work on them. The analysis of the complete diallel for ambulation scores is given as an example of the method, and shows low dominance with high heritability for this character. That for defecation scores is less precise, due to large non-heritable components, but suggests higher dominance and moderate heritability. The suitability of the method to this type of investigation is stressed.

PART TWO

Experiments in Psychopharmacology

GENERAL INTRODUCTION

OF the papers constituting this part, four are concerned with the presentation of experimental data while the other represents an attempt to integrate some of the findings of the separate experimental studies by the technique of discriminant function analysis. In each paper differences in both interests and emphases may be discerned; some showing more concern with processes and effects as such and others with their implications for the description of personality. It would be incorrect to conclude from this statement that each contributor was not concerned, to some extent, with both aspects, even if one is given greater emphasis than the other. What gives cohesion to this set of very different papers is the systematic framework common to each. This framework has been provided by Eysenck (1957a, 1957b) and constitutes an expansion of his approach to the general problem of objectively describing personality. Two functions characterize the usefulness of such a framework. First and foremost, it serves to orientate and guide research. Secondly, it provides a reference system whereby the diversity of research problems it suggests may be inter-related. We are thus taking Eysenck's system as a general or universal proposition, to use Stephenson's term (1952), and it is instructive to recall here the distinction Stephenson drew between regarding a theory as a general or universal proposition, and as 'rational'.

Regarding a theory as a universal proposition represents an earlier stage of system building, where, according to Stephenson, the value of a scientific theory lies in the fruitful research it engenders. At this level, the negative instance need not be too damaging—in fact, may prove enlightening. The second, or 'rational' level, Stephenson describes as that at which a theory is capable of giving rise to quite specific predictions which may be unambiguously tested.

Very few hypotheses in psychology could claim to be at this more advanced level. Certainly the system underlying the work being reported in this section is not. Constant references in the experimental papers will be made to variables from learning theory, when these are largely unknowns and largely unmeasurable in any precise way. We will refer

[1] We are indebted to the Wallace Laboratories for a grant which made possible the investigations reported in this and the subsequent papers. We are also indebted to CIBA for assistance with the Doriden studies.

to personality parameters and questionnaire measures of them although we know that these measures are almost certainly imperfect. How can we then hope to proceed as if we were based on a fully developed 'rational' theory? Of course, we will have expectations about the outcome of research when we proceed under the conditions of the 'softer', more primitive theory and, indeed, as these expectations are confirmed or not confirmed, the theory can be hardened and developed. At the level of the universal proposition, our situation permits a useful degree of flexibility, both in our research interests and in the significance we attach to experimental findings. We are not faced with the crucial experiment until, as the result of necessarily protracted and diversified research, we have refined our concepts, measuring tools and our experimental techniques.

Eysenck's general standpoint is well known (1952, 1955a, 1955b, 1957a), and will not be dealt with here. The expansion of his approach to the field of drug studies should, however, be mentioned briefly. Proceeding from one of his basic notions, that the neural sub-structure of the behavioural dimension introversion-extraversion is the inhibition/excitation balance of the central nervous system, Eysenck has formulated his 'drug postulate' (1957b). This postulate states that: 'Depressant drugs increase cortical inhibition, decrease cortical excitation and thereby produce extraverted behaviour patterns; stimulant drugs decrease cortical inhibition, increase cortical excitation and thereby produce introverted behaviour patterns.'

One can see immediately from this postulate that, if behaviour patterns, following the administration of a depressant or stimulant drug, were to be concordant with the expected behaviour patterns of, respectively, extraverted or introverted groups, this would support the basic hypothesis, connecting introversion/extraversion with the inhibition/excitation balance.

Some work has already appeared that has a bearing on this postulate; Franks and Laverty (1955), Eysenck *et al.* (1957a, 1957b, 1957c, 1957d), Franks and Trouton (1958) are specific examples, and a number of other references will be found throughout the reports of this section. In much of this work sodium amytal (Amylobarbitone Sodium) has been used as the depressant drug and d-amphetamine (Dextro-Amphetamine Sulphate) as the stimulant. In both cases the choice of drugs has been guided, partly by pharmacological evidence about the nature of the drug's action and partly by the clinical use made of the drug. For example, sodium amytal is widely used to mitigate tension and anxiety states, to promote sleep and generally to sedate disturbed patients (Lindeman, 1932; Sargant and Slater, 1954). Such an action could be interpreted as consisting in a reduction in the degree of introversion ('Dysthymia' as it occurs in the neurotic patient), i.e. the action of the drug is towards an increase in extraversion.

Clinical observations of this sort have suggested the initial researches and the drug postulate based on them. Similar considerations have led to the use of the two drugs in the studies now being reported. These drugs are 'Doriden' (glutethimide—3-phenyl-3-ethyl-2,6-dioxopiperidine) and meprobamate (2-methyl-2-*n*-propyl-1,3-propandiol dicarbamate). No general review of the literature of these two drugs will be offered here. The accounts of experimental studies and clinical trials given (concerning Meprobamate) by Gross (1955), Berger (1956), Osinki (1956), Dickel *et al.* (1957), Friedman (1957), Hollister *et al.* (1957) and Himwich (1957); and by Weston (1956), Howell (1956), Blumberg (1956), and Abbas (1957) (concerning Doriden), demonstrate the way in which these drugs have been used in the reduction of tension and anxiety states and the way in which our investigation of them as depressants has been suggested. In each paper, detailed discussions of the drugs will be found as the need has arisen in the treatment of specific processes or findings. The paper by Holland contains perhaps the most extensive of such discussions.

Certain features common to all investigations should be mentioned here.

Subjects

The subjects were (initially) a group of twenty-four adults consisting of thirteen women and eleven men whose mean age was thirty years, with a standard deviation of $\pm$ 8 years. The subjects were paid volunteers coming from a population which one would expect to be similar to an undergraduate population in point of intellectual level. Due to experimental hazards peculiar to each separate investigation, some subjects in each investigation were wasted. When this occurred the subject was replaced by another from the same population. In total, six subjects were lost in this way, so that only sixteen are common to all reports, with the exception of the subjects whose scores were subjected to the discriminant function analysis. Here, each investigator made up the numbers by extra testing so that results on the same group of twenty-four people could be subjected to this analysis. In no case did the substitution of new scores affect the results being reported in the individual papers.

Procedure

The procedure of each investigation is described in detail in the relevant papers, but the general arrangements were as follows. Two subjects were seen by all investigators on each of three days. On one day Doriden was administered, on another meprobamate, and on the other 'No Drug' was administered. Since there were three treatments, six arrangements accounted for all the possible orders of drug administration. Thus, four subjects received the three treatments in any one of the six possible orders. The subjects were allotted to orders at random, although, for convenience, both subjects seen during any one three-day period received the treatments in the same order. After the administration of the drug the subjects were not allowed to discuss their experiences and followed different schedules of testing.

Two schedules of testing times during the day were settled upon by the four investigators and were designated 'Subject 1' and 'Subject 2'. On the first of the three days one subject was put on the testing schedule for Subject 1 and the other for Subject 2. A subject followed the same schedule on each of the three days. With suitable breaks a testing schedule occupied one day—about eight hours.

Doses

Two 250 mgr. tablets of Doriden were given—one in the morning when the subject arrived and the other some four hours later. The manufacturers advised that this would constitute a mild but effective clinical dose. The same time intervals were followed with meprobamate—one 400 mgr. tablet being administered in the morning and a second four hours later. In the case of both drugs a period of forty-five minutes was allowed to elapse between administration and the commencement of testing. On the 'No Drug' day the subject rested during these delay periods. Placebo tablets were not used since Franks and Laverty (1955) found a 'placebo' effect indistinguishable from a 'No Tablet' treatment in the case of eyeblink conditioning and, furthermore, some practical importance was attached to any effects on psychomotor functions the usual clinical situation of administering a tablet of Doriden might have. There were other formal reasons why possible placebo effects were allowed to be confounded with true drug effects. To balance out practice and order effects required six arrangements of our three treatments. To have achieved the same result with the four treatments necessary to isolate a placebo effect, would have necessitated twenty-four arrangements; in our investigation a quite impracticable requirement. The subjects were not told at any time what to expect from the drugs other than that they were harmless and their effects in no way dramatic. The phrase 'rather like aspirin' seemed to reassure most subjects.

The exigencies of working with volunteers—even paid volunteers—over a period of three days, made the problem of food and liquid intake a difficult one. Subjects were instructed by letter to avoid alcohol during the twelve hours previous to the testing time, to forgo strong beverages like tea and coffee on the morning of testing and to limit their breakfast to as light a meal as would suffice. No tea or coffee was taken during the day and luncheon was also restricted to a light meal. Where it was felt to be relevant, medication disqualified a person from acting as a subject. All volunteers were seen by a physician before receiving a drug, with a view to discovering any contra-indications, and before leaving the laboratories to ensure that they were capable of facing the hazards of London traffic unaccompanied. On the 'No Drug' days, during one of the rest breaks, the subjects filled in the Maudsley Personality Inventory (Eysenck, 1956, 1959). Thus a score for each individual on Introversion/Extraversion and on Neuroticism was obtained.

The aims of the studies presented in this part are then threefold: to observe the effects of the drugs on certain psychological processes; to draw implications for personality theory and, regarded by the authors as of less importance, to relate the effects and processes directly, via the questionnaire, to personality parameters.

R. A. WILLETT

5

THE EFFECTS OF DEPRESSANT DRUGS ON LEARNING AND CONDITIONING

R. A. Willett

THE EFFECT OF DORIDEN AND MEPROBAMATE ON EYEBLINK CONDITIONING AND NONSENSE SYLLABLE LEARNING

IT was pointed out in the general introduction that if, for example, a depressant drug resulted in behaviour patterns concordant with those expected of a group scoring high on extraversion, support would have been brought for the hypothesis connecting extraversion with an exaggeration of the inhibitory potential. Of the many processes where central neural inhibition and excitation levels are believed to play an important role, those involved in conditioning and nonsense syllable learning provide two of the more obvious examples. Conditioning was described and analysed by Pavlov and his associates (1927) in terms of inhibitory and excitatory neural potentials and these or similar concepts have been retained either implicitly or explicitly by later workers. Likewise, the various phenomena associated with the rote learning of nonsense syllables have been accounted for, in analogous terms, by Hull and his associates (1940). If, then, measures of conditioning and rote learning are taken, after the administration of depressants such as Doriden and Meprobamate, it should follow, as a consequence of the drug postulate, that 'extravert' behaviour patterns be disclosed and the primary hypothesis that the extravert is characterized by an exaggeration of the inhibitory potential would be thus supported.

When one considers the amount of research done on conditioning and rote learning and the extent to which various drugs are used, it is a little surprising that one can refer to so few investigations where their relationship has been examined. Both conditioning and rote learning play important roles in general behaviour and the administration of drugs affects general behaviour. One would have thought, in consequence, that the effects of commonly used drugs on these two salient components of general behaviour would have been thoroughly investigated; but such is not the case.

A little research has been done on conditioning and drug effects with animals, yielding some evidence of the depressant action of various tranquillizing and sedating drugs (Settlage, 1936; Dworken *et al.*, 1937; Smith *et al.*, 1956). Hunt (1955, 1957) reports on the effect of a number of drugs on a conditioned emotional response, which drugs included meprobamate. He found little effect of meprobamate on the conditioned response. The studies of Franks and Laverty (1955) and Franks and Trouton (1958), both set up to test the drug postulate, are amongst the very few relevant investigations of drug effects using human subjects that we have discovered in the literature. Both investigations report that significantly fewer conditioned eyeblink responses are elicited from a group receiving sodium amytal than from a control group. One must comment, however, that the authors' claims should be viewed with a little reservation. The group means given in both studies strongly suggest that their conclusions are justified. However, the improper use of a *t*-test, after an analysis of variance has yielded an insignificant *F*-ratio, in the case of Franks and Laverty, and the likewise improper computation of six *t*-tests from four arrays of scores, in the case of Franks and Trouton, renders both findings suggestive only.

A problem which has not properly been faced in much eyeblink conditioning work is that of whether random blinking enters into scoring, as an artefact. This is a particularly urgent problem for those who attempt group differentiations on the basis of eyeblink conditioning. Both Franks (1956) and Spence and his associates (e.g. Spence and Farber, 1953) characteristically contrast a group in which *a priori* one might expect more random blinks, with a group where one might expect fewer. In the case of Spence a high drive (high manifest anxiety) group is contrasted with a low drive (low manifest anxiety) group. In Franks a dysthymic (neurotic introvert) group is contrasted with an hysteric group (neurotic extravert). If one each of these groups indeed showed a higher blink rate there is at least the possibility that an artefact could enter into the scoring to make it appear that these groups gave more conditioned responses. Franks (1956) attempted to control this factor by counting the random blinks in the last minutes of his records. We have counted all random blinks to achieve a more complete picture of blink behaviour than could be obtained from this rather atypical sample of the records.

Rather less work has been carried out on the effect of drugs on the rote learning of nonsense syllables. Hull (1935) examined the effects of caffeine (a cortical stimulant) on the rote learning of nonsense syllables and found few changes, other than an increase in the number of associative errors recorded. Felsinger *et al.* (1953) found no significant difference in the number of trials taken to reach their criterion, when the performance of a group receiving a barbiturate was compared to that of a control group. They did however report one significantly inferior recall measure for the barbiturate group.

Steinberg and Summerfield (1955, 1957) and Summerfield and Steinberg (1957) in well-executed studies report that 'learning was markedly impaired' under the influence of the central depressant *nitrous oxide* and that, with incomplete learning, the observed decrement persisted through subsequent learning, after the effects of the drug had disappeared. These authors also present data which suggest that it is the acquisition of the items which is affected, rather than their availability at the moment of recall. Furthermore, in an investigation comparing the retroactive interfering effect of an interpolated task accompanied by and without the administration of nitrous oxide, they found that nitrous oxide reduced the commonly observed decrement when performance on the original task was resumed. The result they put down to the drug inhibiting the processes of interference during the interpolated task. Willett (unpublished paper), in a study comparing the effects of sodium amytal and dexedrine on nonsense syllable learning, failed to demonstrate any significant difference between the performances of the drug groups and a placebo group, although the group means were clearly separated in the predicted direction.

Burstein and Dorfman (1959) examined the effect of meprobamate on the learning of a list of paired associates of high inter-item competition. They argued that since evidence has been brought in support of the hypothesis that a relatively high anxiety level will interfere with the learning of such a list, meprobamate, if it acts to reduce the anxiety level, should result in the list being learned more readily. A comparison of the performance of some sixty subjects divided into a placebo group and a group receiving 1200 mgr. of meprobamate fulfilled this expectation at the 5% level of significance. The hypothesis from which Burstein and Dorfman proceed is in terms of drive (anxiety level here) being multiplicative with, not only the weak habit strength associated with the correct response, but with the habit strength associated with all the competing responses. Hence with higher drive one would expect greater interference, an expectation in the main substantiated (Montague, 1953; Farber and Spence, 1953; Spence, Taylor, and Ketchel, 1956; Spence, Farber and McFarn, 1956). However, the finding of Summerfield and Steinberg on the reduction of interference effects in the presence of the depressant nitrous oxide suggests that the interpretation Burstein and Dorfman have given is not the only one possible. The action of the meprobamate in their study could also be that of inhibiting interference in a manner similar to that described by Summerfield and Steinberg.

The purpose of the present study was to repeat those of Franks *et al.* (1955, 1958) on eyeblink conditioning, and Willett on rote learning, using the two new depressants and employing each subject as his own control. The drug postulate of Eysenck (see General Introduction) would, in general, lead us to expect evidence of increased cortical inhibition and a level of performance concordant with that expected for the extravert, from the two drug groups. Expected performances for each group are given separately in the ensuing report.

Statistical treatment

The data have been analysed and presented in four ways.

(1) Means and standard deviations of measures are the basic data examined and are presented first.

(2) The significance of mean differences is tested by means of a simple analysis of variance.

(3) Where it is believed that one variable was partly dependent on another, analysis of co-variance has been used. If, for example, we wish to examine whether the drugs decrease the number of associative errors produced during rote learning, we must allow for the fewer number of trials to criterion shown by the 'No Drug' group, otherwise, the number of associative errors in the case of the Drug groups may appear spuriously high, as an artefact of the greater number of trials recorded for these groups. The analysis of co-variance is an analysis of the residual variance of (e.g.) associative errors when (e.g.) the number of trials is held constant.

(4) Regression analysis has been used to estimate the degree of correlation between the performance measures and the questionnaire measures. This procedure produces two product moment correlations, one (the total correlation) between the two whole distributions in question, and a second (correlation within groups) which may be thought of as an average of the correlations within each of the six order arrangement groups. We shall adopt the convention throughout of allowing 'R' to represent the total correlation and '*r*' to represent the within groups correlation.

EYEBLINK CONDITIONING

Apparatus

A detailed description of the procedure and apparatus for the eyeblink conditioning technique followed here has been given by Franks (1956) and by Franks and Withers (1955). Briefly, to summarize this information, the conditioning is carried out in a soundproofed room, divided across its longer dimension by a curtain. In one half of the room the subject is seated in a chair provided with head and arm rests; in the other half, the experimenter sits before the apparatus for delivering the stimuli and recording the responses. The subjects' field of vision is restricted by a three-sided booth, painted a neutral colour and having a small red light in the middle of the panel facing the subject.

The conditioned stimulus was a tone of 1000 c.p.s. delivered at 60 db. above each subject's bi-aural threshold, through a pair of high-quality earphones, heavily padded to reduce ambient noise inside the sound-proofed room. The unconditioned stimulus was a puff of air delivered through a plastic tube at a pressure of 65 mm. of mercury. The two stimuli overlapped in time—the tone lasting 850 msec., the puff being delivered 450 msec. after the commencement of the tone. Both stimuli terminated together. Each stimulus could be delivered alone, or both could be delivered together in a prearranged timing sequence.

The eyeblink response was recorded by means of a photoelectric cell held in the right-hand lens carrier of a pair of spectacle frames which the subject wore. This carrier also held the open end of the plastic tube through which the puff was administered. As an eyeblink caused the amount of light reflected from the eye to alter, a change in the electrical discharge from the cell was produced which, after suitable amplification, moved the ink writing pen of a recording milliameter.

Procedure

Each of the twenty-four subjects described in the general introduction was seen on three occasions—once under Doriden, once under meprobamate, and once without any drug. The treatment orders were so arranged that over all the group, at the end of the experiment, treatments were equally distributed amongst occasions, so that eight people had Doriden on the first occasion, eight on the second, and eight on the third. Likewise eight subjects had meprobamate and the 'No Drug' condition on the first, second, and third occasions. Such a balancing was particularly necessary because there is a known practice effect with the eyeblink conditioning technique. Our experience has been that a stimulus presentation schedule of partial reinforcement, in which eighteen 'test' stimuli are distributed amongst thirty reinforcement 'pairs' of stimuli, results in a good range of conditioning scores and occupies the convenient testing period of half an hour. By a reinforcement 'pair' is meant the delivery of the tone and puff, coupled as described above, and by 'test' stimulus is meant presentation of the conditioned stimulus (the tone) alone. In this investigation each of the three testing occasions consisted of six 'test' stimuli distributed amongst ten 'reinforcement pairs'. The number of times (out of six) in each testing session when the subject responded to the conditioned stimulus was taken as the measure of conditioning on that occasion. No count of the subjects' response to the conditioned stimulus when coupled with the unconditioned stimulus is possible with this apparatus, as the recording speed is judged too slow to separate responses to stimuli coming as close together as the tone and puff do.

On each of the three days one subject was seen in the morning and the other in the afternoon. For the three-day testing period each subject was tested at the same time of day. It was expected that the number of responses to the 'test' stimuli would be significantly fewer for the drug groups than for the 'No Drug' group.

Results

(The group receiving Doriden will be referred to as 'A', the group receiving 'No Drug' as 'B' and the group receiving meprobamate as 'C'.)

Acquisition of conditioned responses

Table 5.1 shows the means and standard deviations of the number of conditioned responses to the 'test' stimuli for each group, the analysis

TABLE 5.1

Comparison of mean number of conditioned responses among the Doriden, 'No Drug', and meprobamate groups

(i)

A	B	C
$\bar{x} = 1{\cdot}63$	$\bar{x} = 2{\cdot}54$	$\bar{x} = 2{\cdot}25$
$s = 1{\cdot}22$	$s = 1{\cdot}87$	$s = 1{\cdot}94$

(ii) Analysis of variance table

	Sum of squares	d.f.	Mean square variance	*F*
Total observed variation	220·61			
Observed variation between treatments	10·53	2	5·27	3·38*
Observed variation between occasions	3·44	2	1·72	1·10
Observed variation between subjects	137·94	23	5·99	3·84**
Residual variance	68·70	44	1·56	

N.B. Henceforth ** will indicate that the *F*-ratio is significant at the 1% level and * that it is significant at the 5% level.

(iii) Analysis of variance tables when treatments are combined in pairs

	Sum of squares	d.f.	Mean square variance	*F*
(*a*) Total variation between treatments	10·53	2	5·27	3·38*
(*b*) 'B' vs (A + C)	5·84	1	5·84	3·74
(*c*) 'A' vs (C + B)	9·54	1	9·54	6·12*
(*d*) 'C' vs (A + B)	0·44	1	0·44	0·003
Residual error variance	68·70	44	1·56	

of variance of the three arrays of scores and a series of comparisons made between the scores of pairs of groups set against a single group.

The data presented in Table 5.1 indicate that Doriden produced a significant decrease in the number of conditioned responses when compared to the 'No Drug' treatment. meprobamate produced a decrease also in the same way but one which did not reach formal significance. Indeed, part iii of Table 5.1 indicates that Meprobamate, although acting in a manner similar to Doriden, was closer in degree of action to the 'No Drug' condition than to the other drug.

TABLE 5.2

Regression of number of conditioned responses on Extraversion (E) and Neuroticism (N) derived from the Maudsley Personality Inventory

(i) Number of conditioned responses and 'E'

A	B	C
R = 0·18	R = −0·18	R = −0·08
r = 0·24	r = −0·08	r = −0·05

(ii) Number of conditioned responses and 'N'

A	B	C
R = 0·07	R = −0·06	R = 0·19
r = 0·09	r = 0·30	r = 0·30

N.B. As with the variance ratios ** indicates a regression significant at the 1% level and * a regression significant at the 5% level.

Table 5.2 indicates no tendency for the number of conditioned responses to be correlated with either 'E' or 'N' in any regular or significant fashion.

In order to look at these coefficients in another way, the subjects were divided into high and low scorers on 'E' and 'N' and their conditioning scores on the 'No Drug' day compared. Tables 5.3, 5.4, and 5.5 show this comparison.

TABLE 5.3

Means and standard deviations on Extraversion and Neuroticism of subjects who scored 'high' and 'low' on these measurements

(i) Extraversion

Low 'E'	High 'E'
N = 13	N = 11
$\bar{x}$ = 17·62	$\bar{x}$ = 34·82
s = 9·43	s = 4·35

(ii) Neuroticism

Low 'N'	High 'N'
N = 12	N = 12
$\bar{x}$ = 12·25	$\bar{x}$ = 31·67
s = 6·08	s = 7·14

TABLE 5.4

Comparison of mean number of conditioned responses between high and low scorers on Extraversion

(i) Means and standard deviations—Extraversion groups

Low 'E'	High 'E'
N = 13	N = 11
$\bar{x}$ = 2·85	$\bar{x}$ = 2·19
s = 1·46	s = 2·21

(ii) Significance of mean difference

t = 0·90 (not significant)

TABLE 5.5

Comparison of mean number of conditioned responses between high and low scorers on Neuroticism

(i) Means and standard deviations—Neuroticism group

Low 'N'	High 'N'
N = 12	N = 12
$\bar{x}$ = 2·92	$\bar{x}$ = 2·17
s = 1·71	s = 1·95

(ii) Significance of mean difference

t = 0·95 (not significant)

As the low regression coefficients of Table 5.2 would suggest, the mean differences on the number of conditioned responses between high and low scorers on Extraversion and Neuroticism are not significant. The direction of the mean difference is for low 'E' and low 'N' to be associated with a slightly larger number of conditioned responses.

Random blink rate

In an attempt to resolve the difficulties associated with blink rate, every random blink on all seventy-two testing sessions was counted in this investigation. To facilitate later computations, the mean number of blinks in the inter-stimulus periods (20 sec. ± 5 sec.) for each testing session was calculated. These means were derived by counting all random blinks excluding those that were in response to stimuli. They are the scores on which the results in Table 5.6 are based.

Table 5.6 shows no indication of any significant difference between the drug groups and the 'No Drug' group in number of random blinks.

From the data presented in Table 5.7 it would appear that there is little evidence that random blinking is related to either of the personality parameters but there is some evidence that random blinking and the number of conditioned responses are concomitant.

TABLE 5.6

Group means of mean number of blinks in the inter-stimuli periods for the Doriden, 'No Drug', and Meprobamate groups

(i)

A	B	C
$\bar{x} = 6{\cdot}98$	$\bar{x} = 8{\cdot}53$	$\bar{x} = 7{\cdot}38$
$s = 3{\cdot}09$	$s = 6{\cdot}04$	$s = 4{\cdot}64$

(ii) Analysis of variance table

	Of squares	d.f.	Mean square variance	*F*
Total observed variation	1671·92			
Observed variation between treatments	30·98	2	15·49	1·87
Observed variation between occasions	0·80	2	0·40	0·005
Observed variation between subjects	1274·96	23	55·43	6·69**
Residual variation	365·18	44	8·29	

TABLE 5.7

Regression of blinks on 'E', 'N', and number of conditioned responses

(i) Mean number of inter-stimuli random blinks and 'E'

A	B	C
R = 0·02	R = −0·06	R = 0·22
r = 0·16	*r* = −0·12	*r* = 0·43

(ii) Mean number of inter-stimuli random blinks and 'N'

A	B	C
R = 0·20	R = 0·07	R = −0·10
r = 0·16	*r* = 0·19	*r* = 0·03

(iii) Mean number of inter-stimuli random blinks and number of conditioned responses

A	B	C
R = 0·38	R = 0·39	R = 0·37
r = 0·70*	*r* = 0·27	*r* = 0·27

Discussion of eyeblink conditioning results

The significance of the principal finding is complicated by the fact that while one of the drugs, Doriden, resulted in a clear depression of the conditioning process, the other, meprobamate, did not. That this result is consistent with many others is made clear in the section by Eysenck in which he deals with the discriminant function analysis of these and other data. It is sufficient here to point out that meprobamate produced the same kind of effect as Doriden, namely a depression of the conditioning process, but this effect differed in degree. In our results this difference was sufficient to cause the mean number of conditioned responses in the meprobamate group to be statistically indistinguishable from the mean of the 'No Drug' group. Previous work by Hunt (1955, 1957) has also shown that meprobamate has little effect on the formation of conditioned responses and Marquis (1957) likewise found only slight changes in a wide range of psychological processes after the administration of meprobamate. Some of these results accord well with the notion of a small but regular depressant action.

Part of the reason for the slightness of the effect of meprobamate in our case may have been the size of dose administered. Burnstein and Dorfman (1959), who found a sizeable effect of meprobamate on inter-syllable interference in a nonsense syllable task, used 1200 mgr. of the drug in one administration, three times the dose we gave at one time and 50% more than the two doses we administered over a period of between six and eight hours. It is also possible that the central action of meprobamate may not be that of the simple general cortical depressant which Doriden appears to be. It is not unlikely, for example, that a drug whose action was selective might not interfere with a relatively low level autonomic response, like the eyeblink, to any great extent but could noticeably affect the performance of a relatively complex task, like the learning of nonsense syllables.

If we allow the drug postulate we are investigating to partake of the properties of a general proposition, as described in the general introduction, then, as a provisional conclusion, we can incorporate the statistically insignificant meprobamate result as being of the same kind as Doriden but as being of different degree. Such a conclusion implies that by changing dosage or some other relevant variable a larger, more convincing effect could be obtained. If this were not found to be the case then the system must, ultimately, be refined or modified to incorporate such a finding.

Although these investigations were not entirely appropriate for correlational studies, one might have expected the regression coefficients between conditioning and extraversion to have been higher than they are. There is some evidence that the sedation threshold of extraverts is lower than that of introverts (Shagass, 1956, 1957; Shagass and Naiman, 1955) and hence one might have expected the more extraverted subjects to have been more drastically affected by the drugs and thus to have produced concomitantly lower conditioning scores. Likewise, one would have expected the 'No Drug' treatment scores to be related to extraversion sufficiently closely to produce significant correlation coefficients. The somewhat small numbers employed, having regard to the probability of a rather low reliability for the conditioning procedure, and the dubious action of the two drugs, could account for the insignificant regression ratios, which were, in fact, found. However, a substantial confirmation of the finding under conditions appropriate to a correlation study would command serious attention.

Turning to the data presented in Table 5.7, only that contained in part iii need detain us. With the exception of one ($r_A = 0{\cdot}70$) none of the coefficients shown here are significant ones. Nevertheless the three 'total correlation' coefficients ($R_A = 0{\cdot}38$, $R_B = 0{\cdot}39$, $R_C = 0{\cdot}37$) pointing to a positive relationship between number of blinks and number of conditioned responses are of sufficient magnitude and consistency to demand some comment.

Blink rate could be related to the conditioning score in a number of ways. It might, for example, be a concomitant of the propensity to form conditioned responses where both blinking and conditioning would be related to some common causal factor. Or blink rate could influence the conditioned eyeblink score by increasing this score accidentally, i.e. the more a person blinks the more chance there is of a random blink being mistaken for a conditioned response.

Of the two possibilities suggested the second seems very unlikely, largely because of the precautions taken during the scoring of the conditioning record to exclude random blinks. A blink was counted as a conditioned response only when it occurred within the period 150–600 msec. after the onset of the conditioned stimulus. The limits were chosen to correspond with a wide range of eyeblink reaction times. A faster reaction time than 150 msec. seemed to us unlikely and one slower than 600 msec., even under the influence of depressant drugs, seemed equally unlikely. These limits mean that for a random blink to be accidentally counted as a conditioned response it would have to occur in the period of 450 msec. associated with each conditioned stimulus in a particular way. Furthermore, although it did not occur in this investigation, where the rate of random blinking is such that there is less than 0·450 msec. between blinks, the subject's record is, customarily, rejected as unscorable. It must be admitted that neither of these precautions completely rules out the possibility that a random blink could be counted as a conditioned response, indeed it is difficult to think of any procedure that would achieve this. However, by adopting this scoring procedure, the likelihood of 'false positives' is reduced to a minimum.

It is much more probable that the person who blinks more rapidly has a lower blink arousal threshold. This could be the basis upon which group differentiation might be achieved. However, a lower blink arousal threshold could be, in itself, an indication of a liability to form conditioned responses easily. It could be, on the other hand, simply an indication of greater responsiveness. If, for example, one could achieve the same differentiation between two groups merely by presenting a series of tones (i.e. conditioned stimuli) as could be achieved between two similar groups employing the conditioning schedule, then it would be obvious that 'responsiveness' would have to be taken into account when arriving at a conditioning score.

It will be observed that the correlation coefficients between blink rate and 'E' and 'N', the personality parameters, are negligible here. Moreover, the *F*-ratio expressing the significance of the difference between the blink rates of the three treatment groups is also very small. Hence it is evident that the significant difference between our three drug groups on the conditioning score cannot be attributed to the relationship between random eyeblinks and the conditioning score. We may conclude then that, for eyeblink conditioning, our expectations that the two depressant drugs would decrease the number of conditioned responses recorded was justified in the case of at least one of the drugs, Doriden, and that this result was most unlikely to have been an artefact of a decreased blink rate.

NONSENSE SYLLABLE LEARNING

Apparatus

The apparatus was similar to the standard, electrically driven memory drum used by Hull (1940) and by Hovland (1938). Six series of syllables were available and the members of any one series were exposed, singly, in discrete steps, so that each was shown for a period of two seconds. Massed practice was adopted with a six-second interval occurring between the last syllable of the series and a 'cue' for the reappearance of the first. The syllables were printed in half-inch block capitals and the whole sheet photographed so that they appeared on white matt paper, evenly illuminated by a lamp incorporated into the drum. Twelve syllables made up a series.

The syllables were chosen mainly from the lists given by Stevens (1951) and an effort was made to choose from syllables of low association values. The subjects spelt out the three letters of the syllables. The usual rules were followed in constructing the lists (Stevens, 1951) and, in addition, with very few exceptions, all syllables in a list began with different consonants and ended with different consonants. Syllables with the same vowel as the middle letter were, again with a few exceptions, placed three syllables apart.

Procedure

The subjects began the nonsense syllable task when their conditioning session was completed. On each of the three days they were required to learn one list of twelve syllables to a criterion of one perfect repetition.

When each subject reached seven syllables correct a rest period was interposed. This period lasted for three minutes and was intended to allow reminiscence to occur. During the rest, the subject's time was occupied in reading out a series of three digit numbers which appeared one at a time on a separate channel of the memory drum. To ensure that rehearsal did not occur, the subjects were required to respond to some of the numbers which were in sequence by continuing the sequence for three more digits. Thus, if 234 showed in the window, the subject was required to say 5, 6, 7. Where the numbers were not in sequence the subject merely read them out.

The method of learning was that of serial anticipation. After one trial, during which the subject spelt out the syllables as they appeared one at a time in the window, they were required to anticipate each separate syllable before it appeared in the window. A 'cue' preceded the first syllable, upon whose appearance the subject was required to anticipate the first syllable. The subjects were given experience of the method on a separate list before commencing the first test list. During this training the following main points were stressed.

(1) The syllables should be spelt out *before* they appeared in the window.

(2) Only one syllable at a time should be anticipated, maintaining the rhythm of the drum.

(3) No special learning system should be employed.

(4) Equal attention should be paid to all parts of the list.

(5) On each trial the subject should attempt to get the maximum number of syllables correct. Guessing was encouraged.

(6) If an error was made or no response forthcoming the subject should read out the syllable aloud from the window.

Once it was clear from the training period that the subject understood the instructions the test period proper was commenced.

The same three lists were used for each three-day testing session—one list per day. As with the eyeblink conditioning one would expect a practice effect from day one to day three, even when different lists had to be learnt. However, since the order of treatments was balanced this practice effect would be balanced out of the drug group comparisons.

Results

Speed of learning measures

The analysis presented in Table 5.8 (ii) indicates that there was no significant difference between the three groups on the number of trials taken to reach a criterion of one perfect repetition. The results shown in Table 5.9 are similarly negative, there being no significant or regular correlation between the learning measure and either 'E' or 'N'.

As with eyeblink conditioning scores, the subjects were divided into

TABLE 5.8

Comparison of Doriden, 'No Drug', and Meprobamate groups on mean number of trials to reach a criterion of one perfect repetition of twelve syllables

(i)

A	B	C
$\bar{x} = 43{\cdot}83$	$\bar{x} = 39{\cdot}04$	$\bar{x} = 44{\cdot}17$
$s = 24{\cdot}83$	$s = 21{\cdot}17$	$s = 23{\cdot}79$

(ii) Analysis of variance

	Of squares	d.f.	Mean square variance	*F*
Total observed variation	40,020·32			
Observed variation between treatments	394·70	2	197·35	1·64
Observed variation between occasions	93·34	2	46·67	0·39
Observed variation between subjects	34,232·99	23	1488·39	12·36**
Residual variation	5299·99	44	120·44	

TABLE 5.9

Regression of mean number of trials to a criterion of one perfect repetition on 'E' and 'N'

(i) 'No. of trials' and 'E'

A	B	C
R = 0·21	R = 0·18	R = 0·06
$r = 0{\cdot}24$	$r = 0{\cdot}08$	$r = 0{\cdot}07$

(ii) 'No. of trials' and 'N'

A	B	C
R = 0·03	R = 0·21	R = −0·20
$r = 0{\cdot}03$	$r = 0{\cdot}08$	$r = -0{\cdot}20$

high and low scores on 'E' and 'N' and their learning scorers on the 'No Drug' day compared. Tables 5.10 and 5.11 show these comparisons.

Tables 5.10 and 5.11 indicate some tendency for subjects with low extraversion scores and with low neuroticism scores to learn more rapidly. As the size of the correlation coefficients in Table 5.9 would suggest, these differences are not formally significant. When the two categories leading to more rapid learning are combined and contrasted with the two associated with slower learning the mean difference is greater although again not formally significant.

It was felt that, although the groups showed no significant difference

TABLE 5.10

Comparison of mean number of trials to criterion of one perfect repetition on nonsense syllable learning for 'high' and 'low' scorers on Extraversion and Neuroticism

(i) Means and standard deviations—Extraversion

Low 'E'	High 'E'
N = 13	N = 11
$\bar{x}$ = 33·15	$\bar{x}$ = 46·00
s = 13·96	s = 24·68

(ii) 't' test of significance of mean differences—Extraversion

t = 1·65 (not significant)

(iii) Means and standard deviations—Neuroticism

Low 'N'	High 'N'
N = 12	N = 12
$\bar{x}$ = 31·67	$\bar{x}$ = 46·42
s = 10·81	s = 25·41

(iv) 't' test of significance of mean differences—Neuroticism

t = 1·68 (not significant)

TABLE 5.11

Comparison of mean number of trials to criterion of one perfect repetition on nonsense syllable learning for subjects scoring low on Extraversion and low on Neuroticism against subjects who scored high on Extraversion and high on Neuroticism

(i) Means and standard deviation

Low 'E' and Low 'N'	High 'E' and High 'N'
N = 7	N = 7
$\bar{x}$ = 27·57	$\bar{x}$ = 51·71
s = 6·93	s = 29·00

(ii) 't' test of significance between means of (i)

t = 1·98 (not significant)

in the number of trials taken to reach one perfect repetition, differences in mode of learning might still exist, particularly in regard to the average slope of each subject's learning curve. A sample of the seventy-two sets of scores was plotted and it was apparent that the resulting curves were in the form of a simple exponential function. The score on each trial (i.e. the number of syllables correctly anticipated) was then put into log form so that the exponential curves could be plotted as straight lines whose characteristics would be readily calculable. In fact, as a matter of convenience, the direction of slope of the curve was reversed, by computing for each trial, 12 – Y, where Y was the number of syllables correct on any one trial. Thus for any individual records, log (12 – Y) was plotted against trial number. This convention meant that since 12 – 12 = 0 and there is no value which satisfies log 0, the last, criterion-reaching trial was not plotted. For each of the seventy-two curves formed by the log (12 – Y) scores, the straight line of best fit was calculated and from the equation for this line each slope value was computed. Then the deviation of each plotted point from its corresponding point on the line of best fit was computed and the characteristic deviation tendency for any curve expressed as the root mean squared deviation.

Tables 5.12 and 5.13 present these data and the relevant analysis of them. Fig. 5.1 shows the mean slopes.

TABLE 5.12

Slopes of straight line curves fitted to individual nonsense syllable learning scores where the number of syllables correctly anticipated on a trial is expressed as log (12 – Y); Y = the number of syllables correct on that trial. All scores have been multiplied by 1000 to clear the decimal places

(i) Means and standard deviations of slopes (×1000)

A	B	C
$\bar{x} = 18$	$\bar{x} = 25$	$\bar{x} = 18$
$s = 12$	$s = 15$	$s = 14$

(ii) Analysis of variance of slopes

	Of squares	d.f.	Mean square variance	*F*
Total observed variation	13,816·61			
Observed variation between treatments	823·74	2	411·87	4·05*
Observed variation between occasions	24·53	2	12·27	0·12
Observed variation between subjects	8496·61	23	369·42	3·64**

(iii) Regressions

Regression of slopes on 'E'

A	B	C
R = −0·15	R = −0·27	R = −0·27
r = −0·29	*r* = −0·15	*r* = −0·31

Regression of slopes on 'N'

A	B	C
R = −0·02	R = −0·22	R = 0·12
r = 0·05	*r* = −0·05	*r* = 0·18

The data presented in Table 5.12 indicate that the mean slope of the 'No Drug' group was significantly steeper than either of those of the two drug groups. Since the slopes of the learning curves represent rates

TABLE 5.13

Root mean squared deviations of plotted points on nonsense syllable learning curves from corresponding points on fitted curve. All scores multiplied by 1000 to clear the decimal places

(i) Means and standard deviations of root mean squared deviations (× 1000)

A	B	C
$\bar{x} = 153$	$\bar{x} = 164$	$\bar{x} = 146$
$s = 33$	$s = 33$	$s = 47$

(ii) Analysis of variance

	Of squares	d.f.	Mean square variance	*F*
Total observed variation	109,753·00			
Observed variation between treatments	4593·00	2	2296·50	2·22
Observed variation between occasions	3362·00	2	1681·00	1·63
Observed variation between subjects	55,443·00	23	2410·57	2·37**
Residual variation	45,455·00	44	1033·068	

(iii) Regressions

Regression of root mean squared deviations on 'E

A	B	C
R = 0·15	R = 0·03	R = 0·09
r = 0·04	*r* = 0·12	*r* = 0·04

Regression of root mean squared deviations on 'N'

A	B	C
R = −0·09	R = 0·19	R = −0·24
r = 0·09	*r* = 0·24	*r* = 0·10

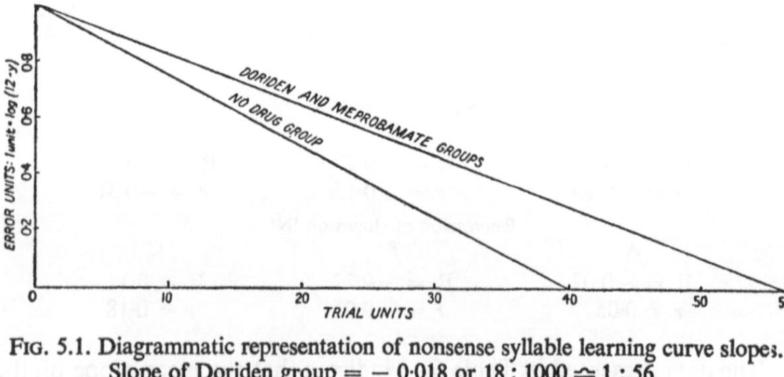

FIG. 5.1. Diagrammatic representation of nonsense syllable learning curve slopes.
Slope of Doriden group = − 0·018 or 18 : 1000 ≃ 1 : 56
Slope of No-Drug group = − 0·025 or 25 : 1000 ≃ 1 : 40
Slope of meprobamate group = − 0·018 or 18 : 1000 ≃ 1 : 56

of learning this result means that both Doriden and meprobamate decelerated the rate of learning the syllables. The regression coefficients did not reveal any regular or significant relationships between the slopes of the nonsense syllable learning curves and either of the two personality parameters. Table 5.13 indicates that there was no significant difference in trial to trial variability between the groups nor was this variable correlated with either of the personality parameters.

Error measures

Three classes of error were distinguished and examined: (*a*) all errors which included simple failures to respond, as well as those of the types (*b*) and (*c*), where (*b*) included all incorrect responses in which also were included (*c*) perseverative and associative errors.

TABLE 5.14

Number of errors of all kinds, including failures to respond, incorrect responses, and associative and perseverative errors

(i) Means and standard deviations—number of errors of all kinds

A	B	C
$\bar{x}$ = 288·04	$\bar{x}$ = 246·46	$\bar{x}$ = 295·500
s = 192·21	s = 147·78	s = 174·00

(ii) Analysis of variance

	Of squares	d.f.	Mean square variance	F
Total observed variation	2,173,434·00			
Observed variation between treatments	34,081·08	2	17,040·54	2·41
Observed variation between occasions	5277·00	2	2638·00	0·37
Observed variation between subjects	1,823,163·33	23	79,267·97	11·22**
Residual variation	310,912·59	44	7066·19	

Table 5.14 indicates that there was no difference between the groups on the tendency to make errors. If one examines Table 5.14 and Table 5.8 it will be seen that some association appears to exist between the number of trials taken and the number of errors made. Thus, strictly speaking, one should control number of trials when comparing number of errors. Since the association between the two variables is positive, there was probably an artificial exaggeration of such differences as do exist between the total error scores of the groups. Nevertheless, the analysis of variance of Table 5.14 (ii) yielded an insignificant variance ratio suggesting that the mean differences are entirely due to chance. In fact, although it is not given here, an analysis of co-variance was carried

out for the total number of errors holding number of trials constant and the resulting *F*-ratio remained insignificant.

We have employed the analysis of co-variance in examining the differences between (*b*) incorrect responses and (*c*) associative and perseverative errors. Both of these could be dependent on either number of trials or total number of errors. The analysis of co-variance is an analysis of the residual variance (of e.g. number of incorrect responses) when (e.g. the number of trials) a related independent variable is held constant. We have used it in analysing the differences in number of incorrect responses and number of associative errors despite the insignificant differences between the two related independent variables because the measures of incorrect responses and associative errors, being of infrequent occurrence and partly dependent on a decision of the subject to guess, were judged to be unreliable. It was felt that any difference other than a gross difference might be obscured.

TABLE 5.15

Comparison of the number of incorrect responses made in each of the Doriden, 'No Drug' and meprobamate groups

(i) Means and standard deviations of number of incorrect responses

A	B	C
$\bar{x} = 43{\cdot}88$	$\bar{x} = 40{\cdot}04$	$\bar{x} = 41{\cdot}21$
$s = 23{\cdot}24$	$s = 25{\cdot}07$	$s = 23{\cdot}76$

(ii) Analysis of co-variance—when number of trials is held constant

	R	d.f.	$\frac{R}{d.f.}$	*F*
$R_1 - R_2$ (Between group variation after adjusting for regression)	1452·78	2	726·39	
R_2 (Within group variation after adjusting for regression)	17,393·85	68	255·79	2·84
R_1 (Total variation after adjusting for regression)	18,846·63			

(iii) Analysis of co-variance—when total number of all errors are held constant

	R	d.f.	$\frac{R}{d.f.}$	*F*
$R_1 - R_2$	1916·52	2	958·26	
R_2	18,272·63	68	278·72	3·57*
R_1	20,189·15			

In essence the technique consists in computing two estimates of the variation amongst the scores of the dependent variable; in this case, number of incorrect responses (Y). Both estimates are of the residual variation in the Y scores, adjusted for their regression on the independent variable, in this case the number of trials. These estimates we are calling R_1, the first estimate of the residual variation obtained when no distinction is made between group means or between regressions; and R_2, the estimate of residual variation obtained when the group means are distinguished. R_1 is thus an estimate of the (adjusted) total variation among all the Y scores, R_2 is an estimate of the (adjusted) variation within the groups of Y scores, and $R_1 - R_2$, an estimate of the variation between the groups of Y scores: a variance ratio of $\frac{R_1 - R_2}{R_2}$ yields a quantity which by reference to 'F' tables indicates whether the group means are significantly different when concomitant '*x*' scores (independent variable) are held constant.

Table 5.15 presents the means and standard deviations of the three groups on the number of incorrect responses made during the nonsense

TABLE 5.16

Comparison of the number of associative and perseverative errors occurring in each of the Doriden, 'No Drug', and Meprobamate groups

(i) Means and standard deviations

	A	B	C
$\bar{x}$	11·75	10·88	11·04
s	9·90	9·08	8·11

(ii) Analysis of co-variance, holding number of trials to criterion constant

	R	d.f.	$\frac{R}{d.f.}$	*F*
$R_1 - R_2$ (Between group variation after adjusting for regression)	17·84	2	8·93	
R_2 (Within group variation after adjusting for regression)	4855·94	68	71·41	0·12
R_1 (Total variation after adjusting for regression)	4873·78			

(iii) Analysis of co-variance holding number of errors of all kinds constant

	R	d.f.	$\frac{R}{d.f.}$	*F*
$R_1 - R_2$ (Between group variation after adjusting for regression)	15·35	2	7·63	
R_2 (Within group variation after adjusting for regression)	4660·94	68	68·54	0·1

syllable learning and the analysis of co-variance of these scores when (*a*) the number of trials and (*b*) the total number of errors of all kinds are held constant.

From Table 5.15 it would appear that when the total number of errors is held constant there is a significantly greater number of incorrect responses given under the drug conditions. This difference is not apparent when the number of trials alone is held constant.

The mean number of associative and perseverative errors occurring among the subjects of the three groups is shown in Table 5.16. These have been treated in an analysis of co-variance, in which, as in Table 5.15, both the number of trials to the criterion and the total number of errors have been held constant. No differences are apparent between the groups on the number of associative errors according to the analyses presented in Table 5.16.

Behavioural oscillations

The count of behavioural oscillations is another measure of variation in performance, although not variation in the trial by trial score of

TABLE 5.17

Comparison of behavioural oscillations in nonsense syllable learning between Doriden, 'No Drug', and Meprobamate group

(i) Means and standard deviations

A	B	C
$\bar{x}$ = 55·29	$\bar{x}$ = 44·42	$\bar{x}$ = 55·00
s = 39·01	s = 30·45	s = 40·72

(ii) Analysis of co-variance of behavioural oscillations holding number of trials constant

	R	d.f.	$\frac{R}{d.f.}$	*F*
$R_1 - R_2$ (Between group variations after adjusting for regression)	321·58	2	160·79	
R_2 (Within group variation after adjusting for regression)	15914·43	68	234·04	0·69
R_1 (Total variation after adjusting for regression)	16,236·01			

(iii) Analysis of variance of behavioural oscillations holding number of errors constant

	R	d.f.	$\frac{R}{d.f.}$	*F*
$R_1 - R_2$ (Between group variation after adjusting for regression)	2224·37	2	1112·18	
R_2 (Within group variation after adjusting for regression)	32,036·97	68	470·98	2·36

number of syllables correctly anticipated, which was the object of computing the root mean squared deviations given in Table 5.13. The behavioural oscillation is a measure employed by Hull (1940, 1943, 1952) and occurs whenever a failure to respond to a syllable follows one or more correct responses to that syllable in the immediately preceding trials. Clearly, again, one would suppose that, other things being equal, there would be a relationship between the number of trials and the number of behavioural oscillations and between the total number of errors and behavioural oscillations. The former is likely to be a positive relationship, the second need not be. Since correct responses must occur for an oscillation to be possible, a large number of errors could lessen the chance of an oscillation appearing. When there are few errors, on the other hand, there will necessarily be fewer oscillations. In fact, in our data, when the distribution of behavioural oscillations against numbers of errors was plotted, a simple linear relationship was seen to obtain. Hence the analysis of co-variance, which presupposes a linear regression between the relevant variables, was an appropriate technique here also. Table 5.17 presents the data on behavioural oscillation.

Table 5.17 indicates that no differences existed between the groups on behavioural oscillations when number of trials and number of errors were held constant.

Reminiscence measures

In its simplest form the phenomenon of reminiscence is an improvement in performance after a suitable rest pause. If the performance is of the

TABLE 5.18

Comparison of differences between first post-rest scores and last pre-rest scores on nonsense syllable learning of the Doriden, 'No Drug', and Meprobamate groups

(i) Means and standard deviations

A	B	C
$\bar{x} = 1{\cdot}92$	$\bar{x} = 2{\cdot}29$	$\bar{x} = 2{\cdot}83$
$s = 1{\cdot}80$	$s = 1{\cdot}62$	$s = 1{\cdot}68$

(ii) Analysis of variance

	Of squares	d.f.	Mean square variance	F
Total observed variation	218·32			
Observed variation amongst treatments	10·50	2	5·25	1·65
Observed variation amongst occasions	15·53	2	7·27	2·31
Observed variation amongst subjects	53·65	23	2·33	
Residual variation	138·94	44	3·16	

type employed here the simplest measure of reminiscence will be to subtract the last score before the rest from the first score after the rest. The size of the difference indicates the amount of reminiscence that has occurred during the rest pause. Of course it may happen that a subtraction of the type mentioned may result in a negative quantity, the first post-rest score being less than the last pre-rest score—a certain degree of forgetting or interference having occurred. Improvement in performance may also show itself as a gain, in reaching some criterion or other, after a rest when compared to an appropriate control group. Hull (1940, 1943) and his associates have interpreted reminiscence as being due to the dissipation of reactive inhibition built up during the pre-rest practice and accumulating to have a suppressing action on manifest performance. If we allow this to be a plausible explanation of reminiscence then from the drug postulate we would expect the drug groups to show reminiscence to a greater degree. Tables 5.18 and 5.19 give two measures of this effect.

TABLE 5.19

Comparison of number of trials from the 'rest' pause to the criterion

(i) Means and standard deviations

A	B	C
$\bar{x} = 25{\cdot}83$	$\bar{x} = 21{\cdot}96$	$\bar{x} = 23{\cdot}21$
$s = 19{\cdot}72$	$s = 13{\cdot}86$	$s = 17{\cdot}17$

(ii) Analysis of variance

	Of squares	d.f.	Mean square variance	F
Total observed variation	21,554·00			
Observed variation between treatments	187·75	2	93·88	1·05
Observed variation between occasions	115·75	2	57·88	0·64
Observed variation between subjects	17,302·00	23	752·26	8·38**
Residual variation	3948·50	44	89·74	

It will be seen from Tables 5.18 and 5.19 that neither of the reminiscence measures demonstrated significant differences between the drug groups and the 'No Drug' group.

It only remains, in Table 5.20, to report the means and standard deviations of the questionnaire measurements of Introversion/Extraversion (E) and of Neuroticism (N). Table 5.20 shows these values and the product moment correlation between (E) and (N).

TABLE 5.20

Questionnaire scores on Introversion/Extraversion (E) and Neuroticism (N)

(i) Means and standard deviations

'E'	'N'
$\bar{x} = 25{\cdot}50$	$\bar{x} = 21{\cdot}92$
$s = 10{\cdot}31$	$s = 11{\cdot}77$

(ii) Correlation between 'E' and 'N'

$$r_{EN.} = 0{\cdot}068$$

Discussion of nonsense syllable data

The principal finding of this investigation was that the depressant drugs decreased the slope of the individual nonsense syllable learning curves when these were compared to those of the 'No Drug' group. If we take degree of slope as indicative of rate of learning, then according to the analysis of this measure both drugs significantly decrease rate of learning. On the other hand, although the same trend is evident when the measure examined is simply the number of trials taken to reach the criterion of one perfect repetition, no significantly poorer learning is evident. This apparent contradiction requires some comment.

The slopes of our fitted straight line curves are determined by the parameters of 'length' and 'height'. In this case 'length' represents the number of trials taken to reach the criterion and 'height' represents the difference in the number of syllables correctly anticipated from the first recorded trial to the penultimate trial. It should be noted that both 'height' and slope are expressed in log scores while 'length' is in terms of raw scores. An analysis of variance of 'length', we have seen, revealed the trend one would expect from a finding of significantly steeper slopes for the 'No Drug' group, but the variance ratio fell short of significance. If the procedure of analysis of variance were quite precise, one might argue that, because 'height' and 'length' determine slope, if slope is different and 'length' is not different, 'height' must be different. However, the procedure is not that precise. Analysis of variance deals with mean values and there is a margin of uncertainty in such a line of reasoning. Provided the expected trends are found in the two independent parameters thus, there is, in fact, no real contradiction in finding a significant difference between the dependent functions, that is, the slopes. In investigating this point, the 'height' for each subject was determined in raw scores and an analysis of variance of the group means carried out. The variance ratio fell just short of significance and the mean values were as would be expected. The 'No Drug' group showed a greater mean 'height'. One further computational point should be mentioned. The within-group variance of the transformed 'height' scores would tend to be more homogeneous than that of the raw scores by virtue of the effect of the log transformation. Hence, it is not surprising that the variance ratio of the transformed scores could be significant, while that of the untransformed scores should fall just short of significance.

Because the analysis of slope involved a transformation and assumptions about the shapes of the performed curves one must place rather more emphasis on the actual scores, even though the assumptions made seem very reasonable. One feels that the way these performance scores arranged themselves, as expected, together with the significant difference between the slopes, being in the manner predicted, adds up to a positive result but one which must be treated with some reservations.

The measure of trial by trial variability in performance was undertaken rather as a result of an impression gained during testing. The inconvenience involved in carrying out the testing 'blind' was judged to be far too high a price to pay for the purely academic advantages this procedure brings with it when quite objective tests are used. Hence the investigator knew each day's treatment and it seemed, at the time, that drug sessions involved much higher variability and variability of a particular kind. Subjects tended to learn nonsense syllables stepwise—i.e. typically they would get two or three syllables correct for a certain number of trials, then suddenly jump to a new and higher level. They might drop on the odd trial but, by and large, their variability would, henceforth, swing about the new level. It was as if the subject were taking rest pauses and then quite suddenly achieving new acquisitions. The drug sessions seemed to produce this variability to a greater extent than the 'No Drug' session. It was hoped that the analysis of the root mean squared deviations might substantiate this observation. However, as can be seen from the data of Table 5.13, it did not.

Error scores during nonsense syllable learning are of two main types: failures to respond at all, and incorrect responses. The latter category could be broken down in a number of ways but two main sub-classes suggest themselves: 'neologisms', syllables similar in form to those in the list but which are not in fact contained in it, and syllables in the list given out of their correct order, either before their position (associative errors) or after their position (perseverative errors). In our analysis we have chosen to group errors into three inclusive groups: total errors of all kinds, incorrect responses, and associative and perseverative errors. The analysis revealed that when the total error tendency was held constant, the drug groups gave more incorrect responses.

In a way this is an unexpected result; one might have imagined that a depressant drug would have reduced the level of response rather than have increased it. On the other hand it is consistent with the finding that extraverts are liable to make more errors, particularly errors caused by impulsiveness (Himmelweit, 1946; Venables, 1956). The same difference would not necessarily have been expected had the total error score been considered, since this score consists of all incorrect responses together with all failures to respond. The characteristic error of the extravert is one of impulsive carelessness and this trait is much more likely to show in a positive error tendency, like giving 'neologisms', than in the negative case of simply saying nothing.

This finding, while consistent with the general theory forming the basis of the investigation, was not actually expected, nor, indeed, did one feel very convinced that a measure like Behavioural Oscillations would be significantly affected. However, one did expect there would be a difference in reminiscence scores and that sizeable, if not formally significant, correlations would have been found between the major scores and 'E' and 'N'.

Reminiscence, as measured here, did not occur. The means of the first post-rest scores, for all groups, were below those of the pre-rest scores. Why this should have occurred is open to question. It is possible that the rest period chosen was inappropriate. It is possible that the criterion applied (seven syllables correct) was inappropriate. In attempting to get a measure of reminiscence in nonsense syllable learning one is faced with the problem of when to introduce the rest pause. We have followed Hovland (1938) in applying a 'number correct' criterion and in so doing ensure that all subjects are at the same relative point on their learning curve. The accumulation and dissipation of inhibition explanation of the reminiscence phenomenon is, however, a 'work' hypothesis and it is difficult to say whether to have reached the same point on a learning curve after different numbers of trials is to have done the same amount of work. It could be argued that, contrary to this doubt, only the act of responding with the correct syllable would be associated with the inhibitory tendencies whose disappearance would allow an improvement in performance to appear. The dissipation of inhibition generated by irrelevant incorrect responses would not affect reminiscence. Furthermore, there is the serious practical difficulty, if one were to advocate the alternative and were to introduce a rest pause after a given number of trials, of deciding where to make the break. Some subjects learn so rapidly that they have returned one perfect repetition before the minimum number of trials likely to produce any degree of inhibition (say fifteen trials), precluding the possibility of reminiscence occurring.

An even more likely cause for the non-appearance of reminiscence lies in the nature of the interpolated task employed. This task, designed to control the subject's attention rather more thoroughly than is possible with the more usual colour naming, proved to be quite difficult and analogous in some ways to the nonsense syllable learning task itself. Despite Summerfield and Steinberg's (1957) finding to the contrary, it is possible that some retroactive interference may have resulted from our interpolated task causing the decrement in performance rather than the expected improvement. The problem can only be settled empirically, using different rest pauses and different dosages.

Finally, one must again mention the absence of any significant or sizeable correlation coefficients between the two personality measures and aspects of performance. On the whole, if one considers only the slopes of the individual learning curves and the number of trials to a criterion, one would have expected subjects with higher extraversion scores to learn more slowly. There should certainly also, if one were to follow Hull and Spence, be a tendency for subjects having higher neuroticism scores to learn more rapidly. If neuroticism is a drive, and drive is a factor multiplicative with others to affect performance, then high drive should go with a high level of performance. This picture is complicated by the ramifications of the Yerkes-Dodson effect which suggests a curvilinear relationship between drive and performance, in which the factors of stress and degree of task complexity play important roles. In fact subjects did appear to find anticipating syllables in a period of two seconds stressful and the task could certainly be regarded as complex. Following the Yerkes-Dodson law then one would expect a high degree of neuroticism to be a disadvantage.

Since the regression analyses revealed such low regression coefficients we did not expect to be able to separate significantly the performance of extraverts (high 'E') from introverts (low 'E') on number of trials taken to reach the criterion but it seemed a fruitful way of taking another look at this data. The same treatment could have been applied to the other measures, of course. The score 'number of trials to criterion' was chosen because it is the most unambiguous measure of performance. Only the 'No Drug' treatment was analysed in this way because the differential effect of drugs on different personalities is still largely unknown. The subjects were grouped on the basis of their 'E' and 'N' scores by calling everyone scoring the mean and above 'Extraverts' or 'the High Neuroticism group' respectively, and those scoring −1 and below 'Introverts' and 'the Low Neuroticism group'. Then, because neuroticism is a multiplicative factor, a group having low extraversion scores and low neuroticism scores was contrasted with one having high extraversion and high neuroticism scores. This grouping was adopted because it was evident that in this relatively complex stressful situation neuroticism should and, in fact, was acting negatively. The results, shown in Tables 5.10 and 5.11, are in the expected direction and the differences, between the groups compared, quite large, although as would be suggested by the low regression coefficients, the variance ratios failed to reach significance. The introverts learned more rapidly as did subjects with low neuroticism scores. Bearing in mind these two findings it is not surprising that stable introverts learnt best of all groups and neurotic extraverts the worst.

In general then we can say that our expectations received some, but by no means incontrovertible confirmation. At the present moment we could be in error at any of a number of places. Our basic hypothesis about personality variables and neural mechanisms could be wrong. Its specific application to the study of drugs could be unjustified. Our choice of drugs could be inappropriate, or the learning postulates we have accepted as explanations of the learning phenomena we are dealing with might also be erroneous. The inconclusive and, in part, contradictory results in this investigation suggest clearly that some elements in our reasoning are incorrect or at least partly incorrect. Only by persistent probing within the field prescribed by our general theoretical position can we hope to come to unambiguous conclusions.

Summary

(1) On three testing days twenty-four subjects received two tablets of Doriden (glutethimide), two tablets of meprobamate and a 'No Drug' treatment. Both drugs were regarded as cortical depressants. The order

of treatments was balanced over the twenty-four subjects to equalize practice effects.

(2) On each day the subject was required to learn a list of twelve nonsense syllables by the method of serial anticipation and underwent an eyeblink conditioning procedure.

(3) On the basis of the hypothesis linking extraversion with cortical inhibitory tendencies it was expected that the depressant drugs would reveal extravert behaviour patterns. More specifically, it was expected that the drug group would have fewer conditioned eyeblink responses and would also show evidence of a decreased rate of learning.

(4) Doriden significantly decreased the number of conditioned responses but meprobamate, although acting in the same way, did not produce a statistically significant effect.

(5) Neither Doriden nor meprobamate significantly increased the number of trials taken to reach a criterion of one perfect repetition on a rote learning task, although the mean scores were separated as expected. When the slopes of the individual learning curves were examined, both Doriden and meprobamate were associated with shallow learning curves, and this difference was a statistically significant one.

(6) Certain secondary effects were examined. The drugs did not effect any change in rate of random blinking. Both drugs significantly increased the number of incorrect responses given during the nonsense syllable learning when allowance was made for the total number of errors recorded.

(7) No reminiscence was found for any of the groups and suggestions as to why this occurred have been offered.

(8) No regular or significant regression coefficients between any of the measures and the questionnaire measures of extraversion and neuroticism were found.

6

THE EFFECTS OF DEPRESSANT DRUGS ON SOME PERCEPTUAL PROCESSES

H. C. Holland[1]

The drugs

LITTLE is known about the action of either meprobamate or Doriden. What information is available suggests that meprobamate must be classed as one of the ataractic drugs which are derived from either phenothiazine, the Rauwolfia alkaloids, benzhydrol, or mephenesin (meprobamate being specifically a mephenesin derivative). Meprobamate is said to be a non-toxic, non-addicting, non-depressant relaxant (Margolis, 1957; Litchfield, 1957; Haizlip and Ewing, 1955), differing from the barbiturates in its site of action, its side effects, and its effect of tranquillization without confusion (Trouton and Eysenck, 1960). Meprobamate has been employed extensively since its introduction in 1956 (Berger, 1956), both experimentally and clinically with normals (Marquis, 1957), anxiety states (Dickel *et al.*, 1957), *petit mal* and behaviour disorders (Litchfield, 1957), and in the study of conditioned fear responses of rats (Hunt, 1957). The main action of the drug appears to be internucial, having a striking effect on the thalamus and sub-cortical structures (Litchfield, 1957). It is said to have little, if any, effect on cortical areas unless very large doses are given, and that the EEG activity associated with it is unlike that produced by barbiturates (Berger, 1956). The side effects of the drug are said to be minimal but may be important for the present experiment. They include drowsiness,

[1] The writer is indebted to the Medical Research Council for a grant which enabled him to take part in this investigation.

dizziness, *ataxia*, and allergic reactions, symptoms which usually disappear when the drug is withdrawn (Berger, 1956). Although the drug has been enthusiastically received by those practitioners interested in the treatment of emotional, mental, and tension states, and extensively used, its actual action on the organism still remains obscure (Himwick, 1957).

The second drug to be used in this investigation is Doriden, which is described in the literature as a rapid-acting, non-barbiturate sedative, and mild hypnotic. It is said to have quieting and sleep-producing properties without the side effects usual in similarly acting barbiturates (Weston, 1956; Howell, 1956; Blumberg, 1956). It has been given clinical trials on several groups of normals and patients including the elderly, the neuropsychiatric, and the epileptic. Groups of prisoners have been sedated by it and it has been used in conjunction with analgesics in first-stage labour (Blumberg, 1956; Abbas, 1957). The action of the drug has been described as nearest to that of phenobarbital but to be shorter acting and with fewer side effects (Gross, 1955).

There are virtually no reports concerning the influence of either of these compounds on the visual mechanisms, particularly in the case of Doriden. With meprobamate the only experimental work which has been traced by the writer comes from Marquis and his group (Marquis *et al.*, 1957), who employed a standard ortho-rater to test several visual functions on fifty subjects, including depth perception, acuity for both near and far vision, and the vertical and lateral phorias. Testing was conducted with treatments of meprobamate, meprobamate and alcohol, placebo and alcohol, and dextroamphetamine sulphate. On none of the visual functions mentioned were there any significant changes attributable to the treatments.

Increases in *ataxia* have been produced in mice and dogs by relatively large doses of Doriden (Gross, 1955), and one of the side effects of meprobamate is slight drowsiness and dizziness (Litchfield, 1957). It was therefore considered important to ascertain if there was any increase in body sway, attributable to the action of the drugs, in a group of human adult subjects.

The effects of drugs on the visual field

The visual field has been defined as that portion of space in which objects are visible at the same moment during steady fixation of the eyes in one direction (Traquair, 1948). A now classical paragraph has described it as an island and the perimetric examination of it as a survey of its outline and contours, where the contours, or isopters, comprise positions of equal sensitivity. The field itself is in a constant state of change due to a number of physiological and psychological factors over which neither the perimetrist nor the subject can exercise any real control. These include at one level such things as physiological nystagmus

(Osgood and Heyer, 1952; Marshall and Talbot, 1940; Marshall, 1942; Talbot and Marshall, 1941), and the various flicks and drifts to which the eyes are subject during the fixational pause, and at another level psychogenically determined mechanisms such as the constant interchange of focal and marginal attention, vigilance, etc. All these extraneous factors must be considered by the perimetrist, but they are not his primary concern. What any investigator of the visual field must do, under these circumstances, is to concern himself with a physical artificiality and to plot the ambit and sensitivity of the stationary eye.

Although perimetric instruments have changed greatly in the last few decades the basic field examination has changed little since the introduction of quantitative methods by Roenne and Bjerrum, who were dissatisfied with the simple outlining of the field by determination of the lowest sensitivity isopter, and who went on to show that the sensitivity gradient of the field could be defined by a series of such lines each representing the perception of a stimulus of a given intensity. Thus any isopter in the visual field must represent the mid-position of two processes, that of excitation and that of extinction (Sharples, 1946; Mann and Sharples, 1946): excitation being the response to an incoming stimulus of given intensity and extinction being the disappearance of that stimulus as it moves along any meridian from the centre to the periphery or from the periphery to the centre.[1] The specific isopter is defined usually on the basis of the visual angle of the test object to which it corresponds.

In the abnormal eye the smooth curve of increasing sensitivity from the periphery to the centre is often pitted with areas of depressed vision due to many different conditions. These may be transient or permanent and they may be due to lesions or excrescences of the retina, the optic tracts, or the visuo-cortical mechanisms (Bender and Teuber, 1946). They go under the general terms of contractions and scotomata. Although these are the concern of the perimetrist and the ophthalmologist in clinical practice, such considerations have been beyond the scope of this investigation, which has been concerned only with general contractions of the field, specifically those which can be induced, by or which follow from, the administration of chemical agents.

The literature is far from replete with examples of induced field contractions, but a section in Traquair (1948) lists among others such agents as quinine, tobacco, several of the arsenical compounds and some of the impurities found in crude alcoholic drinks. These have been

[1] The terms 'excitation' and 'extinction' are used here after Sharples (1946) and Mann and Sharples (1946). In essence the whole process is one of discrimination between target intensity and bowl illumination. In this sense 'excitation' will be defined as a statement that the retinal receptors are sufficient and sensitive enough to permit a judgement of 'different' between target and bowl intensities, whereas 'extinction' will be the point at which resolution of this difference breaks down.

found to be effective in general clinical practice, and it seems that no experimental work supports these observations. Surprisingly few deficiency studies have examined the visual field, but it has been found that anoxia acts to reduce the extent of the field (Birren, 1946; Ikui, 1947; McFarland, 1940, 1943). Some investigators are, however, hesitant in attributing the reduction to the direct effect of the deficiency on the visual mechanisms, and think that a generally depressing effect of anoxia on responses cannot be ruled out (Ikui, 1947).

The present investigation

The design of the present study stems from several sources. In the first place it is probably true to say that when chemical agents have been administered which affect the visual field, they have usually affected the regions of lowest sensitivity, which are in the periphery. This is a simple threshold effect in which the maximum influence of the agent is found at those areas of lowest response potential. In the second place it may be said that when deficiency studies have shown visual field defects they have not only resulted in depression of visual sensitivity but also in a general reduction of reactivity in the organism as a whole. In the third place, we have the drug hypothesis outlined in the introduction to this section, which states that *depressant* drugs will lead to an *increase* in *inhibitory* potentials and a *decrease* in *excitation*, whereas *stimulant* drugs will lead to a *decrease* in *inhibition* and an *increase* in *excitation.* In terms of perimetry and the visual field this hypothesis implies that *the excitation and extinction processes which characterize the specific isopters will be changed in such a way as to alter the extent and gradient (slope) of sensitivity*. An inhibitory drug should reduce and depress the field whereas an excitatory drug should enlarge and raise it.

The above considerations lead to the specific hypothesis to be tested in the present experiment, i.e. if both compounds, meprobamate and Doriden, are basically depressant in character they should act upon the visual field to reduce it and to lower sensitivity. If, however, the drugs differed fundamentally in their effects such similarity of field changes would not be found.

Apparatus (peripheral field)[1]

The perimeter was a commercially available Goldman Spherical Projection type where bowl and target lighting are derived from the same source. The bowl lighting is variable over a very wide range and the bowl target ratio is achieved by filter and photometer screen. Once the basic light bowl ratio has been assessed the target light can be changed in six steps, and there are four colours available. In the present investigation the target size was kept constant at 0·25 mm.[2] and the light at

[1] The editor wishes to thank the Central Research Committee for financial assistance in the purchase of the apparatus.

358 Lux (measured by lightmeter) which gave, with a bowl albedo of 0·7, a reflected intensity of 250 asb.

Method

Because of 'nose plotting' only the left temporal field was investigated. Inner and outer thresholds were determined along fourteen meridians, every 15 degrees with the exception of the horizontal co-ordinate which was missed and readings taken at approximately 88 and 92 degrees respectively.

After the subject had been seated at the instrument and gross adjustments made his right eye was covered by a black surgical patch, his head strapped into the combined chin and headrest, and the depth of penetration of the face into the bowl corrected. This was done in all cases before the final calibration of the instrument was performed because of differential face reflection. Final positioning of the eye was done through the telescopic viewer at the rear of the perimeter from which the subsequent field examination was conducted. At the right hand of the subject was an indicator buzzer activated by a morse key which was used to indicate the appearance or disappearance of the target light, obviating a great deal of head movement due to verbal responses. From the moment that the head of the subject was fixed into the instrument a period of four minutes' light adaptation (at the standard bowl intensity) was allowed before testing began. It could, therefore, be assumed that the subject was light adapted to the background, i.e. bowl illumination. The inner trials were plotted first, followed by the outer threshold assessment. The individual trials, both incoming and outgoing, were randomized.

Results (peripheral field test)

The main results are outlined in Table 6.1. It contains the means of the four variables measured and their standard deviations.

TABLE 6.1

	'No Drug'			meprobamate		Doriden	
Inner threshold	55·78°	4·78°		53·65°	4·55°	53·52°	4·75°
Outer threshold	63·25°	4·51°		65·01°	4·14°	65·50°	4·43°
Mean threshold	59·27°	4·31°		59·22°	4·02°	59·53°	4·33°
Differential threshold	7·74°	1·81°	%	11·30°	2·91°	12·03°	3·00°

The fifth measure to be taken represents the gradient of sensitivity and is the total of the angular positions of four intensity isopters for excitation. A high score on this measure represents high sensitivity and the scores in order as above are as follows: 'No Drug': 229·1; meprobamate: 214·2; Doriden: 214·9. The scores for the individual meridians under each condition are contained in Table 6.2. Table 6.3 gives the means for the four target intensities.

TABLE 6.2

Inner and outer threshold values for the twenty-four subjects on the fourteen meridians for the three treatments

	Control		Meprobamate		Doriden	
1	36·75	41·79	35·83	43·88	35·54	43·42
2	39·42	44.50	38·38	46·75	37·17	46·71
3	42·46	48·46	41·67	51·29	39·71	50·13
4	47·42	54·29	46·21	57·00	45·46	56·92
5	54·33	63·00	53·38	66·38	52·42	64·63
6	61·21	69·67	58·88	71·96	59·33	72·13
7	66.42	75·25	63·71	75·63	64·50	76·71
8	68·24	77·42	65·88	77·92	65·38	79·00
9	69·29	78·58	66·50	79·58	66·25	79·75
10	68·04	77·08	65·67	78·42	65·96	79·88
11	64·38	71·96	60·71	73·67	62·13	77·58
12	60·67	68·46	57·42	68·63	57·75	71·08
13	54·33	61·08	51·67	62·08	52·79	64·46
14	47·58	53·88	45·21	56·08	44·92	55·42

TABLE 6.3

Gradient of sensitivity

		Filter settings			
		0·030	0·096	0·310	1·00
'No Drug'	Mean	26·00	52·63	68·88	81·58
	SD	10·90	7·10	2·54	5·84
Meprobamate	Mean	18·88	48·50	66·79	79·96
	SD	9·72	7·47	6·00	5·45
Doriden	Mean	19·88	48·50	65·33	80·33
	SD	10·65	7·66	5·21	4·96

The figures in the table are the means and standard deviations of the sample, and the three conditions, for the four target intensities. The increased variability of the measure at the lowest intensity is due to a small number of subjects who failed to see the target before the blind spot.

Variability of responses was assessed by separate analysis of variance for each measure and an outline of the analysis is presented in Tables 6.4. to 6.8. In all the measures there are large individual differences which result in significant variances attributable to *people*. These, of course, simply represent idiosyncratic differences in the magnitude of the variables measured and are not the main concern of the investigation. The most important variable is that attributable to the effect of the drugs and is designated in each case as *treatments*. Of secondary but some importance is the other source of variance presented in the outlines. This is due to the *orders* in which the treatments were administered.

An inspection of the analysis of the inner threshold scores shows

TABLE 6.4

Outline of analysis of variance
Standard perimetry—inner threshold

Source	d.f.	SS	m.s.v.	*F*	*p*
Main effects					
Between people	23	1335·04	58·05	10·13	1%
Between treatments	2	77·07	38·54	6·73	1%
Between orders	2	1·42	0·71		n.s.
Residual	44	251·96	5·73		
Total	71	1665·49			

t—ab = 3·319 1%
t—ac = 0·191 n.s.
t—bc = 3·128 1%

a = Doriden
b = No Drug
c = Meprobamate

TABLE 6.5

Outline of analysis of variance
Standard perimetry—outer threshold

Source	d.f.	SS	m.s.v.	*F*	*p*
Main effects					
Between people	23	1128·55	49·07	9·42	1%
Between treatments	2	67·33	33·67	6·46	1%
Between orders	2	11·55	5·78		
Residual	44	229·26	5·21		
Total	71	1436·69			

t—ab = 3·476 1%
t—ac = 0·729 n.s.
t—bc = 2·687 1%

TABLE 6.6

Outline of analysis of variance
Standard perimetry—mean threshold

Source	d.f.	SS	m.s.v.	*F*	*p*
Main effects					
Between people	23	1073·00	46·65	10·08	1%
Between treatments	2	5·61	2·81		n.s.
Between orders	2	3·57	1·79		n.s.
Residual	44	203·73	4·63		
Total	71	1285·91			

that the *treatments* variance is significant at the 1% level, and there is an insignificant variance attributable to *orders*. The same pattern is seen in the outer threshold analysis: *treatments* is highly significant but the order variance is not. A change in the pattern occurs when the mean threshold differences are examined. In this case none of the effects are significant. An insignificant treatment variance is, of course, to be expected of this measure because it is the product of the two divergent scores representing excitation and extinction. The fourth analysis outlines the *changes* in the differential threshold, designating the angular

TABLE 6.7

Outline of analysis of variance
Standard perimetry—difference threshold

Source	d.f.	SS	m.s.v.	*F*	*p*
Main effects					
Between people	23	403·13	17·53	8·39	1%
Between treatments	2	288·48	144·24	69·01	1%
Between orders	2	1·74	0·87		
Residual	44	92·07	2·09		
Total	71	785·42			

t—ab = 10·941 1%
t—ac = 1·766 n.s.
t—bc = 9·176 1%

differences between the outgoing and incoming stimuli. Again in this analysis a very large treatments variance is found, rejecting the null hypothesis at well beyond the 1% level, while the *orders* effect is insignificant. In the final analysis of variance the gradient differences (as defined above) indicate a significant treatment term which is the only one to emerge.

TABLE 6.8

Outline of analysis of variance
Standard perimetry—gradient of sensitivity

Source	d.f.	SS	m.s.v.	*F*	*p*
Main effects					
Between people	23	33,842·17	1471·40	9·34	1%
Between treatments	2	3368·08	1684·04	10·69	1%
Between orders	2	110·08	55·54		
Residual	44	6933·17	157·57		
Total	71	44,253·50			

t—ab = 3·923 1%
t—ac = 0·161 n.s.
t—bc = 4·084 1%

Discussion (field)

The results outlined in the preceding section demonstrate several important points: (*a*) that the field is affected by the drugs used; (*b*) that the effect is on the two processes of excitation and extinction which are the opposite poles of a basic gradient, or continuum of sensitivity; and (*c*) that if these two processes are considered together they cancel each other and have little measurable effect on the position of the common intensity isopter (see Fig. 6.1).

The most important of these findings are those represented under (*b*) and (*c*). They appear to be incompatible with each other and with the basic hypotheses advanced originally. That is to say, the action of the drugs appears to reduce both the excitatory value of the incoming target and, at the same time, increase it for an outgoing target. If the field is defined in terms of the inner limen, results indicate a clear-cut reduction in sensitivity. On the other hand, if they are defined by the

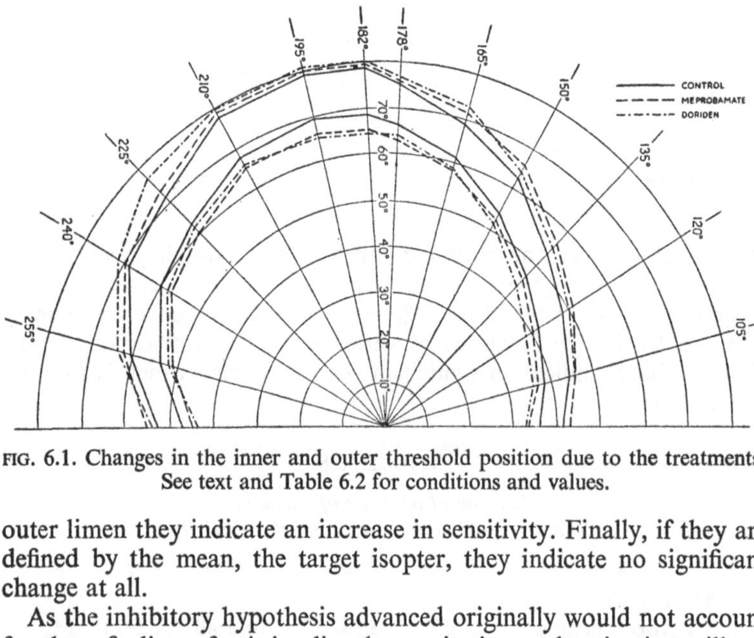

FIG. 6.1. Changes in the inner and outer threshold position due to the treatments. See text and Table 6.2 for conditions and values.

outer limen they indicate an increase in sensitivity. Finally, if they are defined by the mean, the target isopter, they indicate no significant change at all.

As the inhibitory hypothesis advanced originally would not account for these findings, for it implies that excitation and extinction will covary, any explanation must be *post hoc* and speculative. At least two, however, can reasonably be advanced. The first such explanation suggests that there is some change in the psychophysical scale, whereas the second postulates a general slowing of response, which, within the framework of the experimental procedure, gives a false picture of changed sensitivity.

It would be tempting to accept this second type of explanation, which involves the notion of some kind of mental or perceptual inertia, and to conclude by suggesting methods whereby experiments of a similar nature could control for such a possibility. However, to do so would ignore the fact that several other tests involving rapid responses have been administered to the same subjects and have failed to lend support to it. These tests included tasks such as tracking, reaction time, pursuit rotor performance, and auditory vigilance (see other sections of this report). Apart from these facts, the concept of mental inertia is a poor one in terms of explanatory value, suggesting little more than that the system is impaired from optimal efficiency, and delineates little but the conditions of its observation. The only support for this notion stems from the evidence that visual acuity can be increased by 'concentration' (Pirenne, 1957). The first hypothesis implies that there has been some change in the psychophysical scale such that under the drug conditions the sensory 'bits' which comprise it have changed, making it non-comparable with the control. Evidence from psychophysical experiments supports this notion in the demonstration of the non-linearity of JNDs and the applicability of the Weber fraction to only the middle range of intensity dimensions (Woodworth, 1939). Now if it is the case that $\Delta S/S$ is not an unvarying ratio but changes constantly in relation to S, the following question may be posed: Does the depressant effect of the drug reduce the sensory efficiency of the visual system and have the same, or a similar, sensory effect as a reduction in the light intensity of the target? If this question can be answered in the affirmative it leads to a conclusion which goes a little way towards rationalizing several of the results obtained in the investigation. For instance the reduced excitatory value of the constant target light under drug would lead to a larger difference limen; it would also, as a corollary, shift both the upper and lower thresholds, and exert an effect on the absolute threshold.[1]

Flicker perimetry

The critical flicker frequency (CFF) requires little, if any, description to the modern reader. As a psychophysiological phenomenon it has been defined rigorously in terms of its psychophysical as well as its photochemical and neurological components, and excellent and extensive reviews are available (Landis, 1953, 1954). (For peripheral flicker see Abney, 1897; Riddell, 1936; Ross, 1935, 1936a, 1936b, 1936c, 1938; Lloyd, 1952; Alpern, 1953; Hovener, 1954.) In psychology and physiology it has been used as a dependent variable in a great many experiments, and the literature is full of examples of its application. In the behavioural investigations of the influence of chemical agents (Psychopharmacology), particularly those which are thought to affect the brain mechanisms, it is believed to be one of the best developed and most sensitive tests available to the researcher. Indeed, it has been suggested that flicker might be used as a method of standardizing the depressant effects of somnifacient drugs (Landis, 1954). Many researchers, however, believe that caution is required in interpreting CFF as a measure

[1] In a private communication from Sharples to the author he reports that although he has never investigated this problem at photopic levels it is his belief that the difference between the inner and outer thresholds increases in relation to the target intensity.

of the excitatory balance of the CNS. Even the limited field of flicker in relation to drugs has a literature beyond the scope of this paper and it must suffice to say that barbiturates and similar compounds tend to *depress* CFF whereas the aphetamines and so-called stimulant drugs tend to *raise* it (Simonson, 1952; Roback, 1952; Idestrom, 1954). Contradictions do exist to this generalization, for instance caffeine, a stimulant, has been found to depress CFF and the effects of alcohol are still unclear. These contradictions are not surprising if the bi-phasic action of many drugs is taken into consideration. As for the flicker phenomenon itself, it is still uncertain whether the drugs affect the organism towards greater or lesser sensitivity to light or whether it changes some function of the light/dark ratio.

The present experiment is, of course, not an investigation of the flicker phenomenon as such. It is rather an investigation of the effects of two drugs in which CFF has been employed simply as a method of assessing the influence of the main independent variables. For this reason it is unnecessary to specify rigorously the psychophysical conditions, although they are dealt with in the section on the apparatus, and it is sufficient to say that they were kept constant throughout the experiment. (In fact it would probably be more accurate to designate the experimental method as a 'flicker situation'.)

Apparatus (peripheral flicker fusion)

The instrument used in this part of the experiment was a modified Lister moving arm type 315/466. This perimeter has its own illumination source for background and has targets of differing sizes and colours which are changeable. Modification to the instrument took the form of removing the normal target carrier and mounting in its place a small neon bulb type CV988. Placed at 290 mm. the bulb subtended an angle of 1·8 degrees. Flicker was provided by a pulse generator, and the neon activated through a finger key. Owing to the modification the bulb carrier could not be positioned nearer than 4 degrees from the centre spot but from this position to 90 degrees it was continuously variable along any meridian.

Method

The test was administered after the subjects had undergone the standard field perimetry test, the reason being that the Lister perimeter has no provision for the continuous inspection of the eye. It was thought that after some twenty minutes of practice, under supervision, of maintaining fixation on the Goldman perimeter the subjects would be better able to obey the instruction to keep their eyes on the centre. After the subject had been fitted into the apparatus a demonstration was given of both ascending and descending thresholds at the 10-degree position on the 90-degree meridian, as were practice trials. These practice trials were the only way in which the routine differed from day to day. In all fourteen different positions were assessed for CFF from flicker to fusion and fusion to flicker, on the 45-degree and 135-degree meridian at 10, 25, 50, and 60 degrees pa. and along the 90-degree meridian at 10, 30, 45, 60, 70 and 80 degrees pa., all three co-ordinates being in the left temporal field. The method of limits was employed and in the successive 'bursts' of light none was longer than three seconds with a three-second interval between them. Both time intervals were assessed subjectively and were therefore approximate. The frequency was changed in one-cycle steps, during the 'off' periods.

Results (flicker fusion threshold)

The results of testing are presented in Table 6.9, which outlines the mean CFF scores for the treatment groups at the several retinal positions measured. The actual mean values for the fourteen points are shown in Figs. 6.2 to 6.4.

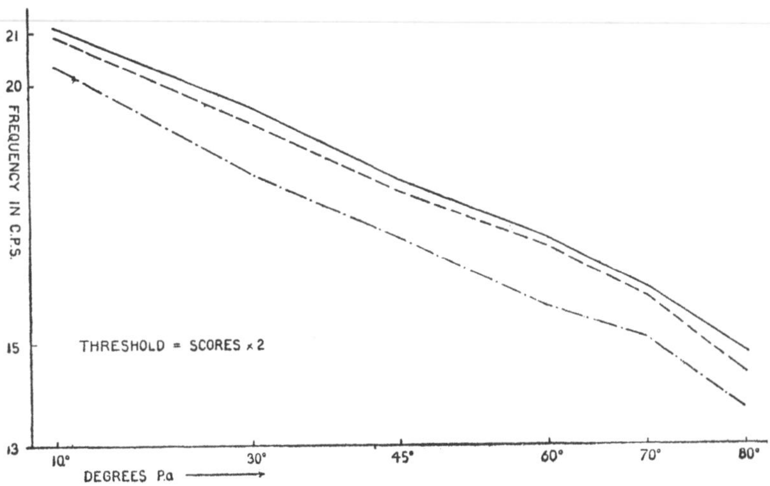

FIG. 6.2. Threshold changes in flicker along the 90° left temporal meridian for the three treatments.

———— Control - - - - - - - - - Meprobamate -·-·-·-·-·-·- Doriden

Three analyses of variance were conducted on the scores and their outlines presented in Tables 6.10 to 6.12. Each score is composed of the mean of the four and six threshold frequencies along the meridian explored. The same general pattern is seen in all of them; significant *F*-ratios being derived for both individual differences and for treatment effects. None of the analyses are complicated by order effects. Examination of the critical ratios (which are appended to the analysis of variance outlines) indicates a rather different pattern from that seen in the

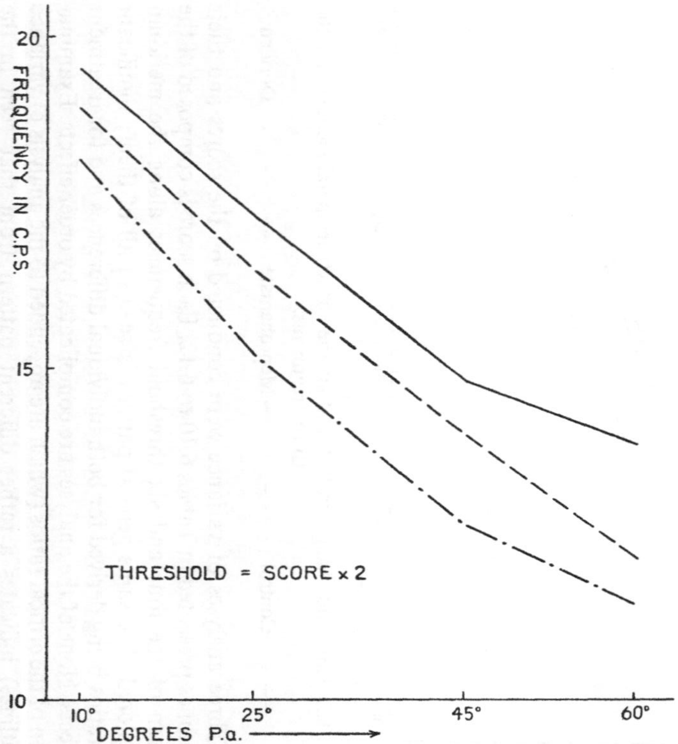

FIG. 6.3. Threshold changes in flicker along the 45° left temporal meridian for the three treatments.

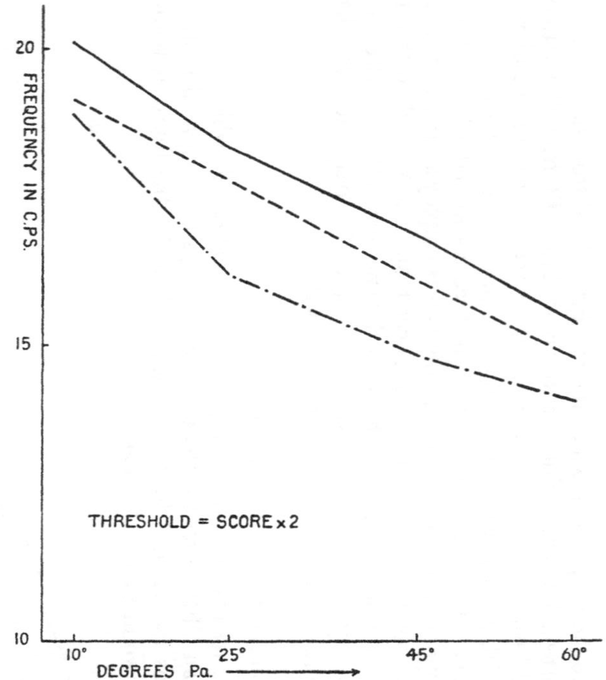

FIG. 6.4. Threshold changes in flicker along the 135° left temporal meridian for the three treatments.

——— Control - - - - - - - - Meprobamate -·-·-·-·-·-· Doriden

TABLE 6.9

Horizontal flicker

TRIAL MEANS /2

	1	2	3	4	5	6
No Drug	21·22	19·55	18·16	17·01	16·12	14·81
Meprobamate	20·97	19·33	17·94	16·90	15·94	14·46
Doriden	20·46	18·31	17·10	15·69	15·19	13·69
135-*degree meridian*						
No Drug	20·06	18·40	16·98	15·44		
Meprobamate	19·15	17·73	16·10	14·98		
Doriden	18·90	16·23	14·81	14·08		
45-*degree meridian*						
No Drug	19·54	17·40	14·88	13·90		
Meprobamate	18·77	16·50	14·02	12·27		
Doriden	18·19	15·52	12·69	11·54		

TABLE 6.10

Outline of analysis of variance
Left temporal field 90-degree meridian

Source	d.f.	SS	m.s.v.	*F*	
Main effects					
Between people	23	3112·82	135·34	2·70	1%
Between treatments	2	536·39	268·20	5·36	1%
Between orders	2	135·22	67·61	1·35	n.s.
Residual	44	2202·06	50·05		
Total	71	5986·49			

t—ab = 3·123 1%   *a* = Doriden
t—ac = 2·519 5%   *b* = No Drug
t—bc = 0·603   *c* = Meprobamate

TABLE 6.11

Outline of analysis of variance
Left temporal field 45-degree meridian

Source	d.f.	SS	m.s.v.	*F*	*p*
Main effects					
Between people	23	2563·11	111·44	3·83	1%
Between treatments	2	733·34	366·67	12·61	1%
Between orders	2	125·84	62·92	2·16	n.s.
Residual	44	1279·15	29·07		
Total	71	4701·44			

t—ab = 4·859 1%
t—ac = 2·262 5%
t—bc = 2·596 5%

preceding experiments. In flicker fusion the differences between Doriden and control and Doriden and Meprobamate are significant in all instances. The differences between meprobamate and control are lower but significant in two cases at the 5% level.

TABLE 6.12

Outline of analysis of variance of scores
Left temporal field 135-degree meridian

Source	d.f.	SS	m.s.v.	F	p
Main effects					
Between people	23	2310·25	100·50	3·98	1%
Between treatments	2	567·93	283·97	11·26	1%
Between orders	2	49·84	24·92		
Residual	44	1110·23	25·23		
Total	71	4038·25			

t—ab = 4·845 1%
t—ac = 2·519 5%
t—bc = 2·326 5%

Discussion (flicker)

The results presented in the preceding section on flicker give rise to several points of interest. They indicate, for instance, that both meprobamate and Doriden depress the CFF threshold. The graphs in Figs. 6.2, 6.3, and 6.4 demonstrate that any depression is fairly uniform along the sensitivity gradient from the centre to the periphery (within the positions measured). Finally they show that the order in which the drugs are administered has no effect on scores.

The overall depression of CFF is to be expected. Both agents have a depressive action as a general feature in addition to their specific effects. The sedative action of Doriden has been outlined in several of the publications alluded to in previous sections; indeed it is described as acting like a barbiturate though having fewer side effects. If this is the case the findings of this investigation are accountable, being consistent with other studies (Simonson, 1952). As pointed out earlier, meprobamate is not as uncomplicated. Its main sites of action appear to be subcortical, particularly in the thalamus, and its cortical effects are reported as being minimal in average doses (Berger, 1956). Nevertheless, its side effects are such that they may well produce the same changes as a straight-forward depressant such as a barbiturate. Another complication with meprobamate lies in its association with anxiety reduction (Dickel, 1957). High anxiety is one of the factors which leads to a reduced CFF threshold (Goldstone, 1955), and while the depressive action of the drug would tend to lower the threshold the anxiety-reducing component should tend to raise it.

The third interesting feature of the findings lies in the apparent uniformity of depression at the different positions tested on the peripheral retina. This is a finding which seems to obviate the possibility of the drugs acting differentially on the photochemical elements involved. Apart from these elements the locus of action of the drugs could be sited in either retina, optic tract, or visual cortex. Any closer specification of the site of action would, for this experiment, be arbitrary.

Finally, the lack of order effects in the analysis indicates the non-existence of practice effects, or the carrying over of any effects from day to day.

Static ataxia

Static ataxia, or body sway when attempting to maintain the body erect, has been known and used clinically for over a hundred years. Its main value has been as a diagnostic sign due to its association with several neurological diseases such as *tabes dorsalis*, chorea, cerebro-arteriosclerosis, and various cerebellar conditions. Apart from these morbid states, *ataxia* is known to be affected by both physical and psychological conditions; fatigue, attention, position of the feet, age, deafness, suggestion and blindness (Eysenck, 1947; Ingham, 1954; Skillicorn, 1955; Edwards, 1942, 1946; Miles, 1922; Killam, 1957). It is also known to be influenced by several chemical compounds including ether, alcohol, pentobarbital, and sodium amytal (Skillicorn, 1955). In the present investigation an attempt has been made to determine the affect of two new agents on the function, Doriden and meprobamate.[1]

Apparatus (static ataxia)

The apparatus for measuring body sway and the technique of administration have been described in detail elsewhere (Ingham, 1954). Briefly, a thread was pinned to the subject at neck level. The thread carried small riders which were displaced from a central position in front of a graduated scale. The test period was one minute during which the subject stood with eyes closed and with heels and toes together, or as near together as was consistent with comfort. The degree of sway was taken as the total displacement of the riders, both forwards and backwards, during the one-minute period. Due to the late introduction of this measure in the test battery only fifteen of the twenty-four subjects of the other experiments were included in the analysis. There may be some slight error in the measurements due to differences in height of subjects.

Results (ataxia)

The mean body sway of the group increased markedly under the drug

[1] Since beginning the investigation the author has become aware of the meprobamate habituation study by Haizlip and Ewing (1958) who found that high dosages (3·2 gm. and 6·4 gm.), in a group of forty-seven patients, led to some 75% of them showing 'staggering gait' or 'inability to walk or stand'.

conditions, but the test failed to discriminate Doriden from mepro-bamate. Values for the treatment groups were as follows: 'No Drug': 1·30″, SD = 0·56″; Meprobamate: 2·12″, SD = 0·96; Doriden: 2·15″, SD = 0·87.

The overall significance of the change from condition to condition was assessed by analysis of variance, the outline of which is presented in Table 6.13. Both *F*-ratios are highly significant at beyond the 1% level of confidence, demonstrating large individual differences and changes due to the treatment effect.

A breakdown of the treatment variance shows *t*-values: 'No Drug'/Meprobamate = 5·529, $p = 1\%$; 'No Drug'/Doriden = 5·732, $p = 1\%$; there was no significant difference between Meprobamate and Doriden.

TABLE 6.13

Outline of analysis of variance
Static ataxia—total body sway

Source	d.f.	SS	m.s.v.	*F*	*p*
Main effects					
Between people	14	25·1027	1·7931	10·84	1%
Between groups	2	6·9528	3·4764	21·02	1%
Residual	28	4·6306	0·1654		
Total	44	36·6861			
t—ab = 5·732 1%					
t—ac = 0·203 n.s.					
t—bc = 5·529 1%					

Discussion (*ataxia*)

The results obtained on static ataxia are of interest from at least two viewpoints: (*a*) there is a small but highly significant change in *ataxia* due to the action of the drugs; and (*b*) the results are consistent with the inhibitory hypothesis. The fact of increased body sway is of importance for several reasons. In the first place it tends to support and confirm, at the human level, studies which have demonstrated impaired balance in animals. With humans at the dosage levels given the impairment under drug is not great, as an inspection of the means will show. Using the control data as the baseline for assessing impairment, sway is increased only by 0·82″ under meprobamate, and by 0·85″ under Doriden. Nevertheless, these proportions represent percentage increases in the order of 60%. The increases are important also when considered in relation to the attitudes of the subjects. Almost all the subjects under Doriden reported feeling muzzy, tired, and to greater and lesser degrees, slightly impaired—and they were. On the other hand, none of the meprobamate subjects felt any deleterious effects of the drug. They did not feel impaired—but were. (Indeed, two subjects fell outright under meprobamate and one under Doriden.) This finding is thought to represent one of the inherent dangers of the tranquillizing group, in that there may be impairment without awareness; until such minimal impairments are known it should be retained for controlled situations only.

Another feature of the results is their support of the initial hypothesis of increased inhibition of the central mechanisms. Although the term 'central inhibition' has tended to be interpreted as cortical inhibition, this is arbitrary and probably springs from the relative freeness of the cortex from gross autonomic complication. Because the sites of action of the two drugs used in the present study have not been clearly delineated it is probably safer to interpret 'central' as implying 'brain' or 'total CNS'.

Some correlational aspects of the investigation

The theory presented in the introduction has outlined the relationship between inhibition and extraversion, and the probably autonomic basis of neuroticism. On these grounds, despite the fact that it is an optimistic venture with such small numbers, it was considered worth while to examine the correlational aspects of the measures taken in relation to criterion measures of both extraversion and neuroticism derived from the Maudsley Personality Inventory (Eysenck, 1957; Jensen, 1958). For obvious reasons the questionnaire was administered on the control day and, therefore, the correlations are between the personality measures and the test measures taken on that day.

The results of the first examination are presented in Table 6.14, and shows the correlations between test and questionnaire variables. None of the coefficients achieve significance and it is consequently meaningless to discuss their relevance to the extraversion theory or the drug postulate.

TABLE 6.14

Table of correlations showing correlation of test scores with extraversion and neuroticism

	Extraversion	Neuroticism
Flicker 45	0·148	0·095
Flicker 90	0·300	0·187
Flicker 135	0·122	0·079
Gradient	0·046	0·235
Outer threshold	0·001	−0·157
Inner threshold	0·036	0·220
Differential threshold	−0·092	−0·146

5% = 0·404
1% = 0·515

The second examination was of the intercorrelation of derived scores and their factorial analysis. As the most profound change in test measures occurred in the differences between the 'No Drug' and the Doriden treatments, a series of scores was derived which reflected this

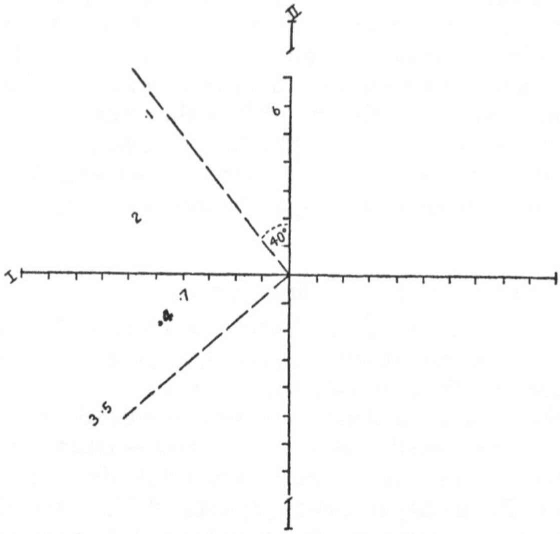

FIG. 6.5. First and second factors, showing also the possible rotation to simple structure.

effect. The matrix of correlations of these scores is presented in Table 6.15. A Thurstone Centroid Analysis of this matrix revealed two factors which have been identified as 'drug effect' and a bipolar factor which

TABLE 6.15

Correlation matrix of change scores

	1	2	3	4	5	6	7
1. Inner threshold		0·434	0·205	0·184	0·229	0·521	0·044
2. Differential threshold			0·297	0·298	0·340	0·158	0·211
3. Flicker 135				0·516	0·806	−0·167	0·447
4. Flicker 45					0·524	−0·120	0·125
5. Flicker 90						−0·253	0·357
6. Gradient							−0·128
7. Extraversion							

5% = 0·404
1% = 0·515

opposes the two tests to each other. The factors obtained (I, II) can be rotated to simple structure as shown in Fig. 6.5 and Table 6.16 (I′, II′), and when this is done the factors are clearly seen as drug effect on the flicker measures and drug effect on the perimetry measures. Extraversion score, the independent assessment of personality, by means of the MPI scale, has a small loading on both rotated factors, the higher being on factor two which is composed of the flicker scores. The initial and rotated factor loadings are presented in Table 6.16. Results suggest a greater drug effect on extraverts in both tests and all measures used.

TABLE 6.16

Tests	I	II	I′	II′	h^2
1. Inner threshold	0·535	0·587	0·794	−0·032	0·6308
2. Differential threshold	0·583	0·191	0·521	−0·324	0·3764
3. Flicker 135	0·748	−0·528	0·077	−0·912	0·8383
4. Flicker 45	0·499	−0·190	0·175	−0·504	0·2851
5. Flicker 90	0·701	−0·482	0·082	−0·847	0·7237
6. Gradient	0·077	0·575	0·490	0·311	0·3366
7. MPI (E)	0·418	−0·091	0·338	−0·262	0·1830

Summary and conclusions

The present investigation has been performed in order to examine the compounds meprobamate and Doriden from two viewpoints: the empirical and the rational. The former examination has been based upon the proposition that the two agents differ in their chemical structure but that their behavioural differences remain obscure. The rational examination has been based upon the established relationship between personality and drug action which has been formally stated as the extraversion/drug hypothesis. Although, in the main, the drug hypothesis advanced by Eysenck has been formulated on differences existing in the performance of chemically 'depressed' and 'stimulated' subjects, it has relevance in the present study because of the basically 'depressive' characteristics of both the tranquillizer and the hypnotic, which, by hypothesis, would be expected to increase cortical inhibition and decrease excitation, thereby changing task performance of those functions dependent upon them.

On the empirical level both drugs have effects on all the tests given. The effect can probably best be generalized as a slight but significant impairment of discrimination. This is exemplified by the increase in the interval of uncertainty on the peripheral field measure, the decrease in CFF, and the increase in *static ataxia*, under the drug treatments. The results are not all in accordance with the generalization of impaired discrimination. No explanation can be advanced for the apparent increase in the visual field under drug when it is plotted from the centre to the periphery, unless a concentration type hypothesis is accepted which appears unlikely if the evidence of other results is considered.

On the rational level the results are generally in accord with the predictions made of them from the extraversion/drug hypothesis,[1] but the simple extraversion hypothesis of poorer discrimination being related to the questionnaire measure taken on the 'No Drug' is not supported. No support was found for the proposition that changes from the control day to the Doriden treatment day (the most profound change) would demonstrate a common single feature.

Perhaps the most interesting finding of the study has been the general failure to demonstrate significant differences between the two drug conditions on the measures taken. (With the exception of flicker fusion.) A clue to this failure is found in the analysis of drug effects conducted by S. B. G. and H. J. Eysenck in Chapter 10. They were able to extract only one significant latent root from their examination of scores from several of the measures in these reports. This finding indicates that for statistical and functional purposes the drugs can be assumed to act along a single dimension of effect and may be treated as variations of the same thing (a 'depressive') as far as molar behavioural changes are concerned.

Although the general tendency is for meprobamate to have less of an effect than Doriden a danger exists in interpreting the degree of functional impairment by the mood of the subject. Both the scores on the experimental variables and the opinion of the author coincide at this point. Few of the subjects failed to report subjective effects following the ingestion of the hypnotic, particularly in the afternoons after the second dose, whereas some of them reported feeling better than usual after taking the tranquillizer. The fact that they were impaired under both drugs indicates that the so-called 'clinical picture' which may be assessed in part from what the patient may say of himself is not a reliable guide to adequacy of performance.

[1] The author has carefully examined three other hypotheses which might be considered applicable to the present investigation. These have been based upon the notions of 'filter factor', noise to signal ratio, and hysteresis. Although the first two offer a somewhat clearer explanation of the peripheral elements involved in the functions measured by the present study they cannot be considered at the present stage as being better than a straightforward inhibition hypothesis. It is likely that they are special cases of a general concept of inhibition permitting a clearer operational definition in specific instances. Cf. Barlow (1957), Stevens (1957, Pirenne (1957), Granger (1959a), (1959b).

7

THE EFFECTS OF DEPRESSANT DRUGS ON VIGILANCE AND PSYCHOMOTOR PERFORMANCE

Emer Treadwell

INTRODUCTION

IT is impossible to predict the psychological effects of a drug with any certainty from a knowledge of its chemical constitution alone, despite the increasing success with which new drugs, designed to meet the needs of psychiatric drug therapy, have been synthesized, especially in the past ten or fifteen years. A very slight variation in molecular structure may completely alter the action of a compound. For instance, two drugs which have identical composition and only a slight difference in structure are Frenquel, an ataractic drug which antagonizes stimulants, and Meratran, an isomer of Frenquel which is however a central stimulant.

Of more immediate importance to the experimental psychologist, however, are the truly enormous variations in the reactions of different individuals to the same drug, and the complexity of the effects of a single drug on the same individual. The first of these two problems makes it imperative to include an assessment of subjects' personalities in any drug investigation (or at least of those aspects of the personality which are believed, on theoretical grounds, to be particularly relevant).

There are many different aspects of the second problem, but the psychologist is chiefly concerned with three manipulable variables which affect it. These are dosage, nature of the tests used, and time (more specifically, the period between administration of the drug and the beginning of testing, and the length of time required for completion of the test).

With regard to dosage it need only be noted here that in a wide range of drugs the relationship between dosage and effect has been found not to be monotonic. Amphetamine in small doses improves performance on a number of associative and other tests, whereas large doses may impair performance on the same tests. However, it is obvious that variations in test results due to a variation in dosage will not usually lead the experimenter to false conclusions about the effects of the drug.

Problems related to the nature of the tests used are more complicated. The meaning of a score on a simple reaction-time test may be interpreted with considerably more confidence than one on a complex reasoning task, while on the other hand the practical (if not the theoretical) value of tests used in the assessment of drug effects has a tendency to vary inversely with the simplicity of the test. Complex tasks therefore cannot be excluded from drug investigations, and of course even seemingly simple tasks may have quite complex factorial structures as the factor analytic studies of Fleishman (1954) and others have shown.

In this context the degree of complexity of drug effects must also be taken into account. The body of established fact concerning the site or sites of action of the various psychotherapeutic drugs is small compared with the great edifice of speculation which has been erected on this still inadequate foundation. What evidence there is suggests that a single drug has not one but a considerable number of effects in different parts of the nervous system, and some of these may be masked or overlaid by others. For example Gottleib (1951) argues that amylobarbitone has a stimulant effect on the central nervous system, which is however masked by the hypnotic effect, and Domino, Fox, and Brody (1955) point out the difficulties of classifying the actions of barbiturates into stimulants and depressants, especially on the basis of 'gross observation'.

These considerations ought to play an important part at the various stages of any project designed to investigate the psychological effects of a drug, but especially in the selection of tests to be used, and in the analysis of test results. Trouton and Eysenck (1960) argue convincingly that tests should be chosen which can be expected, on theoretical grounds, to show differential effects under different drug conditions, and in the investigation to be reported below, the selection of tests was guided, as far as possible, by Eysenck's hypothesis relating depressant drugs to cortical inhibition and the personality dimension extraversion-introversion. The preceding discussion underlines the importance of using tests whose factorial structure and characteristics are already known. It also suggests that the inclusion of tests with moderate amounts of overlapping variance is useful since this facilitates attempts to sort out test factors which are affected by a particular drug or drugs from those which remain unmodified.

The third variable specified above, viz. time, is of especial importance when drugs are administered orally, in the form of pills, as in the present investigation. When taken in this form the drug is absorbed at a much slower rate than it would be if injected directly into the bloodstream, and the body is presented with a *slowly* increasing concentration of the drug. This makes it more likely that qualitative as well as quantitative behavioural changes will occur in the period following the administration of the drug, since different parts of the central and autonomic nervous systems require different minimal concentrations of a given drug before they can be affected. (These qualitative changes may fail to appear altogether when drugs are administered by intravenous injection, which causes the 'main' effect of the drug to occur much more rapidly.) Such changes, being a function of time, must be taken into account in conjunction with the evidence (Fleishman, 1956) that the factorial structure of tests also varies both quantitatively and qualitatively through time, i.e. as a function of practice which is extended in time. In the present investigation, as in all other similar studies, the contribution to total test variance of this variation in drug action over a period of time is unknown, although we attempted to minimize its effect by allowing 40 minutes to elapse between administration of the drug and the beginning of testing, and by placing the longest of the tests last in the order of test administration.

General framework and aims of the investigation

Doriden (glutethimide) is a hypnotic and belongs therefore to the category of central depressants, whereas meprobamate is classified as a 'tranquillizer'. Much has already been written about the difficulties involved in arriving at a psychologically meaningful classification of the psychotropic drugs, and it is generally agreed that current classifications are, at best, provisional. Many workers in the field of psychopharmacology have preferred to ignore these classifications entirely, the connotations of the various labels being as imprecise as they are, and have proceeded instead by making an 'unbiased', i.e. random, choice of drugs whose effects are then studied on a random group of subjects by the application of psychological tests selected equally fortuitously. Trouton and Eysenck (1960) strongly criticize this 'blunderbuss' approach and suggest that a more fruitful alternative is the factorial or dimensional approach.

The present investigation which is concerned with the effects of Doriden and meprobamate on psychomotor performance and on vigilance is an illustration of the latter method of procedure, although for reasons which will become apparent in the succeeding discussion it does not fulfil all the rigorous requirements specified by Eysenck (1957b). Briefly, the dimensional approach requires the administration of a battery or batteries of tests which define meaningful and experimentally demonstrated factors within a precise theoretical framework which is appropriate to the nature of the drugs under consideration.

The theoretical framework for the present study was provided by Eysenck's postulate of drug action in so far as it relates to depressant drugs. This states that: 'Depressant drugs increase cortical inhibition, decrease cortical excitation and thereby produce extraverted behaviour patterns' (Eysenck, 1957b). The appropriateness of the postulate may require some justification, since meprobamate has been described as a tranquillizer rather than a central depressant. At the present stage of knowledge, however, there is little or no basis for drawing any sharp line of demarcation between 'depressants' and 'tranquillizers'.

There are sufficient indications in the literature to suggest that meprobamate, at least in high doses, will act to produce similar effects at the behavioural level to those which would be expected from a central depressant like Doriden. For instance Berger *et al.* (1957) report that in large doses meprobamate antagonizes the stimulants, and that at the same dosage EEG recordings show slowing and spindling at sub-cortical and cortical levels. More direct evidence comes from a study by Reitman (1957). After the administration of larger than clinically recommended doses of meprobamate a group of normal subjects performed significantly worse on a number of psychological tests than they had done under a placebo condition. The tests were selected from Halstead's battery of diagnostic tests of brain damage (Halstead, 1947). This finding gives direct support, on the psychological level, to the suggestion that meprobamate can have central depressant effects, since it is commonly observed that brain damage causes an increase in extraversion and it has been shown that the effects of depressant drugs are similar to the effects of brain damage as far as objective psychological tests are concerned (Eysenck, 1957a). It must be emphasized, however, that all these effects of meprobamate occurred only when doses considerably higher than those normally used clinically were administered, whereas in the present study the dose administered was the standard 800 mg.

The distinction does nevertheless indicate an important difference in the therapeutic roles of the two drugs. Doriden is prescribed clinically in circumstances where it is appropriate that the patient should actually go to sleep, while meprobamate is designed for the ambulant 'patient' who is carrying on his normal day-to-day activities, as is indicated by its description as 'a day-time relaxant'. Therefore, the inclusion of the latter drug in the investigation necessarily had a modifying influence on the choice of tests, since theoretical considerations had to be balanced against the need for gaining information directly relevant to practical problems. The type of practical question to be answered was whether an 800 mg. dose of meprobamate (the normal clinical dose) would cause decrements in performance of a kind and magnitude which would make unsafe the pursuit of such potentially dangerous daily activities as driving a car, and other activities where adequate performance depends upon the maintenance of a high level of alertness together with good psychomotor co-ordination.

The selection of tests. A rigorous application of the dimensional method would have permitted the inclusion only of tests defining experimentally demonstrated factors which were meaningful and relevant within the terms of the drug postulate stated above. However, as already explained this criterion had to be modified in view of the somewhat indeterminate status of meprobamate relative to the category of central depressants; but also because this drug raised additional problems of practical and theoretical interest which lay outside the strict limits of cortical inhibition theory. The final selection of tests represents the best compromise that could be effected within the limits of the testing time available, between the demand for data which would be maximally relevant within the framework of the drug postulate, and the equally important demand that information about other possible aspects of the drugs should not thereby be overlooked. Since this approach to test selection diverges from that advocated by Eysenck (1957a) and would probably not receive his full support, the reasons for adopting it here require some further discussion.

Briefly, the divergence does not spring from disagreement with the principles of dimensional analysis, but rather represents a difference in estimation of the extent to which these principles can usefully be applied in the present instance. Critics of the dimensional approach seem to be correct in pointing out (*a*) that the number of tests at present available which adequately fit the specifications laid down by Eysenck is relatively very small (and in any case too small to supply all the immediate practical information required by practitioners who want to use new drugs therapeutically); and (*b*) that in view of the multiplicity and variety of effects which a single drug may have (depending on physical and psychological factors not all of which are even identifiable), any hypothesis linking a class of drugs or drug effects to a dimension of personality will probably be crude and oversimplified at best, and at worst completely erroneous.

With respect to the first of these criticisms it must be stated that although considerations of practical utility led to the inclusion of some tests in the present investigation whose factor structure is not yet sufficiently understood, it was recognized that, by doing so, the task of interpreting the results was being made more difficult. At a sufficiently advanced stage of knowledge there will cease to be any conflict between the claims of practical applicability and theoretical relevance of results, but this stage has not been reached yet, and in this study we therefore took the calculated risk of attempting to satisfy both claims partially.

The second criticism has been formulated by Eysenck himself (Trouton and Eysenck, 1960), but its force varies according to the amount of knowledge available about any particular drug in which we may be interested. It is particularly applicable to the present investigation, in view of the fact that both Doriden and meprobamate are new drugs whose pharmacology is still in the process of being explored. On the other hand, it is precisely because of such gaps and uncertainties in available knowledge that the dimensional approach is potentially so useful. Provided that positive results are interpreted with the caution they deserve, and that where deductions fail to be verified the opportunity is taken to explore the reasons for this failure, then it becomes possible, by this method, to make inductive leaps with safety, since the method when properly applied is self-correcting and self-modifying.

To summarize, there are still large gaps in our knowledge of the factorial structure of the tests we employ, as well as in knowledge about the sites and modes of action even of well-established drugs, but particularly of new drugs like Doriden and meprobamate. Therefore it may not be unduly pessimistic to expect that one of the most useful results from an investigation like the present one will be a more precise identification of the areas of ignorance which most urgently require further study.

EXPERIMENTAL PROCEDURE AND TESTING SCHEDULE

Full details of the experimental design, the administration of drugs, and the subjects (Ss) who participated in the experiment have been given by Willett in an earlier chapter and will not be repeated here. The tests which were used will be described and discussed in the next section.

All twenty-four Ss performed the four psychomotor tests in the same order on each of the three experimental days. Testing was begun approximately 40 minutes after administration of the appropriate drug on the two drug days and approximately 15 minutes after S arrived in the laboratory on the no-drug day. Half the Ss were tested in the morning and half in the afternoon, but each S completed all four tests in the course of a single morning or afternoon session.

The testing session began with 5 minutes of massed practice on the pursuit rotor. During the 10-minute 'rest' pause before the second period of rotary pursuit practice, Ss were given three 2-minute trials on the triple tester, separated by 1-minute rest pauses. The second period of massed practice on the pursuit rotor was begun exactly 10 minutes after the end of the first practice period and lasted for 5 minutes. A further 5-minute rest pause then ensued before the hand steadiness test was begun. Ss had four hand steadiness trials separated by 10-second rest pauses. The auditory vigilance test was administered $1\frac{1}{4}$ hours after completion of the psychomotor tests and lasted for 32 minutes.

The same test order and, within fairly narrow limits, the same daily timetable was maintained for all Ss under all experimental treatments. The adherence to a strict test order was dictated by a variety of methodological considerations too well known to require discussion, and although this procedure possibly imposes some limitation on the 'generalizability' of the results, it was essential to ensure that any pro-active and retro-active effects between tests should not contribute to the between-subjects variance.

DETAILS AND DISCUSSION OF THE INDIVIDUAL TESTS

Auditory vigilance test

Vigilance is a necessary component of all good psychomotor performance, and it is interesting to note that most of the experimental work on this subject has been stimulated directly by the need to solve important practical problems, as for example the prevention of industrial accidents, and the raising of workers' productivity in the factory without endangering the quality of the products. However, since vigilance is only one of an interacting complex of factors determining the level of psychomotor performance it cannot be studied directly in psychomotor tests.

It is difficult to devise a measure which is both accurate and valid, since vigilance is known to be affected by such factors as level and variety of test stimulation (Baker, 1956; Deese, 1955); environmental conditions (Broadbent, 1953; Frazer, 1953); and motivational fluctuations from whatever cause, including knowledge of results (Mackworth, 1950). In other words the tools used to measure the phenomenon may also alter it. The problem is most acute when the primary interest is in momentary fluctuations in vigilance rather than in the grosser changes which occur over relatively long periods. It has been suggested by Mackworth (1957) that these two kinds of vigilance decrement are interdependent, and are related in the same way as the degree of massing or spacing of practice on learning and performance tasks is related to the final level of efficiency reached within a given time. However, there are reasons for doubting whether the analogy is as close as this, and these reasons will be discussed later in the section. For the moment it is sufficient to note that we have no direct knowledge of the relationship between the two, for the important reason that there is no satisfactory technique for obtaining a continuous record of vigilance. A large number of inspection tasks presenting Ss with a rapidly succeeding series of signals have been used, and have shown that vigilance improves as the rate and number of signals increases. They have also revealed wide individual variations in the frequency with which momentary drops in efficiency occur. The data from these tests help to define the problem, although this type of task is itself unsuitable for answering the questions posed in the present investigation: e.g. how frequent, and serious, are the drops in vigilance which occur in the not uncommon everyday situation where signals appear at relatively long and irregular intervals, and how will the normal level of efficiency in this situation be affected by depressant drugs?

It follows from what has just been discussed that the most satisfactory way of obtaining the estimates of vigilance we require is to use a task in which signals occur infrequently and at irregular intervals; in which the response required from S is simple and does not involve the learning of a new skill; in which knowledge of results is minimal; and in which the test situation does not artificially either increase or diminish the environmental supports to the maintenance of vigilance which are normally present in a real-life situation. (The last requirement argues against administering the test in a completely soundproof room, for example.) One of the main, but unavoidable, disadvantages of this method is that for comparatively long periods of the test time we do not know what the vigilance level is. Momentary drops are probably occurring which in a real-life situation may or may not have serious consequences, depending on chance factors. However, the disadvantage from a purely practical point of view is comparatively easily overcome. By increasing the number of Ss tested we can increase the accuracy of the quantitative estimates of the effects produced by the various drugs under investigation, because the fluctuations in vigilance are uncorrelated in time between individuals.

Description of the test

The stimulus material consisted of a tape-recording of a random series of digits, which were read out at a constant rate of one per second. Interspersed at irregular intervals in this regular sound sequence were a number of signals, a signal being defined as three successive odd digits. The frequency with which signals occurred was approximately six every 5 minutes, the time interval between signals ranging from 3 seconds to 1 minute 41 seconds with a mean interval of 58 seconds. The test proper lasted for 30 minutes and was preceded by a 2-minute practice period which was included to ensure that all Ss understood the instructions. In the instructions, which were pre-recorded on the test tape, Ss were told to respond to every signal, as soon as it occurred, by tapping the table-top once with a pencil. They were warned that a signal might occur at any time and that it was therefore necessary to pay close attention throughout the test. The test score was the number of signals missed and this was computed separately for each 5-minute period.

This auditory vigilance test is a shorter and simpler version of a test designed and used by Bakan (1959) in an experimental study of the relationship between extraversion-introversion and vigilance. Before discussing his results, which are of great theoretical interest in the present context, it will be useful to attempt a theoretical analysis of the processes involved in vigilance test behaviour.

Analysis of vigilance test behaviour

In the test described above S is presented with a regular series of auditory stimuli which are physically very little differentiated from one another. He differentiates them by following the test instructions which require him (*a*) to identify each succeeding stimulus as an odd or an even number and (*b*) when the number is odd to recall the identity of the two preceding stimuli. Thus, as long as S is obeying the test instructions each stimulus, whether it forms part of a signal or not, contributes an increment of reactive inhibition (I_R). S's behaviour may be envisaged as a kind of hunting behaviour, the goal of which is the detection of signals. Every time a signal is detected reinforcement therefore occurs. However, the effect of this reinforcement is not clear. The habit of attending is already well established in S's repertoire when the test begins, and no further increments of $_SH_R$ will be added to it by these reinforcements. The only 'learning' that can possibly be initiated is the formulation of hypotheses about the occurrence of further signals, but these hypotheses will not be reinforced, and cannot improve performance, since the signals are distributed at random in the display series and S has already been given this information in the instructions.

The role of the reinforcements is almost certainly one of preventing or delaying the extinction of the attending response, and it must be noted that they occur in an irregular pattern (partial reinforcement) which is known to be particularly effective in preventing extinction. The processes which occur when an already asymptotic habit receives further reinforcements and the reasons for the effectiveness of partial reinforcement schedules are both highly controversial subjects, and it would be unprofitable to try to analyse these features of the vigilance test any further in the present context.

The only one of the test processes therefore which seemed clear-cut enough to form a basis for the formulation of expectations about the effects of depressant drugs on test performance was the build-up of I_R already mentioned. The analysis of this factor can now be taken further.

I_R will increase to the point where it is equal in strength to the positive drive (D) when a rest pause will occur. During the rest I_R is dissipated and conditioned inhibition ($_SI_R$) is formed. The taking of a rest means that S is no longer making the necessary discrimination between successive stimuli, i.e. the stimuli become dedifferentiated and signals occurring during this period will therefore not be detected. The more signals missed the less reinforcements there are and therefore the faster the process of extinction of the attending response.

This feature of vigilance test behaviour represents an important difference between the typically passive vigilance task and a psychomotor task, which is always more active. The difference lies essentially in the amount of sensory feedback which the task can provide to indicate when S is failing (one aspect of knowledge of results) For example, when S's performance on the pursuit rotor worsens because he is forced to take an involuntary rest pause, the pattern of sensory feedback from his own movements changes, and this probably helps to curtail the length of the pause by causing disinhibition. In the vigilance task, on the other hand, a rest pause tends rather to augment the tendency of not responding: the dedifferentiation of stimuli which takes place when inhibition reaches a certain level will then require the intervention of an environmental 'distractor' unconnected with the task to act as a disinhibitor and thus stop the process. If no distractor intervenes, the dedifferentiation of stimuli (which represents a high-level neurophysiological block) may be followed by a kind of sensory adaptation comparable with what happens, for example, when we cease to be aware of the regular ticking of a clock. This is one possible reason for the drowsiness which Ss often report in vigilance tests, and for the fact that Ss occasionally fall fast asleep.

The behaviour described above corresponds, in terms of neurophysiology, to changes at the level of the 'central arousal system' of Moruzzi and Magoun (1949). This arousal system can be thought of as representing a second major pathway by which all sensory excitations reach the cortex, and its activity has been shown to be necessary to all organized cortical activity. This is particularly relevant to the prediction which was made concerning the effect of Doriden and meprobamate on vigilance behaviour, since only in the case of Doriden does the pharmacological evidence indicate clearly that the drug has a particular effect in the appropriate sub-cortical areas. Sigg, Schneider, and Holland (1957) report that subanaesthetic doses of Doriden caused the threshold for brain-stem arousal to be elevated in the cat, and the thalamo-cortical recruiting response slightly increased. At higher doses the brain-stem arousal response was blocked and the thalamo-cortical recruiting response was disorganized.

Statement of experimental expectations

Since Doriden and meprobamate both have central depressant properties they will be expected to accelerate the growth of inhibition, and the implications of this for vigilance performance, together with the neurophysiological considerations discussed above, led to the following expectations: Vigilance performance under Doriden will be significantly lower than under the 'no-drug' condition; vigilance performance under meprobamate will be lower than under the no-drug condition but possibly higher than under Doriden.

Previous experimental findings

The work of Bakan previously mentioned (Bakan, 1959) lends strong support to the general hypothesis that factors which increase cortical inhibition will lower the level of vigilance performance. He was principally interested in the effect of the introduction of a secondary task on the level of performance of a primary vigilance task. The primary task was substantially the same as the task used in the present investigation, while the secondary task consisted of detecting a different signal (the number 6) every time it occurred in the display series. The introduction of this second task thus had the effect of markedly increasing the frequency with which the signals occurred. Dividing his Ss into an 'extravert' and an 'introvert' group he found that within the first 32-minute period of his 80-minute test extraverts performed less well than introverts on the primary task alone (1-tail U-test. $p = 0{\cdot}03$). With the addition of the secondary task this difference between the two groups disappeared, extraverts now detecting primary signals with the same success as introverts did without benefit of the secondary task. Improvement in the extravert score occurred over the first 32-minute period following the introduction of the secondary task, while the introverts only reached a correspondingly significant level of improvement after 64 minutes, although their overall performance was still slightly better than in the extravert group.

According to Eysenck's theory of extraversion-introversion extraverts build up reactive inhibition more quickly than introverts and dissipate it more slowly. Comparisons between extravert and introvert groups are thus equivalent, with respect to the theory, to comparisons between a 'depressant drug' group and a 'placebo' or 'no-drug' group. The difference between Bakan's two groups on the primary task may be interpreted as being due to the fact that the faster accumulation of inhibition caused extraverts to take more rest pauses, miss more signals and therefore more reinforcements, and led to more precipitate extinction of the attending response. The secondary task improved the performance of the extravert group because signals now occurred at much shorter time intervals, yielding more reinforcements before I_R had sufficient time to force Ss to rest. Introverts did not show a corresponding improvement in the first 32 minutes because they were already performing at or very near the maximum level allowed by the test without benefit of the secondary task.

A repetition of Bakan's experiment, somewhat modified, was carried out by Claridge (cf. Vol. 2) who compared the performance of normal subjects, dysthymics (neurotic introverts) and hysterics (neurotic extraverts) during a 30-minute period of work on the primary vigilance task, followed by 10 minutes on the primary plus the secondary task. As expected dysthymics had significantly fewer errors than hysterics on the primary task, this difference disappearing after the introduction of the secondary task. Fig. 7.1 is a graphical representation of his results.

In conclusion we may note that the results of other studies dealing with the effects on vigilance of a variety of depressant and stimulant drugs have consistently tended to support the hypothesis that vigilance is impaired by the depressants (drugs which act to increase central inhibition) and is improved by stimulant drugs (which increase central excitation and raise the tolerance level for inhibition.) For example Felsinger, Lasagna, and Beecher (1953) report that male college students showed significant impairment in performance on a 9-minute

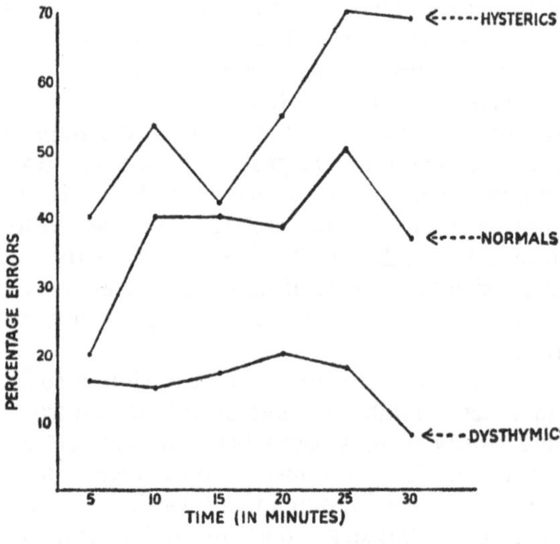

FIG. 7.1. Thirty-minute auditory vigilance test.

attention test as long as 5½–8 hours following the administration of one of the barbituric depressants, pentobarbital sodium, and Mackworth (1950), using his Clock Test of visual vigilance, showed that the marked decrease in vigilance which is normally observed after 30 minutes' continuous work, can be effectively prevented by the administration of 10 mg. of amphetamine sulphate.

Vigilance test results in the present experiment. Despite a number of complaints about feelings of drowsiness, and the fact that on two occasions Ss fell asleep in the latter part of the test (one S under Doriden and another under meprobamate), the general level of performance was nevertheless high.

Performance under each of the three treatment conditions is shown graphically in Fig. 7.2. The superimposed graphs show that, as expected, performance was best under the no-drug condition, worse under meprobamate, and worst of all under Doriden. All three graphs show more errors in the second half of the test than at the beginning, but the increase in error is no greater under the drug conditions than under no

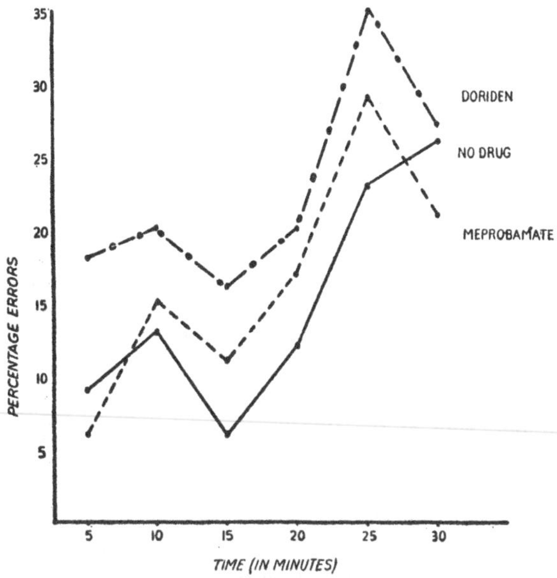

FIG. 7.2. Auditory vigilance test.

drug. The mean error scores for the whole test are: No drug, 4·3; meprobamate, 4·8; Doriden, 6·2.

Table 7.1 gives the results of an analysis of variance of the error scores, and shows that the differences between treatments are not statistically significant. Since the task did not involve the learning of any new skill it is not surprising that the differences between Days are also non-significant. The highly significant differences between Ss give an indication of S reliability $\left(r = \frac{F - 1}{F} = 0{\cdot}78\right)$

TABLE 7.1

Vigilance test error scores: analysis of variance

Source of variance	Sums of squares	d.f.	m.s.v.	*F*-ratio	Significance
Subjects	1153·208	23	50·139	4·53	$p < 0{\cdot}001$
Treatments	41·583	2	20·791	1·88	n.s.
Days	46·333	2	23·166	2·09	n.s.
Residual	486·751	44	11·06		
Total		71			

Since Extraversion (E) and Neuroticism (N) (p. 107) were available for all Ss, the possibility that the non-significance of the differences between treatments might be due, in part, to an interaction between the effects of the drugs and individual personality differences, was checked. There were no significant correlations between E and N scores and the drug effects (the latter being assessed by computing two sets of 'change' scores, i.e. no drug v. meprobamate and no drug v. Doriden). As a further check on the relationship between vigilance decrement and personality differences the error scores of the six most extraverted Ss were compared with those of the six most introverted, and similarly with the six highest and six lowest scorers on the N scale. There was no evidence of a differential effect of the drug treatments on high as compared with low scorers on either of the personality variables, but a significant difference was found between extraverts and introverts with respect to the *total* vigilance decrement which occurred over the three experimental treatments. The difference was in the expected direction, extraverts having a higher mean error score than introverts ($t = 2{\cdot}55$. 1-tail t-test. $p < 0{\cdot}02$). Ss with high N scores had more errors than low N scorers under each of the three experimental conditions, the overall difference between the two groups yielding a t-value of 2·2 (2-tail t-test. $p = 0{\cdot}05$).

The difference between extraverts and introverts, which is in line with the findings of Bakan (1959) quoted above, is meaningful in terms of a difference in cortical inhibition between these two groups. The difference between the high and low N groups on the other hand is attributable to a difference in the anxiety-arousing potentiality of the test situation for one group as compared with the other. Although Ss with high E scores are similar to Ss with high N scores with respect to the number of signals missed during the vigilance test, their actual behaviour in the test situation differed markedly. The former group was under-responsive whereas the latter was over-responsive, being in fact the only section of the experimental sample who made false responses (i.e. by tapping the table in the absence of a signal). They were also inclined to make verbal comments on their performance, apologizing to the experimenter for making mistakes, criticizing the general level of their performance and so on. Their detection of genuine signals was poor, therefore, because of the interference caused by irrelevant and/or incorrect responses. It is noteworthy that the performance of this group on the no-drug day was actually worse, although not significantly so, than on either of the drug days, in contrast with the extravert group who made fewer errors on the no-drug day than on either of the other two days (see Table 7.2).

Before leaving the vigilance test, another possible reason for the non-significance of the differences between treatment groups should be mentioned. This is the presence of the experimenter in the testing room. Previous experiments have shown that vigilance decrements are much greater when the experimenter is absent than when he is present throughout the test. He provides a stimulus which is not 'irrelevant' in the same sense as other non-task stimuli are. When S's attention wanders from the task the sight of the experimenter ought to be much more effective in redirecting his attention to the vigilance test than other environmental stimuli, because of the causal relationship between the experimenter's presence and the activity in which S is currently engaged. Since the degree to which non-task stimuli impinge is a function of the

TABLE 7.2

Mean vigilance error scores of four extreme groups

Treatment	High Extravert. group (Ss = 6)	High Neurot. group (Ss = 6)	Low Extravert. group (Ss = 6)	Low Neurot. group (Ss = 6)
No drug	7·1	7·3	1·8	1·8
Meprobamate	8·0	4·5	4·0	3·3
Doriden	8·8	7·0	5·5	2·0

degree of vigilance decrement it is therefore quite possible that the presence of the experimenter served to reduce differences between performance in the various treatment conditions. There is some direct evidence in the test data to support this argument. Fig. 7.2 shows that an improvement in performance occurred under all three treatments in the third and again in the sixth 5-minute period. These two periods coincide with two points in the test at which the scoring booklet used by the experimenter had to be turned to a new page, and although this was done as unobtrusively as possible, so as not to distract S, some Ss undoubtedly noticed the movement. Thus improvement in performance occurs during the two periods in the test in which Ss are most likely to pay attention to the presence of the experimenter.

Hand-steadiness test

A hand-steadiness test is one of the most popular candidates for inclusion in any battery of tests employed to investigate drug effects in human subjects. Its popularity, one suspects, derives mainly from its simplicity in administration rather than from any clearly formulated theoretical rationale. This is reflected in the frequent failure to offer any adequate and meaningful interpretation of the results even when these show clear-cut differences between treatment groups. As a result we still know very little about the determinants of hand steadiness and the factors responsible for its deterioration.

It has frequently been observed that hand steadiness and general fine motor co-ordination tend to be decreased in neurotics as compared with normals, but there is also some slight evidence to suggest that hysterics (neurotic extraverts) show more impairment than dysthymics (neurotic introverts). Petrie (1946) found a small but significant difference in this direction between an hysteric and a dysthymic group on the O'Connor Tweezers test, which is a simple manipulative test in which Ss can choose their own rate of work, but in which a 'reckless approach' (i.e. the sacrifice of accuracy to speed) is penalized. However, this test is not a hand-steadiness test as such, although highly loaded on that component, and no parallel personality difference has ever been established with a conventional hand-steadiness test.

The available evidence about the effects of stimulant and depressant drugs on this function is not helpful. Animal experiments have shown that although deterioration of motor co-ordination is a characteristic effect of sedative-hypnotic drugs, centrally stimulating drugs can also produce this effect (Gross, Tripod, and Meier, 1955). Furthermore, a deterioration of hand steadiness and general motor control in human subjects can be induced by the administration of drugs with predominantly autonomic action. This is a well-known effect of adrenalin and other sympathomimetic drugs. Basowitz, for example, showed that minimal doses of adrenalin can produce a highly significant deterioration in hand steadiness (Basowitz, Korchin, and Oken, 1955). As a result of some recent work on two tranquillizing drugs, reserpine and chlorpromazine, Toman, Everett, and Jeans (1957) have put forward a speculative neurophysiological hypothesis linking an expected extraverting effect of these drugs with their known tendency to produce tremor and deterioration of motor control in general. Unfortunately, however, their hypothesis is not specific enough to be experimentally useful within the context of the present investigation.

One probable reason for the generally confusing results which have been obtained is that hand steadiness is not unitary, but has two different, identifiable components. Evidence from high-speed photography (Travis, 1929) supports the factor-analytic findings of Seashore in this respect (Seashore, Dudek, and Holtzman, 1949). Lindquist (1941) distinguished between a large, slow tremor component whose 'initiation and conduct is dependent upon the integrative functions at the cortical level', and a fine rapid tremor which is superimposed on the first and results from 'the imbalanced state of neuromuscular activity and, contrary to earlier concept, is considered as being causally dissociated from cortical activity'. There is also evidence that amplitude and frequency of tremor are inversely related (Travis and Hunter, 1931).

On the basis of these findings a more rational method of scoring steadiness performance was worked out by Hauty (1954) which, it was hoped, would give detailed and meaningful information about the effects of various drugs on motor performance. The method, which applies to the stylus and graded aperture type of apparatus, produced some interesting results in Hauty's study of the effects of a central stimulant, Dexedrine, and Seconal, a barbituric depressant. Using six groups of eleven subjects each, who were given either 5 mg. Dexedrine, 10 mg.

Dexedrine, 100 mg. Seconal, 200 mg. Seconal, a placebo or no drug, he found that the barbiturate reduced fine tremor but adversely affected co-ordinative activities, whereas Dexedrine increased fine tremor but did not significantly affect co-ordination. Doubling the dose of stimulant had no significant effect but the larger dose of depressant led to a further significant reduction in fine tremor and also increased gross tremor. The placebo group showed significantly greater tremor than the no-drug group ($p < 0{\cdot}05$).

If each individual's performance had been evaluated in terms of a single steadiness score the group differences would have been obscured, suggesting the erroneous conclusion that the effect of the stimulant and the depressant drug was the same. The net effect at behavioural level can and often will be the same for stimulant and depressant drugs, because of the inverse relationship between the two components of steadiness. This is an important datum in its own right and in a practically oriented investigation may be all that it is necessary to establish, but the value of practical information of this kind, in terms of its 'generalizability', will be relative to the method used to establish it. The chief value of analytical studies like Hauty's is that, by supplying new information about the effects of drugs on the separate part functions, they make it possible to generate meaningful hypotheses about the effects expected at behavioural level. Although it has been shown that the separate part-functions which determine hand-steadiness scores are not only theoretically distinguishable but also to some extent experimentally separable, nevertheless the greatest possible refinements in hand-steadiness apparatus cannot accomplish more than an alteration or series of alterations in the relative contributions of the two components to any test score; at the behavioural level the components cannot ever be completely separated. Whilst the ultimate concern is always to predict and control performance at this latter level, this can only be accomplished effectively via an analysis of the part-functions.

Returning to Hauty's drug findings, the differences reported appear to mean that the deterioration of hand steadiness brought about by the depressant is due to interference or inhibition at the cortical level, whereas the stimulant lowers the overall performance level by virtue of its peripheral side effects. This suggests that stimulants ought to improve overall performance in Ss who have a high basic level of cortical inhibition (i.e. extreme extraverts), but should not improve the performance level of ambivert and introvert Ss. (This hypothesis has not, however, been tested experimentally.)

Before leaving Hauty's results the curious finding that the placebo group showed significant impairment in hand steadiness compared with the no-drug group requires some comment. The author's speculation that this is due to apprehension or anxiety in the placebo group may be correct, but in view of much clinical evidence that placebo is often markedly successful in reducing anxiety symptoms in patients it could equally plausibly be argued that the difference between the no-drug and placebo groups ought to be in the opposite direction.

The effect of anxiety on hand steadiness is of particular interest in relation to meprobamate since this drug is used in the treatment of anxiety symptoms, and being an interneuronal blocking agent is claimed to be particularly effective in the treatment of muscular spasm. The experimental studies of meprobamate have so far yielded rather conflicting evidence with respect to its effect on anxiety symptoms. Marquis and Kelly (1957) found no deterioration in hand steadiness in normal subjects following the administration of 800 mg. meprobamate, but an index of palmar sweating was significantly higher under meprobamate than under placebo in their study. Laties (1957), on the other hand, reports that palmar sweating is significantly reduced by meprobamate. There is no ready explanation for these contradictory results.

Confining the discussion to hand steadiness alone, it would be useful to know whether the deterioration in performance which is observed in anxiety states is mainly due to an increase in fine tremor or in gross tremor, or both. This question has not yet been investigated (and of course the relative contributions of these two components will vary with the type of apparatus used to measure hand steadiness), but there is some support for the hypothesis that the deterioration is mainly due to peripheral rather than central factors. First, the results of a large number of recent experimental studies of the effects of anxiety stress on performance and learning have interpreted anxiety as a drive variable, and have shown in general (*a*) that performance efficiency is a curvilinear function of drive strength, and (*b*) that optimal drive strength tends to be an inverse function of the difficulty of the task. If these laws are applicable to the hand-steadiness test then this, being a very simple task, ought to benefit from the heightened drive produced by moderate anxiety. However, the opposite tends to occur. This fact, taken in conjunction with findings showing that slightly more complex motor tasks bear out the above prediction *despite* the interfering effects of increased tremor, palmar sweating, etc. (Freeman and Geise, 1940; Maltzmann, Smith, and Brooks, 1956), suggests that deterioration of performance on the hand-steadiness test is due to an increase in fine tremor, peripheral in origin. Furthermore, one of the findings in the Marquis and Kelly study lends support to the argument (Marquis, Kelly, Miller, Gerard, and Rapaport, 1957). They report that hand steadiness was impaired under a placebo + alcohol condition, but not under meprobamate or meprobamate + alcohol, and they add the comment that meprobamate seems to counteract the alcohol effect. This may mean that the deterioration observed under alcohol is due to interference with the co-ordinative component of hand steadiness at the central level (alcohol being a central depressant); a deterioration which is compensated by an improvement in the fine tremor component due to a decrease in test induced anxiety under meprobamate + alcohol.

The preceding arguments are admittedly speculative, but in the absence of sufficient experimentally established evidence concerning the factors which affect hand steadiness they provide the only alternative basis for formulating expectations about the effects of Doriden and meprobamate on test performance. The predictions which follow from our discussion are:

(*a*) Hand-steadiness error scores will be higher under Doriden than under the no-drug condition.

(*b*) Hand-steadiness error scores under meprobamate will not differ significantly from the no-drug score.

No specific prediction was made about the effects of Doriden in comparison with meprobamate on this test.

Description of the hand-steadiness test

The apparatus consisted of a rigid vertical brass rod centred in an open frame of polished black wood. The frame supported the rod from above and below, while the back wall of the frame provided a high contrast background for the rod. The rod was 24″ long and had a regularly and gradually increasing circumference from 0·6″ at the top to 1·2″ at the base. A metal ring of 1·5″ inner circumference, attached to a handle 6″ long, could be moved freely up and down the length of the rod. Everytime the ring touched the rod an electric counter was activated, which thus automatically recorded the number of hits made. The apparatus stood upright on a table which was 30″ high.

S was instructed to stand directly in front of the apparatus. Because Ss varied quite widely in height and in arm length, it was decided that the best way to control these differences, without making an elaborate series of measurements and adjustments to the apparatus, was to allow each S to choose his own 'most comfortable distance' from the rod. Ss were however specifically instructed to hold the ring handle by its end, and as far away from the ring itself as possible. They were also forbidden to support their preferred hand or arm in any way during the test.

Each S had four test trials, two in the downward and two in the upward direction, with 10-second rest pauses between trials. The rate of work was not controlled exactly, but Ss were instructed to move the ring at a moderately fast rate, actively controlling its movement at all stages. It was found particularly important to stress the necessity for *active* control especially in the two downward trials, since otherwise the task could be simplified by S allowing the ring to be carried quickly from top to bottom by its own weight.

The score was the average number of contacts per trial.

Results of the hand-steadiness test. The average intercorrelation of the four hand-steadiness scores was high in all three treatment conditions: in the no-drug condition $r = 0{\cdot}76$, under meprobamate $r = 0{\cdot}72$, and under Doriden $r = 0{\cdot}71$. There was no consistent trend of improvement or of decrement from the first to the fourth trial so the four scores were combined to give a single mean score for each S under each experimental treatment.

The mean error scores for treatments are as follows: No drug, 78·5; meprobamate, 74·75; Doriden, 77·4. The results of an analysis of variance carried out on the error scores is given in Table 7.3. It confirms that these differences between treatments are well within the limits of chance variation. The expectation that there would be no difference between performance under meprobamate and under the no-drug condition is thus borne out by the data, but the prediction that Doriden would cause a deterioration in performance is not.

TABLE 7.3

Hand-steadiness error scores: analysis of variance

Source of variance	Sums of squares	d.f.	m.s.v.	*F*-ratio	Significance
Subjects	33,073·112	23	1437·961	7·29	$p<0{\cdot}001$
Treatments	181·028	2	90·514		
Days	2494·528	2	1247·264	6·33	$p<0{\cdot}001$
Residuals	8672·444	44	197·10		
Total	44,421·112	71			

A subjective impression that Doriden tended to increase the variability of performance was not supported by statistical analysis: the standard deviation of the scores obtained under no drug, meprobamate, and Doriden are $23{\cdot}5 \pm 3{\cdot}5$, $21{\cdot}9 \pm 3{\cdot}2$, and $28{\cdot}5 \pm 4{\cdot}2$ respectively, but these do not differ significantly from one another.

The practical conclusion to be drawn from these results is quite clear: under the particular conditions of drug administration and test procedure obtaining in the present experiment there is no deterioration of hand-steadiness performance under either meprobamate or Doriden. The interpretation of the results is not so simple, however.

The fact that Doriden did not produce the expected deterioration in performance does not invalidate the hypothesis that this drug increases cortical inhibition, nor does it even mean that the drug has no effect on motor co-ordination. Holland (p. 152, above) found a significant increase in static ataxia under Doriden and also under meprobamate using the same Ss and on the same days as the present experiment. There is a crucial difference between his ataxia test and the hand-steadiness test, however; the regulation of fine muscle movement which is of predominant importance in the latter test is not required in the ataxia test. It will be remembered that Ss were not prevented from supporting themselves (e.g. by leaning against the table or wall) during the performance of the hand-steadiness test, provided that the hand and arm used in moving the ring up and down the brass rod were not supported in any way. Moreover, in the static ataxia test Ss' eyes were closed, whereas they were of course open during the hand-steadiness test. In short, the relative freedom of movement allowed during the performance of the latter test gave Ss ample opportunity to compensate for the kind of co-ordination deterioration measured by Holland's test.

There still remained an important co-ordinative component in hand-steadiness performance, however. This corresponded to the upper part of the vertical brass rod, where the difference between the diameters of the rod and the ring was maximal, and where Ss had to work with their hand at or above shoulder level.

It was argued in the preliminary discussion of the test that the co-ordinative component would be adversely affected by the depressant action of the drugs on cortical centres, this effect being obscured in the case of meprobamate by the concurrent improvement effected in the fine tremor component due to the anxiety-reducing action of the drug. The close similarity of the results for Doriden and meprobamate suggests that a similar cancelling out of effects may have taken place in both cases. Two notable features of the test data point to this conclusion. The first is the unexpectedly high *F*-ratio for Days in the analysis of variance table. The mean scores for days are 84 on Day I, 77 on Day II and 69·6 on Day III. This steady improvement in performance over the three days is unlikely to be wholly due to improvement in skill through learning, since there was no evidence of a comparable improvement over the series of four test trials within each day. This suggests that the improvement in performance may be a function of simple familiarity with the test situation. It may therefore be attributed to a decrease in fine muscle tremor which would occur as the test becomes less anxiety-provoking. The second noteworthy feature which suggests that anxiety may play an important part in performance is the fact that hand-steadiness performance, in contrast with the other three tests used in this experiment, was actually worse under the no-drug condition than under either of the drug treatments.

Since it is known that anxiety symptoms may sometimes be as effectively reduced by the administration of a placebo, as by a tranquillizer for example, the relatively good performance of Ss under both drug treatments as compared with the no-drug condition may be due to the placebo effect of taking a pill, apart from any more specific effects which the drugs might be expected to have in this respect.

These suggested explanations for the high level of hand-steadiness performance under Doriden and meprobamate were checked by comparing the mean scores of the six Ss from each of the two extremes of the Neuroticism Scale distribution, the expectation being that the difference between the two extreme groups would be greater under the no-drug condition than under either of the drug treatments. More specifically, if a high level of anxiety leads to higher error scores on this test, through an increase in fine muscle tremor, then high-N scorers ought to have significantly worse performance than Ss low on N. Also, if anxiety is reduced by taking a pill, then an improvement in performance ought to occur in the high-N group under both the drug conditions, and the difference between the high- and low-N groups ought to be reduced in consequence.

The results are fully consistent with these expectations. When the differences between treatments are compared for the high-N and low-N groups separately, the only significant differences are in the high-N group. The mean no-drug score in this group is significantly worse than the corresponding Doriden or meprobamate scores. Doriden vs. no drug gives a *t*-value (correlated *t*-test, 1-tail) of $2{\cdot}41 > p < 0{\cdot}05$. For meprobamate vs. no drug $t = 2{\cdot}27 > p < 0{\cdot}05$. The differences between the high- and low-N groups under Doriden and meprobamate are not significant, but under the no-drug condition the difference is just significant at the 5% level ($t = 2{\cdot}10$, 1-tail *t*-test). The actual mean scores are given in Table 7.4.

TABLE 7.4

Mean hand-steadiness error scores of high- and low-N groups

	No drug	Meprobamate	Doriden
High-N group (Ss = 6)	91·7	77·5	79·5
Low-N group (Ss = 6)	72·8	72·7	71·0

The complex psychomotor tests

In the vigilance and hand-steadiness tests we were dealing with factors which are important components of skilled psychomotor performance. The triple tester and pursuit rotor tests, which will be discussed in this section, are both complex skills in their own right and as such are more directly comparable with the psychomotor tasks which form part of the normal pattern of everyday activities. Since the names of these tests do not give sufficient indication of their nature, a description of each of the tests will be a necessary preliminary to further discussion.

Description of the pursuit rotor

The apparatus consisted of a turntable 10″ in diameter which revolved clockwise at a constant speed of 60 r.p.m. A metal disc 0·7″ in diameter was set flush with the surface of the turntable, the distance between the centre of the disc and the centre of the turntable being 3·25″. A light articulated metal stylus, 7″ in length from the tip of the handle to the right-angled bend, activated one of two automatic recording chronometers whenever the tip of the stylus was in contact with the metal disc or 'target'. Recordings were made of the length of time contact was maintained between stylus tip and target during successive 10-second periods, an automatic device switching the recording between the two recording chronometers every 10 seconds. The recording apparatus formed a separate unit from the test apparatus, and during the test was not visible to S. The turntable had a wooden base 6″ in depth, and stood on a 30″ high table, so that the work surface was 36″ above floor level.

The instructions required S to stand upright in front of the apparatus, holding the stylus lightly in his preferred hand. As in the administration of the hand-steadiness test S was allowed to choose his own 'most comfortable distance' from the apparatus. His task was to pursue the rotating target with the stylus, trying to maintain maximum contact between the two. It was forbidden to lift the stylus off the surface of the turntable during the work period. S was asked not to press down heavily on the stylus, thus bending back the handle, but to keep the handle parallel with the turntable surface. The correct movements were demonstrated by the experimenter at the beginning of the testing session. Finally, S was instructed to start and stop work instantly on receiving the appropriate signal.

There were two continuous work periods of 5 minutes each, separated by a 10-minute rest. The score was the length of time during which the stylus was on target.

Description of the triple tester

The apparatus consisted of a brass drum rotating in the forward direction, i.e. towards S. A sheet of Ivorine was marked out as a helical road along which holes were punched in a serpentine pattern. The brass surface of the drum was completely covered by the Ivorine except where the punched holes exposed it. A bronze ball, moved sideways on a rack, was steered along the road by means of a steering wheel, S's task being to hit as many of the exposed brass dots as possible. Each hit was recorded on an electric counter, the score being the total number of hits per trial. A trial was defined as one complete 'journey' from the starting point to the end of the road, the starting and finishing points being clearly marked by red lines.

The bronze ball and rack are not controlled directly by the steering wheel, but are moved through the operation of an integrating gear, thus producing a time-lag between S's response to the pattern of dots and the corresponding response of the bronze ball. This feature of the apparatus was explained to S in the preliminary instructions in order to control any possible effect on performance of individual differences in general mechanical knowledge. Variations in score attributable to this characteristic of the apparatus were thus confined to variables relevant to the investigation, e.g. vigilance, which was importance in determining the effectiveness of anticipatory responses.

S's task was further complicated by the fact that at various points along the road, the route defined by the brass dots forked into two, the alternative routes running roughly parallel for a short time before converging again. A firm decision was necessary at these choice points if performance was not to become disorganized, and this decision was made difficult by an apparent but indeterminate difference between the number of dots along the alternative routes. There was in fact no consistently greater opportunity of increasing the score by choosing one path rather than the other, the illusory difference being perceptually created by means of differences in the pattern of placement of the dots along the alternative routes. The choice points produced significant differentials in score only between those who made a choice and those who oscillated uncertainly between the two routes. Subjective reports indicated that this feature of the test was not found to be stressful, but served rather to maintain motivation at an advantageously high level.

S sat in a low chair directly in front of the apparatus which stood on a table 30″ high. The height of the seat was adjusted to S's requirements. The apparatus was fully explained and demonstrated before testing began. Each S had three 2-minute trials, separated by 1-minute rest pauses.

Characteristics of psychomotor performance curves

The pursuit rotor has been the most frequently used, among a variety of tracking and tracing tasks, in experimental investigations of the characteristics of psychomotor performance curves, and is therefore especially useful in the study of drug effects on psychomotor behaviour, where systematic deviations from the 'norms' of performance are to be expected.

Performance curves in which psychomotor proficiency scores are plotted against continuous work time typically show a fairly steep initial incline after which the curve flattens out and then declines, without necessarily having approached asymptote at its highest point. After a period of 'no work', or alternative activity, performance resumes at a level appreciably higher than the pre-rest level (reminiscence); there is usually a very short-lived steep rise in the curve (warm-up), after which it continues to rise more gradually until it flattens out again and declines.

In terms of Hullian theory the flattening out and subsequent decline in the curve with continued work are due to the build-up of two inhibitory factors, I_R and ${}_SI_R$, which subtract from the positive habit strength (${}_SH_R$) thus lowering effective reaction potential (${}_S\bar{E}_R$). (Jones (1958) has pointed out an inconsistency in Hull's treatment of I_R and ${}_SI_R$ and proposes a modification of the equation for ${}_S\bar{E}_R$, in which I_R

subtracts from positive drive (D) and $_{S}I_{R}$ subtracts from $_{S}H_{R}$, $_{S}\bar{E}_{R}$ being a multiplicative function of the resultant net drive and net habit strength.)

The post-rest improvement in performance (reminiscence) is held to be due to the dissipation of I_{R} during rest, while the warm-up phenomenon, which was neglected by Hull himself, is, according to Eysenck (1956a), due to the extinction of $_{S}I_{R}$ in the immediate post-rest period.

There is conclusive evidence to show that work decrement phenomena cannot be explained entirely or even largely in terms of peripheral muscular fatigue, but on the contrary are effects of centrally generated inhibition. This evidence has been adequately reviewed elsewhere, e.g. McGeogh and Irion (1952), and need not be repeated here.

Eysenck (1957a) has shown how work decrement and all the various phenomena related to it, e.g. superiority of distributed over massed practice, reminiscence, post-rest warm-up, can be accommodated within a modified Hullian theory in which the two basic explanatory concepts are central (or cortical) excitation and inhibition. His drug postulate (Eysenck, 1957b) which has already been discussed leads to the general prediction that psychomotor performance will be lowered by drugs which have a depressant action in the CNS, and this, together with the converse that stimulant drugs will correspondingly improve performance, has been borne out in a number of drug investigations (Eysenck, Casey, and Trouton, 1957). The general prediction cannot be expected to apply uniformly to all tasks under all experimental conditions however, the outcome in any given situation depending on the relevance of both the main and the subsidiary drug effects to the requirements of the specific task.

Analysis of the differences between the triple tester and the pursuit rotor task

The decision to include both the pursuit rotor and the triple tester in the present battery was in fact governed by the consideration that while they had important factors in common, which moreover they share with most psychomotor skills, the balance or relative weights of the various factors differed considerably from one to the other. Comparisons between the two might thus be expected to throw additional light on the ways in which the depressant drugs affect psychomotor performance. The similiarities and differences which it seemed most important to take into consideration before attempting to formulate any precise expectations about the effects of meprobamate and Doriden on each of the tests will now be discussed.

(*a*) Hand steadiness: This is a performance factor common to both tests. The co-ordinative or gross tremor component of hand steadiness would appear to be equally important in each, and therefore both tests should be adversely affected by the deterioration in this component expected under both drug treatments. On the other hand the fine tremor component should affect only the pursuit rotor. The steering wheel of the triple tester is unresponsive to weak hand movements, but on the pursuit rotor contact between stylus and target is easily disturbed by slight 'irrelevant' movements of the type caused by tremor.

The relationship between hand steadiness and performance on the pursuit rotor is well illustrated in an experiment carried out by Brengelmann (personal communication) in which extraverts and introverts were given practice on a pursuit rotor with a target of variable size. The extraverts were inferior to introverts in performance when the target was small, due to the fact that extraverts had a greater tendency to make small oscillatory movements which caused them frequently to lose contact with the target, even when their rotatory movements were accurate enough to keep them in the target area. The difference between the two groups narrowed as the size of the target was progressively increased.

The oscillatory movements described above cannot be exclusively identified with the fine tremor component of hand steadiness, but probably also include a small co-ordination component. Since this is an aspect of pursuit rotor performance which is not shared by the triple tester, and one which was expected to be adversely affected by the two drugs used, it is therefore possible that pursuit rotor performance will show a greater deterioration under the drug conditions, than triple tester performance.

(*b*) Vigilance: Vigilance is a function of perceptual monotony; the simpler and less varied the stimulus pattern the sooner will attention waver. Similarly it is known that vigilance is more successfully maintained when knowledge of results is available than when it is absent, efficiency of task performance being proportional to the degree of completeness of the knowledge available. In both these respects the pursuit rotor task is more difficult than the triple tester. The repetitive unvaried nature of the former task stands in marked contrast to the latter, where S is presented with a complex pattern of visual stimuli requiring a correspondingly complex series of motor responses, which in their turn produce a highly differentiated succession of kinesthetic feedback cues. In addition, the recording instrument used with the pursuit rotor operated silently, whereas the triple tester electric counter clicked audibly whenever a hit was scored. These auditory cues added a further dimension to the pattern of stimulation, increased S's knowledge of results and constituted a reinforcing factor which probably served to maintain test motivation at a high level. A final factor which might be expected to have a differential effect on vigilance level was the difference in the duration and spacing of practice on the two tasks.

The analysis so far indicates that the basic vigilance level ought to be high in triple test performance and low on the pursuit rotor, under the no-drug condition. Meprobamate and Doriden were each expected to reduce the general level of vigilance. Therefore, the difference between the two tasks with respect to the amount of support they give to the maintenance of an adequate level of vigilance suggests that deterioration of performance under the drug conditions ought to be more marked on the pursuit rotor than on the triple tester.

The foregoing discussion may have overemphasized the difficulty of maintaining vigilance during pursuit rotor performance. It should therefore be added that even a very monotonous psychomotor task provides S with a greater variety of stimulation than does a pure vigilance task. Normal Ss not infrequently fall asleep in the course of a long vigilance test, but except under conditions of abnormal fatigue this does not happen in psychomotor tasks. It appears therefore that task stimuli are able to sustain a minimal level of vigilance; a level which possibly defines a lower limit beyond which the variables which reduce vigilance become ineffective, except under the abnormal fatigue condition mentioned above. The changing factor structure of the task as practice continues must also be taken into consideration. Although the conditions of practice on the pursuit rotor are potentially extremely detrimental to the maintenance of vigilance, it is possible that this effect is neutralized in the later stages of practice by changes in the pattern of component factors. Factor analyses of rotary pursuit have shown that as practice continues the variance contribution of a factor specific to the task increases at the expense of more general factors, of which vigilance or attention is known to be one.

Effects of the drugs on work decrement phenomena

Having examined the ways in which the main differences between the two psychomotor tests were expected to interact with the drug action, thus modifying the predicted decremental effect of the latter, it now remains to discuss this decremental effect of the drugs in relation to the various work decrement phenomena which can be measured in psychomotor tasks. These phenomena have already been listed and interpreted in the section dealing with the general characteristics of psychomotor performance curves.

(1) *Depression of performance due to the build-up of reactive inhibition:* Kimble and Horenstein (1948) have shown that a 90-second period of massed practice is sufficiently long to allow the build-up of a measurable amount of I_R. Pre-rest practice on the triple tester continued for 2 minutes and on the pursuit rotor for 5 minutes, so that although practice did not proceed without break for the entire course of either test it was sufficiently massed to raise I_R to a level adequate to produce 'work decrement' in the no-drug group. The introduction of the two drugs was predicted to result in a significant lowering of the overall performance score on both tests below the no-drug level (other

factors being equal) because of the depressant characteristics of these drugs; by lowering the tolerance threshold for I_R they would induce a greater number of involuntary rest pauses which would decrease the score directly (S not working) and indirectly by creating the conditions necessary for the production of $_SI_R$.

(2) *Reminiscence:* The triple tester was not suitable for the measurement of reminiscence because each 2-minute practice period yielded only a single overall performance index. The study of this phenomenon was therefore confined to the pursuit rotor.

The formulation of a prediction with respect to the effect of meprobamate and Doriden on reminiscence presented a special problem, the nature of which can best be illustrated by quoting the results of some previous experiments on reminiscence effects (*a*) in extraverts and introverts and (*b*) in normal groups who were treated with stimulant and depressant drugs prior to testing.

(*a*) Eysenck (1956*b*) reported a small but significant positive correlation between a questionnaire measure of extraversion (1956*c*) and reminiscence scores obtained in pursuit rotor performance, while Treadwell (1956) found significant differences in reminiscence scores on a track-tracing test between extreme groups of extraverts and introverts who had been selected on the basis of scores obtained on the T scale of the Minnesota Extraversion-Introversion questionnaire (Evans and McConnell, 1941). In addition, more indirect evidence for the same kind of relationship between the reminiscence effect and extraversion, comes from Broadbent's investigations into individual differences in vigilance decrement phenomena (Broadbent, 1958). In two experiments he obtained significant correlations between relative degree of improvement over a rest period in a vigilance task, and an index of level of aspiration on the triple tester, the latter measure being almost identical with one which Eysenck (1947) had previously found to differentiate significantly between neurotic extraverts and neurotic introverts. Broadbent also found, in these experiments, that the absolute amount of decrement with work periods was correlated with the relative degree of improvement over a rest period, and in a later experiment with a similar type of task he obtained a significant correlation between amount of decrement and an extraversion questionnaire score.

(*b*) Eysenck, Casey, and Trouton (1957) compared the pursuit rotor performance of groups of normal subjects who had received pre-medication consisting of either 10 mg. of d-amphetamine sulphate, 4·5 grains of sodium amylobarbitone or a placebo. There were significant differences in the overall performance of the various groups but no differences in reminiscence. Inspection of a graphical representation of the results (*op. cit.*, p. 647) reveals that while reminiscence occurred under all drug treatments there was also a strongly marked tendency for the groups to maintain the same positions relative to one another from the immediate pre-rest period into the post-rest period. Reminiscence measures were taken at two different stages of practice but on each occasion the amounts for the four treatment groups were highly similar.

Although it may be rash to conclude, without further empirical evidence, that this reminiscence-effect discrepancy between extraverts and introverts on the one hand, and stimulant and depressant drug groups on the other, will hold under all experimental conditions, nevertheless the results just quoted require some explanation.

Before proceeding to a more detailed analysis of the problem, one possible simple explanation which might suggest itself at this point will be mentioned and very briefly discussed. Assuming for the moment that we ought to expect stimulant and depressant drugs to produce differences in reminiscence parallel with those reported in extraverts and introverts, then the failure of the amytal group to show more reminiscence than the control group in Eysenck's study might be accounted for by the following hypothesis: The depressant drug may simply slow down the rate of I_R dissipation so much that a significant amount still remains to be dissipated at the end of the rest interval, thus artificially attenuating the reminiscence effect. However, this possibility must be rejected in view of the results of another recent study which was concerned with the effects of Doriden on pursuit rotor performance. In this investigation a whole day was allowed to elapse between the pre-rest and post-rest practice periods, but the reminiscence scores of depressant drug and placebo groups were still closely similar (Eysenck: personal communication). This experimental result indicates that the effects of depressant drugs on behaviour cannot be entirely attributed to a rise in the level of cortical inhibition.

An analysis of the reminiscence measure itself will help to clarify the problem raised by the drug study results. Reminiscence is operationally defined as the difference in score between the first post-rest and the last pre-rest trial. The pre-rest score, which is an index of the size of the effective reactive potential ($_S\bar{E}_R$) immediately prior to the rest pause, is subtracted from the post-rest $_S\bar{E}_R$ index. The result is usually expected to be a positive quantity (although reminiscence has become deservedly famous as the 'now-you-see-it-now-you-don't' phenomenon), indicating that after rest practice resumes at a higher level. Using the Jones (1958) modification of Hull's formula for effective reactive potential: $_S\bar{E}_R = (D + I_R)(_SH_R + {_SI_R})$, we can see that differences in reminiscence may be due to variations in any one, or several, of four distinct components; since depressant drug groups do not show more reminiscence than control groups, and moreover, continue to perform at a relatively low level 24 hours after administration of the drug, it appears that $_SH_R$ is the component most directly relevant to the present problem.

Positive habit strength ($_SH_R$) is an important component of the reminiscence score. Hull's account of this construct typically does not include any statement about variations in $_SH_R$ due to individual differences. However, among the variables which govern (*a*) the rate of growth, and (*b*) the upper limit of the curve of habit strength, there are at least two which he assumed to be determined by experimental conditions of practice and therefore constant for all Ss performing under the same set of conditions, but which recent neurophysiological evidence suggests may vary as a function of individual differences in cortical excitation and which may also be varied by the action of stimulant and depressant drugs. According to Hull's Postulate IV, $_SH_R$ is a simple positive growth function of number of reinforcements, but he qualified this account by adding that 'an adequate statement of the primary law or laws of learning would . . . take the form of an equation in which $_SH_R$ would be expressed as a joint function not only of number of reinforcements but of the quantity and quality of the reinforcing agent, and of the temporal relationships of stimulus to response, and of response to goal object' (Hull, 1943).

Variations in 'the quantity and quality of the reinforcing agent' may certainly occur independently of the experimental manipulation of external rewards. Neilsen, Doty, and Rutledge (1958) have recently confirmed previous reports that electrical stimulation of certain regions of the CNS is itself rewarding and animals will actively seek stimulation, and Fuster (1957) has shown that performance of a learned visual discrimination in monkeys is improved with respect to both speed and accuracy, as a function of stimulation of the reticular formation. In other words increased excitation is associated with improved performance apparently because an increase in non-specific stimulation provides additional reinforcement for the establishment of concomitant stimulus response connections. This evidence indicates that Ss with a high basic excitatory threshold and Ss under the influence of a depressant drug may acquire a smaller increment of $_SH_R$ per reinforcement than Ss with a low basic excitatory threshold or Ss under stimulant drug medication.

The temporal relationship of stimulus to response is another part determinant of the upper limit of the $_SH_R$ curve, the limit being 'a negative growth function of the degree of asynchronism of stimulus and response when both are of short duration' (*op. cit.*, p. 178). Here again individual differences come into play. For example, Lindsley (1957) and Lansing, Schwartz, and Lindsley (1956) have shown that the probability of S responding to a stimulus occurring at a specific point in time, as well as 'the efficiency of response' if a response is made, is closely related to the phase of the alpha activity in which the stimulus falls. Lansing (1957) reached the conclusion that the maximum potential speed or efficiency of response was realized only when the stimulus message arrived in the cortex at an optimal excitability period in a certain phase of the appropriate sensory alpha wave, and the motor discharge originated in the motor area in a similar optimal phase of the motor alpha wave. Individual differences in the timing of successive phases of the 'excitability cycle' have not yet been directly investigated, but on the basis of what is already known Lindsley (1957) has suggested that this may be the neurophysiological basis for inter-individual differences in the formation of habits.

Interpersonal variations of the kinds suggested refer to excitatory mechanisms and would be functionally independent of differences in inhibitory thresholds and rates of growth of inhibition.

The postulation of individual differences both in the rate of habit acquisition and in the asymptotic value of $_{S}H_{R}$ is therefore quite consistent with Hull's theoretical formulations and compatible with Eysenck's postulate of individual differences in cortical inhibition (Eysenck, 1957a).

The absence of a differential reminiscence effect in the drug studies reviewed above may now be explained as follows: The immediate pre-rest performance of all groups is depressed by the combined effects of I_R and I_{SR}, and the dissipation of I_R over the rest period therefore results in improved performance in all of the groups (reminiscence). However, the pre-rest performance of the depressant drug groups is additionally lowered by a retardation of the growth of $_{S}H_{R}$ caused by the effect of the drug on central excitatory mechanisms. This effect, being permanent, persists over the rest period and causes the depressant drug group to resume practice at the same *relative* position as they held prior to rest.

If the difference between the two sets of data had been confined to the reminiscence effect alone then the distinction drawn between lowered excitation (in the case of the drug data) and heightened inhibitory effects (in the case of the extravert-introvert data) might appear arbitrary. However, the emphasis which has been given to the effects on excitatory processes in the drug studies is justified by other features of the experimental data apart from the reminiscence effect.

Within the first five minutes of pursuit rotor practice the divergence between the performance curves of extraverts and introverts does not become significant at any point (although Oakley (1958) found that the *trends* of his two performance curves were just significantly different at the 5% level within the first 5-minute period of massed practice). The separation between the drug groups in the same period is on the other hand quite marked. This separation is further increased as practice continues and the effect remains even after 24 hours' rest, whereas the corresponding differences between extraverts and introverts never become so great and do not show the same stability or permanence. These contrasting characteristics of the two sets of curves are directly predictable from the hypothesis used to account for the reminiscence effects discussed above. Thus, if depressant drugs decrease the magnitude and/or the number of $_SH_R$ increments below the normal level, then performance should be depressed from the very beginning of practice; the effect should increase steadily as practice continues and should be of a permanent nature. Depression of performance due to the build-up of I_R on the other hand will not be effective until a certain amount of I_R has accumulated; the increase in the effect with continued practice will probably be erratic because of the complicating effects of involuntary rest pauses and the generation of $_SI_R$, and the effect will disappear either partially or completely, after a rest pause.

The preceding discussion helps to answer a question which the earlier part of this analysis may have suggested: i.e. whether the various behavioural differences between extraverts and introverts which have been attributed to differences in cortical inhibition might not in fact be due to differences in basic excitatory levels. Some of the differences in learning and conditioning between the two groups could equally well be ascribed to differential build-up of I_R or to differential rates of acquisition of $_SH_R$, but the inhibition postulate accounts for more of the empirical facts more parsimoniously. The conclusion nevertheless leaves the question of possible additional differences in excitatory levels between extraverts and introverts quite open.

Similarly, although the presence of a differential reminiscence effect may be accepted as evidence for underlying differences in I_R levels, the absence of such an effect in the drug study data does not mean that depressant drugs do not cause increases in inhibition. It is quite possible that depressant drugs lower the threshold of inhibition and also raise the excitation threshold but that the behavioural effects of the latter obscure those of the former. The increase in reminiscence which would normally be expected to follow as a result of higher pre-rest levels of I_R in the depressant drug group, would almost certainly be cancelled out by the effect of the correspondingly lower $_SH_R$ values in this group, since reminiscence is a multiplicative function of I_R and $_SH_R$.

With respect to the present investigation the prediction was made that the meprobamate and Doriden groups would both show a reminiscence effect but that the mean reminiscence scores of these groups would not differ significantly from that of the no-drug group.

Complex psychomotor tests results: triple tester. The most striking feature of the triple tester data is the wide variations in score between individuals. The effects of practice were also marked. Scores improved rapidly from trial to trial but there was no differential rate of increase under the various treatment conditions. Successive trial scores showed high intra-subject consistency, the average intercorrelation between trials on the no-drug day being 0·91, while the overall reliability, estimated from the *F*-ratio for Ss in the analysis of variance table, was 0·88.

In analysing the effects of the experimental treatments a single index of performance was therefore used. This was the average score over three trials for each S under each experimental condition. The mean performance scores for the various conditions are: No drug, 74·4; meprobamate, 69·8; Doriden, 69·5. The differences between treatments, although in the expected direction, were thus very small, and an analysis of variance showed them to be insignificant. The results of the analysis are given in Table 7.5.

TABLE 7.5

Triple tester scores: analysis of variance

Source of variance	Sums of squares	d.f.	m.s.v.	*F*-ratio	*p*
Subjects	81,177·9188	23	3529·4747	37·15	$p < 0{\cdot}001$
Treatments	564·9714	2	282·4857	2·97	$p < 0{\cdot}1 > 0{\cdot}05$
Days	15,183·475	2	7591·7375	79·91	$p < 0{\cdot}001$
Residual	4180·0377	44	95·0		
Total	101,106·4029	71			

It was noted in the preliminary discussion of the triple tester that the intrinsic interest of this test, and in particular, the variety of stimulation it provided, was expected in some degree to mitigate the potentially decremental effects of the two drugs. In contrast with the pursuit rotor task, Ss who concentrate on achieving a high degree of accuracy in their response to the immediate stimulus (target), are likely to have a much lower performance score on the triple tester than Ss who set themselves the relatively easier task of following the general direction of the 'road' to be followed, relegating precision of response to a position of secondary importance. Only at the higher level of skilled performance, after the grosser anticipatory adjustments have been mastered, does it become of primary importance to respond to the immediate stimulus pattern with a fine degree of accuracy. In other words, in the intermediate ranges of skill S is not penalized for the relatively 'slap-dash' type of response which tended to be characteristic of Ss under the influence of the two depressant drugs.

A number of wartime studies of the effects of sleep deprivation on combat performance confirm general observation in everyday situations that persons suffering from a moderate degree of general fatigue are able to perform a task for which they are highly motivated just as well, if not better (due to a decrease in anxiety), than they would when not fatigued, provided that quick decisions and very fine adjustments of response are not essential to successful performance.

One other possible contributory cause of the relatively high level of triple tester performance in the two drug conditions when compared with the no-drug condition was the degree of distribution of practice in this test. As reported above, there were three 2-minute practice periods separated by two 1-minute rest pauses. The length of a single practice period was in fact determined by the apparatus, 2 minutes being the time required to traverse the road from beginning to end. However, this 2-minute period has a special significance within the context of an inhibitory theory of performance decrement in psychomotor skills. There is evidence from a number of experiments that under normal conditions reactive inhibition (I_R) first reaches its asymptote of growth after 90 seconds to 2 minutes' massed practice on the pursuit rotor. This upper limit or 'critical level' of I_R is directly related to the positive drive level (D); the higher the motivation, the greater the tolerance for I_R. When $D - I_R = 0$ an involuntary rest pause (I RP) is taken, during which I_R dissipates sufficiently to allow S to resume practice. The reduction of the negative drive I_R also provides reinforcement for a habit of not responding, and conditioned inhibition (${}_SI_R$) thus begins to grow.

In the triple tester situation motivation was undoubtedly high, and considerably higher than during pursuit rotor performance. Therefore, although both depressant drugs increased the inhibitory potential it is quite probable that the critical level of I_R was not reached within the 2-minute practice period. The ensuing 1-minute rest would probably not be long enough to allow all the accumulated I_R to dissipate, but since I_R dissipation is a negatively accelerated function of time the major part would have disappeared before the beginning of the second practice period. In short, the two factors of high motivation and distribution of practice were largely effective in compensating for the increase in inhibitory potential due to the administration of Doriden and meprobamate. A comparison between the triple tester results, and those for the pursuit rotor which will now be reported, supports this general argument, although a further experiment would have to be performed in order to decide which of the two variables is the more effective in counteracting the effects of the drugs, high motivation or distributed practice.

Pursuit rotor results. Fig. 7.3 illustrates the mean performance trends under each of the three experimental conditions. The plotted points represent the percentage of time on target in successive 30-second periods of massed practice throughout the test, which consisted of two 5-minute periods separated by a 10-minute rest interval. Time on target was recorded separately for each 10 seconds of practice time.

It was expected (*a*) that both drugs would cause performance decrements which would be greater towards the end of practice than in the early stages, (*b*) that a significant amount of reminiscence would occur under each of the experimental conditions, and (*c*) that the amount of reminiscence would be the same under all three conditions.

An index of improvement in performance was computed for each S under each of the experimental conditions. This was the difference between mean time on target during the first and the last 2 minutes of practice. A preliminary analysis of the sets of twelve 10-second scores obtained in the first 2 minutes alone showed that, not unexpectedly, there were no differences between treatments at this stage of practice. It also showed that these initial learning scores had very low reliability, due, without doubt, to the fluctuating factor structure of the test in the early stages of learning. Although the initial learning scores, and also

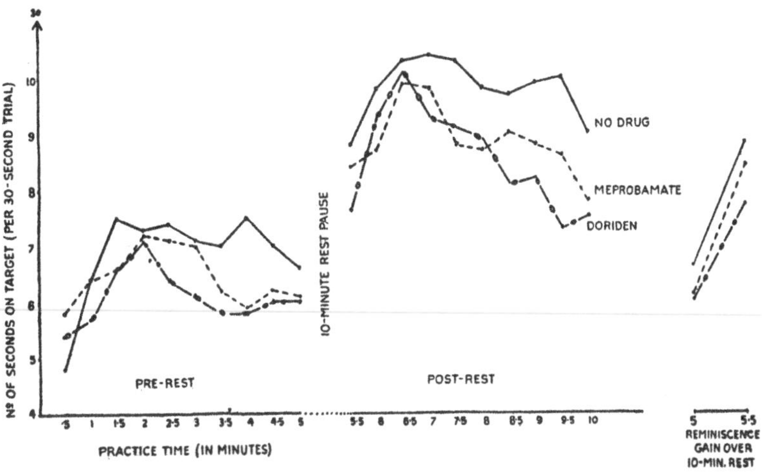

FIG. 7.3. Rotary pursuit performance.

the index of improvement, are therefore of doubtful value from the theoretical point of view, since their heterogeneous factor structure makes it impossible to interpret them meaningfully in terms of specific processes, yet for the purpose of answering practical questions about the effects of Doriden and meprobamate on psychomotor performance their use is quite defensible.

TABLE 7.6

Pursuit rotor index-of-improvement scores: analysis of variance

Source of variance	Sums of squares	d.f.	m.s.v.	*F*-ratio	*p*
Subjects	2557·18	23	111·18	1·14	n.s.
Treatments	518·59	2	259·29	2·67	$p < 0{\cdot}1 > 0{\cdot}05$
Days	931·16	2	465·58	4·80	$p < 0{\cdot}05$
Residual	4270·44	44	97·05		
Total	8277·37	71			

The mean index-of-improvement scores were: No drug, 11·97; meprobamate, 8·18; Doriden, 6·47. The differences between treatments are in the predicted direction, and the results of an analysis of variance, reproduced in Table 7.6, show that although the differences fail to reach the 5% level of significance, they are significant well beyond the 10% level. Since the trend of the obtained differences was as predicted, and as the difference between Doriden and meprobamate was non-significant, a one-tail *t*-test was used to test the no-drug treatment against Doriden and meprobamate combined. The difference between these means was significant at the 5% level. (Correlated $t = 2{\cdot}02, p = 0{\cdot}05$.)

In order to test the prediction that the greatest difference between treatments would occur in the later stages of practice, an analysis of variance was carried out on the scores obtained in the last 2 minutes of practice alone. The mean performance scores again rank themselves in the same order with respect to the experimental treatments, being 39·0 in the no-drug condition, 33·0 under meprobamate, and 31·0 under Doriden. The *F*-ratio for treatments is 4·67, which has a probability value less than 0·05. The full results of the analysis are given in Table 7.7.

TABLE 7.7

Pursuit rotor performance in ninth and tenth minutes of practice: analysis of variance

Source of variance	Sums of squares	d.f.	m.s.v.	*F*-ratio	*p*
Subjects	8802·16	23	382·70	4·79	$p < 0{\cdot}001$
Treatments	745·72	2	372·86	4·67	$p < 0{\cdot}05$
Days	5400·01	2	2700·00	33·80	$p < 0{\cdot}001$
Residual	3515·08	44	79·89		
Total	18,462·97	71			

Although these results show that the administration of 800 mg. of meprobamate or 500 mg. Doriden may cause statistically significant decrements in psychomotor performance in normal Ss, the absolute amount of impairment is still slight, and as the triple tester results indicate, the drug effects may be effectively counteracted by an increase in level of motivation and/or by a work schedule in which practice is distributed rather than massed.

Pursuit rotor reminiscence results. The conventional, uncorrected reminiscence measure was used, i.e. the difference in score between the last pre-rest and the first post-rest trial. As can be seen in Fig. 7·3, performance improved after the 10-minute rest pause under all three experimental conditions, the mean reminiscence scores being +3·05, +2·58, and +2·05 under no drug, meprobamate, and Doriden respectively. In each case the difference between the mean score on the last pre-rest trial and mean score on the first post-rest trial was significant at the 5% level (2-tail *t*-test for correlated measures). This result confirms the first reminiscence prediction. An analysis of variance of the three sets of reminiscence scores confirmed the second prediction, that the amount of reminiscence would not differ significantly under the three treatment conditions. Table 7·8 gives the results of this analysis.

TABLE 7.8

Pursuit rotor reminiscence scores: analysis of variance

Source of variance	Sums of squares	d.f.	m.s.v.	*F*-ratio	*p*
Subjects	20·4679	23	0·8899		n.s.
Treatments	0·4050	2	0·2025		n.s.
Days	2·6961	2	1·3480		n.s.
Residual	51·3664	44	1·170		n.s.
Total	74·9354	71			

Summary of results and conclusions

Some of the implications of the relatively slow rate of absorption of perorally administered drugs were pointed out in the preliminary discussion. Since each of the tests was always performed at the same time relative to the time of administration of the drug (within the limits of a range of variation of approximately 10 minutes), the observed drug effects are therefore a function of the interval between drug- and test-administration, and a different test order might possibly have produced different results. As there is no way of quantitatively assessing the effects of this variable, or potential variable, from the data of the present experiment, it is therefore not possible to compensate for it by statistical manipulation of the data.

However, a comparison of the performance means for each of the four tests under each of the three treatment conditions provides some relevant qualitative information. Mean differences between treatments, although uniformly small, showed a consistent trend in the direction which had been predicted: the no-drug treatment produced the highest mean performance on all tests (with the expected exception of the hand-steadiness test, in which meprobamate yielded the best mean performance); Doriden produced the greatest mean decrement, while meprobamate was intermediate between the other two treatments. This substantial agreement between data collected at intervals ranging from 40 to 130 minutes after drug administration suggests that the influence of drug absorption rates on the obtained test results is quantitative rather than qualitative.

While each of the four tests used in this study gave a set of results which can be legitimately and meaningfully interpreted without reference to the results yielded by the other three tests, nevertheless a much wider degree of generalization, and a fuller evaluation of the effects of the two drugs, is possible when the results of the separate tests are interrelated. When this is done it becomes clear that the absence of significant decrements in some of the tests where decrements were expected does not indicate that the original hypothesis was wrong, but is attributable rather to the effect of interactions between the depressant action of the drugs with other variables in the test situations which tended to compensate or counteract these depressant effects. The specific variables having this compensatory effect were not the same in the various tests. Thus for example in the less complex tests, hand steadiness and auditory vigilance, a comparison between high- and low-neuroticism sub-groups within the experimental sample indicated that the effects of Doriden and meprobamate on performance vary according to S's position on the Neuroticism continuum. In the two complex psychomotor tasks, on the other hand, no direct relationship was found between the drug effects and scores on Neuroticism or on Extraversion. However, when the performance changes which occur under the depressant drug conditions on the pursuit rotor are compared with the corresponding triple tester data it can be seen that the drug effects vary with variations in such test parameters as, for example, degree of monotony of stimulus patterns, or degree of distribution of practice.

In order to gain a more general estimate of the effects of the drugs on psychomotor performance it was therefore decided to combine S's scores on all four tests and to carry out an analysis of variance on the resultant set of composite scores. The standard score equivalents of the following four measures were used: (*a*) the average error score per trial on the hand-steadiness test, with the arithmetical sign reversed; (*b*) the total number of signals detected during the course of the auditory vigilance test; (*c*) the average number of hits per trial on the triple tester; and (*d*) the index-of-improvement score on the pursuit rotor.

TABLE 7.9

Analysis of variance of composite standard scores

Source of variance	Sums of squares	d.f.	m.s.v.	F-ratio	p
Subjects	290·7475	23	12·6412	5·64	$p<0{\cdot}001$
Treatments	16·9718	2	8·4859	3·79	$p<0{\cdot}05$
Days	10·5922	2	5·2961	2·36	
Residual	98·6760	44	2·240		
Total	416·9876	71			

The mean standard scores for treatments were found to be +0·58 in the no-drug condition, +0·02 under meprobamate, and −0·46 under Doriden. The results of the analysis of variance, which are given in Table 7.9, proved these differences to be significant beyond the 5% level. Thus when performance on all the tests is considered together the expected differences between treatment conditions are found to be present, at an acceptable level of statistical significance.

8

THE EFFECTS OF DEPRESSANT DRUGS ON PALMAR SKIN RESISTANCE AND ADAPTATION

Irene Martin

IF palmar skin resistance reflects behavioural arousal, as Duffy has argued (1951, 1957), then it should be affected by central depressant or stimulant drugs. There is no clear evidence on this point (Laties, 1957; Marquis *et al.*, 1957) and the present experiment was therefore carried out to consider the effect which meprobamate and Doriden might have upon a number of measures of skin resistance; the results will be given in this section.

Alterations in skin resistance occur largely as a function of sweat-gland activity, brought about via sympathetic innervation of the autonomic nervous system. As far as is known the two drugs used have no direct effect upon the autonomic nervous system but it is well recognized that this system has functional connections at many levels with the central nervous system, and may, therefore, be affected by central depressant drugs.

As Eysenck (1957a) has pointed out, depressant drugs may be regarded more precisely as potentiating reactive inhibition (I_R) which builds up in time, as, for example, when an individual is making a series of responses to repeated stimuli. Eventually the subject ceases to respond to the stimulus (i.e. has adapted) when inhibition reaches a certain level, but if a period of time is allowed for disinhibition to take place, the response, in the present case the GSR, can be evoked again (Porter, 1938). Habituation then is a simple form of *learning not to respond*, and one in which inhibitory processes play a large part.

It is thus an interesting topic for investigating drug effects. Decreasing responsiveness in time is a commonly observed feature of most successive readings of skin resistance; both of basal skin resistance, which usually shows a steady rise during a period of recording (indicating decreasing arousal, or more precisely decreasing sympathetic nervous system activity), and of the specific short-term changes to stimuli, the GSRs, which are superimposed on the basal readings (Coombs, 1938; Davis, 1930, 1932, 1934; Davis *et al.*, 1955; Duffy and Lacey, 1946; S. B. G. Eysenck, 1956; Mundy-Castle and McKiever, 1953; Seward

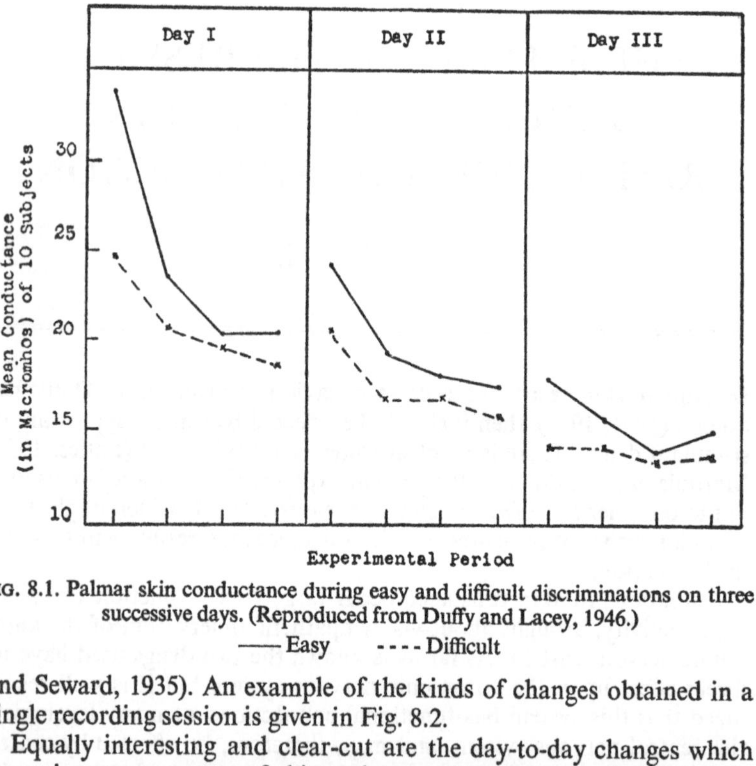

FIG. 8.1. Palmar skin conductance during easy and difficult discriminations on three successive days. (Reproduced from Duffy and Lacey, 1946.)
—— Easy ---- Difficult

and Seward, 1935). An example of the kinds of changes obtained in a single recording session is given in Fig. 8.2.

Equally interesting and clear-cut are the day-to-day changes which occur in measurements of skin resistance. Exposure to stimulation on one day will certainly affect reactions on subsequent days; an example of this can be seen in Fig. 8.1, reproduced from Duffy and Lacey (1946), which clearly shows the day-to-day effect on palmar skin conductance.[1]

These three types of changes, that is (i) basal resistance within a session, (ii) GSRs within a session, and (iii) changes in both over successive days, were investigated in the present experiment, details of which will now be given.

[1] Conductance, being the reciprocal of resistance, is represented in the graph as *declining* with decreasing sympathetic activity.

Method of measurement

Apparent skin resistance was measured continuously over a period of 15 minutes, approximately 1–1½ hours after oral administration of the drug. The psychogalvanometer provided an overall coverage up to 1 megohm, and delivered a very small constant current of 10 μA.

Electrodes were brass, 1″ in diameter, strapped dry to the palms by means of rubber bands (the palms first being cleaned with acetone). Checks with these electrodes in a saline solution over a period of an hour showed that errors due to polarization were smaller than 1 kilohm, a figure well below the minimum measuring unit of 2 kilohms which was adopted.

Since the nature and intensity of the disturbing stimulus is known to exert a significant effect upon adaptation, two types of stimuli were used: the first a series of twenty tones (100 db. 980 c.p.s.) spaced at intervals of 30 seconds, and the second a series of questions (presented at a similar time interval) dealing with the presence of neurotic symptoms within the subject. Subjects received the stimuli through headphones while seated in a sound-proof, dark room, separated from the experimenter and apparatus.

Procedure

After 3 minutes' recording during rest the series of tones was presented to the subject, and followed by a 3-minute relaxation period. At this point the door of the sound-proof room was opened, the earphones were removed, and the subject given a speaking tube to hold so that communication in the next part of the experiment (the series of questions) could be effected from outside the sound-proof room. Subjects were instructed to respond briefly to the questions.

This procedure was repeated on three consecutive days, one day with Doriden, one day with meprobamate, and one day with no drug (see page 107 for a description of the sample and the experimental design).

In summary, the main effects considered in the first place were those arising from (i) the absorption of drugs, and (ii) habituation both throughout a single session and from day to day, upon reactivity measured by skin resistance to two types of stimuli. In a follow-up experiment, using one of the drugs, the effect of different time intervals between stimuli upon rate of adaptation was also investigated.

Temperature, humidity, and time of day

Several studies (reviewed by Venables, 1955) have reported significant relationships of skin resistance to temperature and humidity, and it was necessary to take account of these variables.

Fortunately, it was possible to keep the temperature of the experimental room reasonably constant at 65° F., and the mean temperature did not vary by more than 0·5° F. over the three days. Similarly, there was little variation in humidity measurements, which average 45·5%. These figures are *below* those quoted by Venables (1955) as having an effect on skin resistance.

Time of recording was held constant between 11 a.m. and 12 noon.

Results

The results will be presented in two parts, the first dealing with measurements of skin resistance during tones stimuli, and the second with readings obtained during the questions.

(1) *Tones stimuli*

A large number of readings in kilohms resistance was obtained from each subject on each occasion, and from these untransformed measurements the following variables were derived and submitted to analysis of variance:

(i) mean level of skin resistance for each session,
(ii) an estimate of the slope which these readings of basal resistance might take throughout the series, and indicating a rise or fall in resistance,
(iii) a measure of the curvature which might exist in this slope.

The results of the analyses of variance carried out on these three variables are given in Table 8.1, where it can be seen that Variable (i)

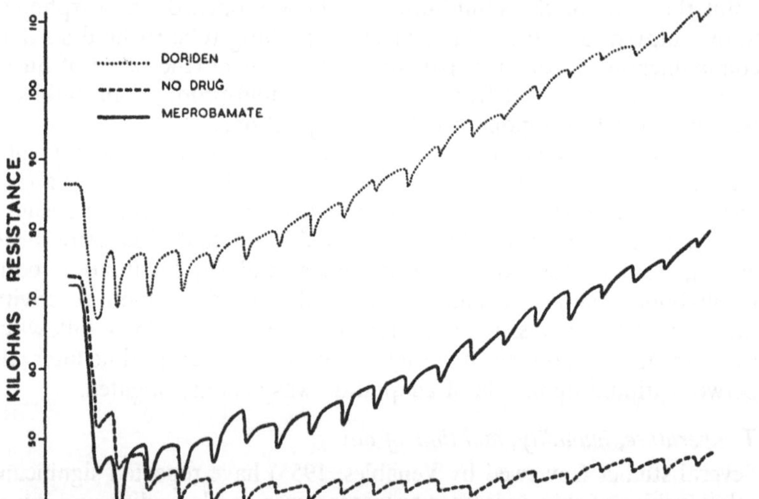

FIG. 8.2. Measurements of palmar skin resistance during twenty tones stimuli under three conditions—Doriden, no-drug, and meprobamate.

has significant *F*-ratios for all three effects, subjects, treatments and order, whereas only order and subject effects are significant for Variable (ii). Non-significant *F*-ratios for all effects were obtained on the estimate of curvature.

TABLE 8.1

Analyses of variance

Tones		d.f.	m.s.v.	*F*
(i) Mean level of skin resistance				
Total observed variation	77,468,977	71		
Observed variation between subjects	53,218,612	23	2,313,853	6·23*
Observed variations between treatments	3,682,820	2	1,841,410	4·96†
Observed variation between days	4,233,316	2	2,116,658	5·70*
Residual variance	16,334,229	44	371,232	
(ii) Estimate of the slope				
Total observed variation	443,053,088	71		
Observed variation between subjects	254,886,510	23	11,082,022	3·12*
Observed variation between treatments	7,622,286	2	3,811,143	1·07
Observed variation between days	24,114,180	2	12,057,090	3·39†
Residual variance	156,430,112	44	3,555,230	
(iii) Estimate of the curvature				
Total observed variation	291,128	71		
Observed variation between subjects	93,146	23	4050	0·95
Observed variation between treatments	3917	2	1958	0·46
Observed variation between days	6514	2	3257	0·76
Residual variance	187,551	44	4262	

* Significant at or beyond 1% level. † Significant at or beyond 5% level.

Table 8·2 gives the actual mean measurements obtained for separate treatments and days, and shows that meprobamate and Doriden alike raise level of skin resistance. The effect of order, which gives rise to significant *F*-ratios for both variables, shows level and slope of skin resistance to be higher on successive days.

If basal skin resistance reflects degree of arousal the results may be interpreted as showing lower levels of arousal under Doriden and meprobamate. Changes within a session (the estimate of slope) are not differentiated by the drugs, although there is a tendency for the slope to be higher under meprobamate, as can be seen in Fig. 8.2, which illustrates the course of skin resistance changes under the different treatments on day 1.

TABLE 8.2

Tones

(i) Mean level of skin resistance for treatments and order. (Units in kilohms resistance; N = 8 in each cell.)

	Days 1	2	3	Totals
Doriden	90·6	85·8	86·7	263·1
No-drug	46·8	78·3	76·7	201·8
meprobamate	61·4	98·6	121·0	281·0
	198·8	262·7	284·4	

(ii) Estimate of the slope of skin resistance for treatment and order. (Units represent average increment in kilohms per 30/seconds; N = 8 in each cell.)

	Days 1	2	3	Totals
Doriden	1·90	1·37	1·60	4·87
No-drug	−0·43	1·70	3·69	4·96
meprobamate	1·35	2·76	3·92	8·03
	2·82	5·83	9·21	

Other measures obtained from the records were the frequency and amplitude of each GSR to the tones. In the past, the problem of how to handle data on GSRs has been vigorously debated, and many suggestions have been made about the best measuring units and statistical techniques to use—for it is universally found that amplitude of GSRs is closely related to level of pre-stimulus skin resistance. (In the present experiment there is a correlation of 0·627 between amplitude of the first GSR on each day and the associated pre-stimulus level.) Yet the variety of transformations which have been suggested have served not only to multiply this problem (see S. B. G. Eysenck, 1956) but also have been shown to be unstable, and, as Lacey (1956) has argued, have no rational basis.

In the present data significant relationships exist not only between basal resistance and amplitude of GSRs but also between other variables; mean basal skin resistance and the slope of resistance throughout the session are related, as are both of these with number of GSRs given in the series. No statistical treatment could be applied to all these variables simultaneously, and since it was not considered useful to submit the GSR data to various elaborate transformations for making responses independent of basal resistance, only two possibilities were left. These were to analyse response measures knowing that they depend heavily upon initial resistance, and to present them in graphical form without reference to statistical significance levels. Both were undertaken.

TABLE 8.3

Analysis of variance

Tones

Skin resistance: stress level

		d.f.	m.s.v.	*F*
Total observed variation	68,486,095	71		
Observed variation between subjects	42,725,488	23	1,857,630	5·16 *
Observed variation between treatments	4,850,246	2	2,425,123	6·74 *
Observed variation between days	5,084,127	2	2,542,063	7·07 *
Residual variance	15,826,234	44	359,687	

* Significant at or beyond 1% level.

An analysis of variance was carried out (see Table 8·3) using a simple measure of responsiveness, namely $x - y$, where x is the basal resistance

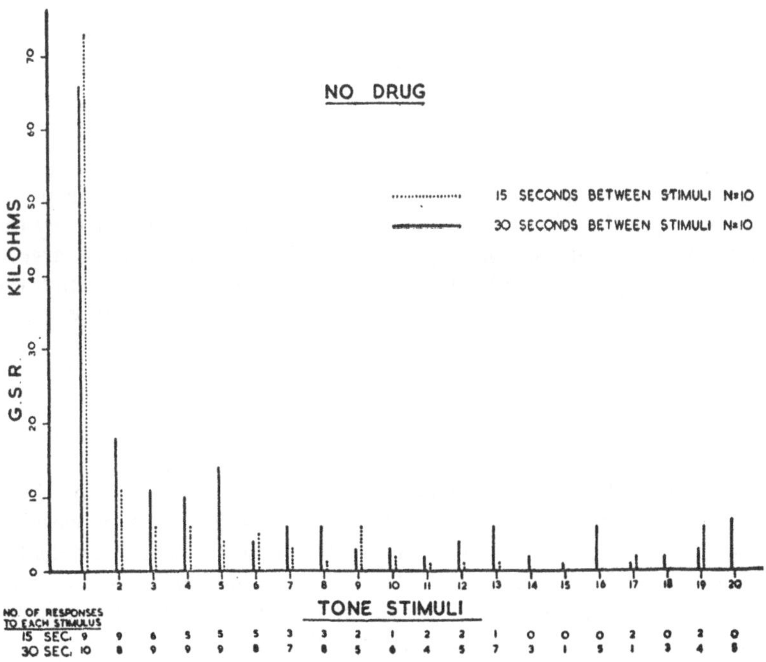

FIG. 8.3. Average amplitude of GSRs to tones with 15- and 30-second intervals.

before a stimulus, and *y* is the minimum resistance recorded to the tone stimulus (the stress level); where no response occurred the basal resistance reading, *x*, remained unchanged. The results of this stress level analysis must be interpreted in the light of its known dependence upon initial level, but nevertheless they are of interest in themselves for they show that all effects—individuals, treatment and order—are highly significant; as would be expected, the stress level, measured in kilohms resistance, reached under no-drug conditions is much lower than that obtained under the two drugs. The significant *F*-ratio for order implies that the effect of the tones is greater on day 1 than on successive days.

The graph indicating the diminishing amplitude of GSRs throughout the 30-second tones stimuli is given in Fig. 8.3; it is in agreement with Coombs' (1938) findings that adaptation of the response proceeds rapidly at first and then slows down. (The figure also shows amplitude of GSRs to the 15-second stimuli used in the second study, to be discussed later in this section.)

On this same topic a factor of great interest was observed, namely an apparently *changing* relationship in time between basal skin resistance and amplitude of the GSR. The positive relationship between size of response and base level was initially high, but it dropped during the series in the following way:

		No. of responses
Stimulus 1	$r = +0{\cdot}627$	72
Stimulus 10	$r = +0{\cdot}409$	35
Stimulus 20	$r = +0{\cdot}099$	28
		(Total no. of Ss = 72)

It appears that resistance usually increases during a session and also that as the series of stimuli progresses the likelihood of a response occurring to the stimulus declines. The first response, evaluated by the subjects as a strong startle response, is in almost every case the largest, and is closely related to background level—when resistance is high the response (in kilohms) appears to be large, and when resistance is low the response is small. Later on in the series the amplitude of the GSR is decreased, and in fact the response may cease to occur at all whatever the resistance level. But GSR adaptation is enhanced when mean resistance is high and when it rises throughout a session, even though it occurs to some extent when basal levels remain steady.

Similar findings have been previously reported: the results of Davis *et al.* (1955) led them to conclude that as tissue resistance is increased so the threshold is raised, and to suggest that under some conditions the local state of skin tissue modulates the response process. To what extent this modulation takes place is of far-reaching significance in the interpretation of this sort of experimental data.

Although *successive* GSRs demonstrate adaptation in terms of lower amplitudes, the *first* GSR in any series seems to represent a simple, strong startle response. This element of startle is very marked in response to the first stimulus on the first day, when the subject has no idea of the nature of the tone stimulus, but it is also present in the responses to the first tone on days 2 and 3, since the period elapsing between days allows a degree of disinhibition to occur. The absolute size of the first GSR is, as has been shown, closely related to preceding basal level; and so a simple percentage ratio was calculated on the first startle responses in order to consider the effect of drugs upon a measure of GSR relatively independent of basal readings. A significant difference was found between the Doriden and no-drug percentage ratios, the responses under Doriden being smaller ($t = 4{\cdot}65$), but there was no significant difference between meprobamate and the no-drug condition.

But even this simple measure of percentage change was used with some misgivings. The basic data are pre- and post-stimulus levels, and Lacey (1956) has convincingly argued, first that computing percentage or algebraic change is a redundant step, and next that correlations between such changes and initial level are extremely difficult to interpret. He has put forward a method for calculating 'autonomic lability scores' which are independent of basal level, and it will be seen later that these were obtained from the data of the second study.

It was stated above that two measures of the GSR were derived from the data, one of amplitude—discussed above—and one simply of

TABLE 8.4

Number of GSRs occurring to tones stimuli
(N = 8 in each cell.) Twenty stimuli per person

	Day 1	2	3	Totals	't'
A. Doriden	85	86	74	245	
					A & B = 4·35†
B. No-drug	128	105	125	358	
					B & C = 4·10†
C. Meprobamate	122	70	53	245	
	335	261	252	848	

† Significant beyond the 1% level.

the frequency of occurrence of a GSR. Under the conditions of the experiment a change of two kilohms or more occurring within the 10-second period following a stimulus was counted as a GSR. The counts obtained are given in Table 8.4. They, too, are affected by the drugs: the total number of responses occurring under Doriden and meprobamate is significantly lower than the total no-drug responses. And again the effect of day-to-day habituation is very clear, as can also be seen in Table 8·4. The greatest drop in responsiveness is from day 1 to day 2; after that the decrease is slight. It would be of interest to establish the nature of the adaptation curve taken over a number of days for, theoretically, conditioned inhibition should be developed in time, so that the response would cease to occur at all.

Summary

(i) The drugs raise level of skin resistance, and reduce the number of GSRs given to tones stimuli.

(ii) The effect of order is highly significant upon practically all the variables.

(iii) Basal skin resistance is greatly reduced by the first stimulus, which induces a strong startle response, but it climbs again throughout the session (see Fig. 8·2).

(iv) An intricate set of relationships was demonstrated between the measures; further, some of these relationships change in time. The most interesting is probably the connection between rate of adaptation and background level of skin resistance.

(2) *Questions stimulus*

Physiologists have deliberately avoided the investigation of palmar sweat gland activity because of the influence of 'psychic' elements on the response. This kind of sensitivity has, on the contrary, made the region of special interest to psychologists, and attempts have been made to relate palmar sweat-gland activity to such things as the 'significance' of verbal stimuli to the individual (hence the use of the technique in lie-detection experiments).

In the present study interest was focused on the degree of reactivity to two quite different types of stimulus, one a series of twenty tones and the second a series of ten questions. The questions, spaced at 30-second intervals in keeping with the presentation of the tones stimuli, were given to the subject after previous instruction to reply with single words—'yes', 'no', 'sometimes', etc. The questions were derived from a neuroticism rating scale described by Eysenck (1947); they were as follows:

(1) Do you frequently feel anxious and worried about things.
(2) Would you describe yourself as an irritable person.
(3) Are you on the whole a sociable person.
(4) Do you often feel depressed.
(5) Are you given to feelings of inferiority.
(6) Do you suffer from insomnia.
(7) Do you suffer from headaches.
(8) Have you always plenty of energy.
(9) Are you inclined to worry about your health.
(10) Do you often feel tense, unable to relax.

The questions always followed the sensory stimuli, a fact which must be remembered in the evaluation of the results. The subjects remained seated, as before; at the completion of the auditory stimuli they were allowed a short rest while the instructions were given. During this period of conversation with the experimenter the skin resistance of practically all subjects dropped by a very great amount and rarely recovered during the questioning period. (The subjects were not told the nature of the questions beforehand.) Many subjects volunteered the information that they were sleepy or relaxed at the end of the auditory stimuli, which had little arousal value late in the series. In almost every case the mean resistance during questioning is very much lower than that obtained during the tones (even when tone means are based on the first twelve readings to make them comparable with the questioning means): indeed, there is so little overlap in the two groups of measurements that significance tests were not applied. Similarly, the slope of the readings is lower during the questions. No doubt the fresh stimuli occurring with the break in the experiment served to arouse the subjects and revive their attention, and it is likely that resistance, once lowered by the interruption, persisted at a low level simply because the subject was thoroughly awakened, and not by virtue of the arousal value of the questions. It is not possible to decide which explanation is true, since the order of the two types of stimuli was fixed: it could have been balanced only by greatly elaborating the experiment.

There are few systematic studies comparing reactions to verbal stimuli with those to sensory stimuli (see Darrow and Solomon, 1934; Hoch, Kubis, and Rouke, 1944; Kubis, 1948; Paintal, 1951; and Jost, Ruilman, Hill, and Gulo, 1952). The most relevant study is by Davis (1934), who compared skin resistance changes over five successive days in response to noise, music and mental work; he found that the size of the reaction became progressively smaller to the noise, remained constant for the mental work and increased to the music.

Changes in the tones and questions measurements from day to day were examined by comparing the *F*-ratios for order, as follows:

	Tones	*Questions*
Mean resistance	$F = 5.70\ (<1\%)$	$F = 6{\cdot}65\ (<1\%)$
Estimate of slope	$F = 3{\cdot}39\ (<5\%)$	$F = 2{\cdot}46$ (n.s.)

These are very similar for both types of stimuli, and obviously a properly balanced experimental design is needed to provide conclusive evidence on this point of differential adaptation rates.

These *F*-ratios, together with those obtained for drug effects on the questions measurements, can also be seen in the analyses of variance in Table 8.5. All main effects are significant for the measure of mean resistance, but none for the estimate of slope.

On this occasion, specific GSRs to each question were not measured; the subject was holding the speaking tube which sometimes gave rise to movement artefacts on the records, particularly about the time of occurrence of the GSR. While basal readings were rarely affected by

TABLE 8.5

Analyses of variance

Questions		d.f.	m.s.v.	*F*
(i) Mean level of skin resistance				
Total observed variation	15,128,309	71		
Observed variation between subjects	9,787,532	23	425,545	5·09*
Observed variation between treatments	551,595	2	275,797	3·30†
Observed variation between days	1,111,107	2	555,553	6·65*
Residual variance	3,678,075	44	83,593	
(ii) Estimate of the slope				
Total observed variation	2,723,847	71		
Observed variation between subjects	1,075,814	23	46,775	1·41
Observed variation between treatments	23,625	2	11,812	0·36
Observed variation between days	163,394	2	81,697	2·46
Residual variance	1,461,014	44	33,205	

* Significant at or beyond 1% level. † Significant at or beyond 5% level.

movement, the GSRs were not always clearly separable from this artefact.

Summary

(i) Mean level of skin resistance during questions is affected by drugs and by order.

(ii) None of the effects was significant upon the estimate of slope.

(iii) Level and slope of skin resistance (in kilohms) were lower during questions than during tones.

THE INTER-RELATIONSHIP OF MEASURES

(1) *Between measures of skin resistance*

This aspect of the data was secondary to the main effects of drugs and order, but as anyone working in this field will recognize, it forms an important problem in the understanding of psychophysiological data.

Relationships were assessed by means of regression analysis, and the outcome is a number of regression coefficients between functions, (i) with all groups combined, and (ii) with each group treated separately and providing a mean *r* within groups. (The groups represent different orders in administering the drugs.) Table 8.6 gives the coefficients obtained between mean resistance and estimate of the slope for each of the three days; only on day 3 are the coefficients significant, and then

TABLE 8.6

Tones

(i) Regression analysis of two variables of skin resistance:
(*a*) mean level of skin resistance and
(*b*) estimate of slope

	r (all groups combined)	*r* (within groups)
Day 1	0·354	0·018
Day 2	0·121	−0·190
Day 3	0·576†	0·530*

(ii) Correlations between number of GSRs given to stimuli and
(*a*) basal level of skin resistance
(*b*) estimate of slope

	All days combined *r*
(*a*) GSRs and basal resistance	−0·500†
(*b*) GSRs and estimate of slope	−0·521†

* Significant at the 5% level. † Significant at the 1% level.

highly so, showing that high mean resistance tends to be associated with a rapidly rising resistance throughout a session. Correlations between these measures and number of GSRs given to stimuli (all subjects combined) are also given in the same table; again the relationship is very

TABLE 8.7

Questions

Regression analysis of two variables of skin resistance:
(*a*) estimate of slope and
(*b*) level of skin resistance

	r (all groups combined)	*r* (within groups)
Day 1	−0·266	−0·268
Day 2	0·381	0·308
Day 3	0·175	0·221

A correlation of 0·406 (all groups combined) is required for significance at the 5% level.

A correlation of 0·456 (within groups) is required for significance at the 5% level.

significant, high mean resistance and steep positive slopes tending to be associated with few GSRs. Apparently in such cases the threshold is raised so that a GSR is *less* likely to occur. Conversely, when resistance and slope are low, a response is *more* likely to occur.

Regression coefficients for the two measures of mean level and slope during the questioning period are given in Table 8.7, but none of these is significant. The small negative correlation on day 1 suggests that subjects with higher resistances tend to become more aroused, rather than relaxed, during the questions. Such a factor, by producing negative slopes, might explain the non-significant effect of the drugs on the measure of slope.

(2) *Between measures of skin resistance and the questionnaires*

As frequently occurs in measurements of skin resistance, the variation between individuals is extremely large, and presumably reflects our lack of knowledge at the present time of factors which should be controlled. How much of the variance is contributed by peripheral and how much by central factors we are hardly in a position to say, although there is evidence that both play a part.

An explanation of individual differences in terms of central excitation/inhibition processes has been proposed by Eysenck (1957a) in connection with his dimension of introversion-extraversion. A questionnaire measuring this dimension and also that of neuroticism was given to all subjects, and scores of extraversion and neuroticism obtained from it. Regression analyses were then carried out between these scores and the various measures of skin resistance, but none of the resulting coefficients was significant.

There are three major findings from this experiment. These are: (i) the drugs significantly increase skin resistance, (ii) the effect of order (adaptation) is highly significant on almost all measures of skin resistance, and (iii) rate of adaptation is dependent upon basal level of skin resistance.

Immediately following this experiment a second was planned, partly to see if the findings would hold with a second sample, and partly to extend our understanding of habituation and drug effects as reflected in measurements of skin resistance.

Certain modifications were incorporated into this second study. The first was the introduction of a new galvanometer.

Apparatus

The new galvanometer consists of a valve voltmeter, the deflections of which are directly proportional to changes in apparent resistance. In this instrument four valves are employed, in two pairs. The 'active' pair comprises a high input resistance cathode follower, D.C. coupled to an output valve; the 'passive' pair is complementary and establishes constant conditions irrespective of supply voltage changes. Considerable negative feed-back is employed, amplification of about only one and a half being required. Calibration resistors are provided to give mid-scale deflections on each of twelve ranges, giving an overall coverage up to

1 megohm.[1] Electrodes were dry, german silver, and strapped to the palms as before; current was 10 μA.

Placebo

A second modification was the use of a placebo. No placebo had been given to the subject on the first study's no-drug day. In the second experiment it was given on every no-drug occasion for both control and experimental subjects.

Experimental aims and design

One matter which seemed to require clarification in the earlier experiment (and one obscured by the design employed there where all subjects received drugs on two out of the three days) was whether the normal course of changes in skin resistance over the days was affected in any way by the drugs. To investigate this point it was necessary to introduce a control group who received *no drugs at all* during the period of the experiment (in this case, two days). The experimental group received a drug on day 1 only. The two groups could then be compared (*a*) for differences due to the drug on day 1, and (*b*) for differences in *amount of change* from day 1 to day 2, when both groups received a placebo. In this way it was possible to consider not only the *immediate* effect of a drug but also its effects upon subsequent measurements.

Only one drug—Doriden—was used on this occasion, and the dosage was increased to 375 mg.

A further factor of importance was the extent to which drug and habituation effects might be altered by using different time intervals between stimuli. Two further groups of subjects were therefore used in an experimental procedure similar to that described above in all respects but one: intervals between stimuli were only 15 seconds instead of 30 seconds. Following the earlier work of Coombs (1938) it was predicted that more rapid adaptation would ensue with the shorter time interval—a result which would also be expected from the idea that reactive inhibition is built up more quickly with massed stimuli.

Subjects were seated in the same sound-proof, dark room, separated from the experimenter and apparatus, as described previously, and stimuli (tones and questions) were applied in the same manner. On this occasion the subjects were all normal women, paid volunteers, with an age range of twenty to forty-five years.

To summarize, the overall design of the experiment was as follows:

(N = 10 in each group)

	30-second intervals			*15-second intervals*	
	Day 1	Day 2		Day 1	Day 2
Group 1:	Placebo	Placebo	*Group 3:*	Placebo	Placebo
Group 2:	Doriden	Placebo	*Group 4:*	Doriden	Placebo

[1] My sincere thanks go to John Curtis who designed and built this instrument.

Temperature and humidity

Mean temperature and humidity were slightly different in the second study, which followed the first and was carried out during the summer months. They were 67·3° F. and 44·5%. There was very little difference in these measures between groups or days, and no overall correlation with basal skin resistance.

Results

Variables derived from the data were of the same kind as those obtained in the first experiment, namely mean resistance level, estimate of slope, and number of GSRs. In addition, autonomic lability scores were calculated (Lacey, 1956).

Effect of Doriden on day 1

The nature of the statistical analysis was rather different since, as can be seen from the design given above, the drug treatment occurs on day 1 only. A form of analysis of variance was therefore used, the scheme of which is outlined in Table 8.8.

TABLE 8.8

General scheme of analysis

Total variance of dependent variable (day 1)	$= Vy$
Total variance of independent variable (day 2)	$= Vx$
Accounted for by dependence on independent variable	$= Wxy^2/Vx$
Residual variance	$= \frac{Vy - Wxy^2}{Vx}$

The procedure is carried out: (1) ignoring known effects, (2) taking known effects (i.e. drug, time interval and interaction between them) into account, and the two residual variances are compared to determine whether the reduction in the size of the residual variance from (1) to (2) is significant.

The first analysis, carried out on mean resistance level during tones, is given in Table 8.9. The overall F is 1·99 which is not significant, showing that all the main effects—drug, time intervals, and interaction of these two—do not significantly affect this measure. The same type of analysis was carried out on three other measures: (i) the slope of resistance during tones, (ii) mean resistance during questions, and (iii) slope of resistance during questions. The Fs obtained were not significant (see Tables 8.9 and 8.10).

Two considerations led to some further probing of these data: the first that the results of the earlier experiment had been clear-cut, and led us to have certain expectations about the direction of the outcome of any subsequent experiment, and secondly that preliminary t-tests on some data of the second experiment had shown that some of these effects

TABLE 8.9

Analyses of variance

Level of skin resistance during tones

		d.f.
Residual variance in day 1—no distinctions	192,991,602	38
Residual variance in day 1—all distinctions (i.e. drug, time interval and interaction)	164,813,261	35 (*a*)
Accounted for by distinctions	28,178,341	3 (*b*)

m.s.v. from (*a*) = 4,708,950

m.s.v. from (*b*) = 9,392,780 $F = \frac{(b)}{(a)} = 1{\cdot}99$ (n.s.)

Slope of skin resistance during tones

Residual variance in day 1—no distinctions	634,428,444	38
Residual variance in day 1—all distinctions	572,700,691	35 (*a*)
Accounted for by distinctions	61,727,753	3 (*b*)

m.s.v. from (*a*) = 16,362,870

m.s.v. from (*b*) = 20,575,918 $F = \frac{(b)}{(a)} = 1{\cdot}49$ (n.s.)

TABLE 8.10

Analyses of variance

Level of skin resistance during questions

		d.f.
Residual variance in day 1—no distinctions	53,674,753	38
Residual variance in day 1—all distinctions (i.e. drug, time interval and interaction)	45,964,882	35 (*a*)
Accounted for by distinctions	7,709,871	3 (*b*)

m.s.v. from (*a*) = 256,996

m.s.v. from (*b*) = 131,328 $F = \frac{(b)}{(a)} = 1{\cdot}957$ (n.s.)

Slope of skin resistance during questions

Residual variance in day 1—no distinctions	15,833,478	38
Residual variance in day 1—all distinctions (i.e. drug, time interval, and interaction)	14,230,722	35 (*a*)
Accounted for by distinctions	1,602,756	3 (*b*)

m.s.v. from (*a*) = 534,252

m.s.v. from (*b*) = 406,592 $F = \frac{(b)}{(a)} = 1{\cdot}314$ (n.s.)

were, by a 1-tail test, of satisfactory significance. A further analysis was therefore made on resistance level during questions between Groups 1 and 3, by breaking down the *F*-ratio so that each effect could be considered separately (see Table 8.11).

Even with this breakdown of the F, neither drug nor interaction effect achieves significance much beyond the 10% level, although both are greater than that of the time interval. The numbers of subjects in each group are unfortunately small, and it is very likely that with larger numbers the differences would reach a higher level of statistical significance.

TABLE 8.11

Analysis of variance: distinguishing treatments

Level of skin resistance during questions

		d.f.
Residual variance accounted for by all distinctions	7,709,871	3
Distinguishing drug: no-drug		
Accounted for by distinction (d_1)	= 3,453,782	1
$F = 2{\cdot}54$ (n.s.)		
Distinguishing 15 seconds: 30 seconds		
Accounted for by distinction (d_2)	= 445,461	1
$F = 0{\cdot}31$ (n.s.)		
Interaction: the drug/time interval		
Total distinctions—$d_1 - d_2$	= 3,810,628	1
$F = 2{\cdot}83$ (n.s.)		

Changes from day 1 to day 2

A series of *t*-tests between day 1 and day 2 readings was carried out, first on all the four groups combined and then on each separately; the results are given in Table 8.12. The overall '*t*'s (i.e. on the four groups combined) are in general rather low, but reach significance at the 5% level for two out of the four measures. Inspection of the separate '*t*'s on each of the four small groups, however, reveals a consistent tendency for the placebo groups to have a greater *increase* in resistance from day 1 to day 2 than the drug groups.

In the case of the placebo groups a definite prediction could be made from all previous work that day 2 measurements would be greater than day 1, and the use of a 1-tail *t* seems justified. With the drug groups it was not possible to predict the direction of day 2 readings, and the 2-tail *t* is therefore appropriate. From Table 8.12 it can be seen that, as before, the effect of order is clear-cut and quite statistically significant for both 30- and 15-second placebo groups, with day 2 readings higher than those of day 1 as expected. This is not so for the drug groups; indeed, the means of day 2 readings for these groups are often lower than those of day 1 (but not significantly so).

While the drug is having its effect there is slightly decreased arousal (increased skin resistance). But the 'learning-not-to-respond' which occurs during a single experimental session and which in the no-drug condition is followed by higher resistance and greater positive slopes on *subsequent days* is demonstrably affected by the drug. In this respect the experimental group is at a disadvantage compared with the no-drug

TABLE 8.12

Table of 't's obtained from mean differences (in kilohms resistance) between day 1 and day 2
(The + and − signs indicate the direction of the differences from day 1 to day 2)

		Level of s.r. during tones	Slope of s.r. during tones	Level of s.r. during questions	Slope of s.r. during questions
No-drug group[1]	Group 1	(+)2·75†	(+)1·70	(+)1·86*	(+)2·65†
	Group 2	(+)2·15*	(+)2·19*	(+)1·50	(+)1·73
Drug groups[2]	Group 3	(−)0·42	(−)0·61	(−)0·02	(−)0·53
	Group 4	(+)1·14	(−)0·76	(+)0·79	(−)1·26
Overall t (all four groups combined)		(+)2·022*	(+)2·168*	(+)1·684	(+)0·996

[1] For Groups 1 and 2 (no-drug groups) it was predicted that the readings would be greater on day 2, and 1-tail t-tests were applied. With d.f. = 9 a t of 1·85 is significant at the 5% level, and a t of 2·262 is significant at the 2·5% level.

[2] No prediction was made concerning Groups 3 and 4, and 2-tail 't's are appropriate. With d.f. = 9 a t of 1·85 is significant at the 10% level, and a t of 2·262 is significant at the 5% level (2-tail test).

* Significant at the 5% level. † Significant at the 2·5% level.

subjects, whose learning on day 1, presumably indicating at least semi-permanent changes within the nervous system, enables them to respond *less* to the general stimulus aspects of the situation on day 2.

Effect of time interval and drugs on GSRs

It was predicted that a 15-second interval would produce more rapid adaptation (fewer GSRs) than a 30-second interval between stimuli. This was found to be so at a high level of significance ($t = 4{\cdot}889$, $p < 0{\cdot}001$). These results support the hypothesis that reactive inhibition builds up more quickly with the shorter time interval between stimuli, thus producing more rapid adaptation. Doriden appears to have no effect on the number of GSRs given by either group on day 1. Three groups (the two placebo and the 15-second experimental) give *fewer* responses on day 2 than on day 1, as expected, but one (30-second experimental) gives the same number. As with basal resistance, there is therefore a tendency for the drug to affect the second day's readings, but only in the 30-second group.

Rate of adaptation in the first study (30-second intervals only) appeared to be related to the mean resistance level; correlations were −0·500 between number of GSRs and basal resistance, and −0·521 between number of GSRs and slope. The corresponding figures in the second study (30-second no-drug group) were −0·306 between responses and level, and −0·485 between responses and slope. But in the 15-second no-drug group lower and non-significant correlations were obtained, namely, −0·147 between responses and level, and −0·169 between responses and slope.

There is no immediate explanation for these different relationships. The whole matter is one requiring more extensive investigation, for in the first experiment *overall* correlations were obtained, which included subjects with and without drugs. Different correlations between rate of adaptation and level of arousal might exist in normal and drug states, and they should be obtained on larger numbers of subjects than the small groups used here if more conclusive evidence is to be obtained.

The relationship of amplitude of GSR with basal level diminished in a very clear-cut way throughout the series of twenty tones in the first study. One of the surprising results of the second was the failure to confirm the diminishing correlation to zero throughout the series. There is a drop in the size of the correlation from +0·88 (N = 80) on the first stimulus to +0·63 (N = 27) on the tenth, but the latter is still significant beyond the 0·01 level. Inspection of the original measurements of the second experiment revealed that about four or five of the subjects were giving very large responses throughout the series of stimuli up to the twentieth, although their basal resistances were high. This was not observed in the earlier set of data, in which only one subject showed a tendency to continue responding in this way.

On this occasion, autonomic lability scores were calculated, following the method proposed by Lacey (1956); the regression equation, derived from the regression of stress level on initial level, enables an individual's GSR to be considered in terms of its deviation from the expected GSR of a group with the same basal resistance, and the resulting measure of change is independent of basal resistance. All groups were combined, and autonomic lability scores obtained from the first GSR given on the first day. Scores of the experimental subjects were compared with those of the placebo group, with the prediction that the response would be smaller during the drug. A *t* of 1·66 was obtained which, on a 1-tail test, was not quite significant at the 5% point (which requires a *t* of 1·73).

Relation of skin resistance measures to personality questionnaires

Regression analyses were carried out between level of skin resistance during tones and questions, and the measurements of extraversion and neuroticism obtained from the questionnaires. Only one correlation reached an acceptable level of statistical significance, namely between level during questions and extraversion (within groups); $r = +0{\cdot}336$, significant at the 5% level. Obviously further support for this is needed in view of the zero correlation obtained between the same measures in the earlier experiment.

Correlations were also computed between the personality measures and autonomic lability scores, but these were found to be non-significant.

In summary, the main findings of the second experiment were as follows:

(i) The effect of Doriden on level of skin resistance was significant at about the 10% level. No effect on number of GSRs was observed.

(ii) Rate of adaptation is much more rapid when intervals between stimuli are short.

(iii) Although Doriden does not greatly affect the measurements on day 1 there is a clear effect on the differences between day 1 and day 2 measurements. Readings (in kilohms resistance) are significantly *higher* in the control group on day 2 than on day 1, whereas they are lower, or the same, in the experimental group.

Discussion

In the first experiment Doriden and meprobamate increased the level of palmar skin resistance and reduced the number of GSRs given to a series of stimuli. Two predictions arising from rather differently oriented theories with different degrees of precision are thus supported: one by Duffy that level of skin resistance reflects degree of behavioural arousal, and one by Eysenck that depressant drugs potentiate inhibitory processes (I_R) such as occur during adaptation. The findings of the second experiment were not so clear in these respects, although all in the predicted direction. (This was probably due to the small numbers of subjects used, and raises the issue, only too well realized, of the regrettably large variances which are encountered in this type of experimental data. The possibility of a placebo effect must also be considered.)

'Theories' of arousal, activation, or energy mobilization, have not reached a highly systematized stage of development, and at the present time are rather loose accounts of certain limited aspects of behaviour, with both behavioural and neurophysiological implications. Behaviourally, the terms denote a continuum ranging from wakefulness to sleep which is measurable, Duffy has argued, in the prevailing levels of autonomic and skeletal muscle activity; the neurophysiological counterpart is studied by recording changes in the electrical activity of the brain before and following stimulation, a technique which has greatly advanced the understanding of the arousal systems of the brain.

In this latter connection the data of Sharpless and Jasper (1956) and Gastaut *et al.* (1957) on changes in electrical 'activation patterns' during repeated stimulation are both interesting and relevant. It seems that all new signals which cause an alerting reaction act on the lower and less differentiated part of the reticular system, producing *generalized* desynchronization of electrical activity which is suppressed after a few repetitions, but that the repeated signal, robbed of its alarm quality, acts on the part which is higher and more specialized, provoking a *localized* desynchronization (Gastaut *et al.*, 1957).

In line with these suggestions it was observed in the skin resistance experiments that the *onset* of a series of stimuli (i.e. the first tone and the introduction of the questions) produced a great drop in the level of skin resistance. These changes apparently reflect the subject's arousal to novel stimuli, and may well arise in some poorly differentiated part of the brain associated with general arousal. Subsequent stimuli produce more moderate reactions until adaptation is complete, at which stage the response ceases to occur. Sharpless and Jasper also observed that electrical activation disappeared from all regions with repetitions of the stimulus.

Interesting though such data are, they have not been integrated with psychological findings into any useful theoretical structure from which specific, purposeful, experiments can be planned. On the other hand, purely behavioural theories such as those of learning are already well developed and expanding; reasonably precise predictions can be made from them, and they provide for the unification of many diverse facts and laws (Eysenck, 1957a).

Unfortunately, psychophysiological research workers have never clearly seen their subject within this sort of behavioural framework, and have tended more often to turn to neurophysiological work for enlightenment. This is in some ways a pity. Psychophysiology obviously cannot ignore the connections with neurophysiology, and it should, moreover, benefit from them. But above all it needs a behavioural framework to provide a more sharply defined purpose if experiments being carried out in this field are to have greater impact on general psychology.

The experiments which have been reported in this section were not originally planned or deduced from learning theory, although it seemed clear that there must be simple connections between adaptation and learning. In summing up the literature and considering the significance of the findings, however, it seemed fruitful to turn to existing behavioural theory, and undoubtedly many of the functions studied in psychophysiology could well be understood in terms of the main concepts employed in learning situations. To illustrate this, if GSR adaptation is explained in terms of increasing reactive inhibition (I_R) then a number of simple hypotheses emerge, some of which were tested in the experiments reported here. One is that I_R builds up more rapidly when stimuli are massed, another that I_R should dissipate in time, both confirmed by the results. Again, extraverts should adapt more quickly (since according to Eysenck (1957a) they build up I_R more rapidly) although experimental data failed to confirm this.

There are, needless to say, individual differences in rate of adaptation; in some subjects with high mean resistance and more rapidly increasing slopes of resistance, the threshold is apparently quickly raised so that only few responses are given. If degree of arousal is adequately measured by palmar skin resistance, then the adaptation process relates to it. But it will be recalled that the original correlation between rate of adaptation and basal skin resistance was obtained on all the subjects combined, i.e. including those with and without drugs. Since the relationship appears to have important theoretic implications it is imperative that it should be more precisely defined. Is it, for example, the same in the drug as in the no-drug state? Is it affected by changing stimulus conditions, e.g. by varying the intensity, or time intervals between stimuli? Further experiments, by providing a clearer understanding of the nature of the relationship, should lead to a more accurate assessment of the influence of basal levels of skin resistance (or arousal) upon the adaptation process.

If the more rapid adaptation of GSRs under depressant drugs is explained *behaviourally* in terms of increasing inhibitory potential, the difficulty arises of explaining, in like terms, the effect of the drugs on basal skin resistance. Both are mediated by the sympathetic division of the autonomic nervous system and vary as a result of sweat gland activity, but each has different time characteristics. Basal resistance changes are slow and gradual, whereas GSRs are relatively quick, with latency and recovery times of only a few seconds. In the latter, inhibitory potential is built up as a result of constant elicitation of the GSR; the former, if increasing resistance can be likened at all to an inhibitory state, is akin to the *generalized* inhibition (or negative drive) associated with subjective feelings of boredom and sleepiness. In this connection Malmo (1958) has suggested that physiological measures such as level of skin resistance may be used to assess amount of drive, and he has suggested that there may be a close connection between the concepts of drive and arousal.

The second experiment carried the investigation of drug effects a step further. The results showed that Doriden taken on day 1 affects the level and slope of skin resistance on day 2. These, when no drug is given, are significantly higher (in kilohms) on day 2; but following Doriden, are the same or slightly lower. The usual interpretation of increasing levels of skin resistance over successive days is in terms of reduced arousal or 'energy mobilization' brought about by greater adjustment to the total situation. Apparently (i) arousal is lower while the drug is having an immediate effect, and (ii) the normal change from day 1 to day 2 is in some way affected by the subject's receiving a depressant drug on day 1.

Whether these findings extend to the GSR data is not clear, since 30-second GSRs were about the same in number on day 2 (following the drug) as on day 1, whereas 15-second GSRs showed the usual decrease. In the case of GSR adaptation the prediction made by Eysenck (1957a, p. 238) could be applied: namely, that if learning takes place while the subject is having a depressant drug he should produce higher reminiscence scores *after an interval* than subjects having a placebo treatment. (The argument is that inhibition builds up more rapidly under the depressant drug and so dissipates to a greater extent during the interval.) It would therefore be expected that Doriden subjects would give *more* responses on the following day than the placebo subjects, and this tendency was, in fact, observed.

Quite clearly, more extensive investigations along these lines are required, with larger numbers of subjects, so that the effect of drugs upon specific factors can be more clearly ascertained. Although there will be obvious difficulties in fitting psychophysiological data into existing behavioural explanations—the role of basal levels of autonomic activity is a case in point—nevertheless the way is clear for the development of a number of precise experimental designs.

Relationship of GSR to pre-stimulus level

To conclude, it is worth while giving some attention to an important matter which has been encountered time and time again in this type of research—the relationship between the amplitude and occurrence of GSRs and pre-stimulus levels. The findings which have just been reported clearly have implications in the search for transformations which partial out effects of basal readings, a search which has hardly touched upon the real problem—that of ascertaining why this relationship holds and under what conditions it changes.

The present results show that relationships between both size of response, its threshold, and basal resistance, change as a function of (i) position of the response in the series, and (ii) time intervals between stimuli. Initially, resistance level is positively and highly related to amplitude of response; as Davis (1930) has pointed out, in cases of initial high resistance there is considerable polarization of cells, and a raised threshold. A stimulus, such as the very loud tone used, which is able to pass the threshold of a large number of cells will produce a reaction of great magnitude and lower the threshold. *As the series of stimuli progresses, however, resistance rises and the threshold is raised; responses are less likely to occur but when they do are smaller in amplitude, and may be only slightly correlated with basal resistance.* Presumably these changes in threshold can occur at both peripheral and central levels.

The importance of reaction threshold was recognized by Hull, who employed the term $_SL_R$ in his system of behaviour, but it has since received little serious attention. The findings of neurophysiological experiments may possibly be used with profit to reinstate this neglected concept of behaviour theory.

9

THE EFFECTS OF DEPRESSANT DRUGS ON REACTION TIMES AND 'SET'

Irene Martin

A GREAT deal of work has been carried out in the past on the human reaction time, but in spite of this there are a great many aspects of it which have received little attention, and about which no clearcut evidence is available. The effect of drugs upon reaction time is one of them.

There are two important reasons for considering drug effects on RT. The first is the application of such information to everyday matters where speed of reaction plays a significant part. The second concerns the general task of investigating the type and nature of drug effects, and in this context the study of RT should prove useful; for it is basically a very simple function which can be elaborated in many ways to increase the role of central processes (as, for example, in the choice RT).

There has been no systematic analysis of drug effects upon specific measures of RT in any single set of experiments; unfortunately, those reported in the literature deal with diverse chemical agents under a variety of RT situations (e.g. Abramson *et al.*, 1955; Cheney, 1936; see also Teichner, 1954, and Woodworth and Schlosberg, 1954, for references to this work). Moreover, as Teichner points out, many of the earlier studies did not have the advantages of modern statistical procedures, and so are difficult to evaluate.

The measure of reaction time obtained in the present study was that of pressing a telegraph key with the preferred hand upon hearing the signal to respond (a 70 db. 1000 c.p.s. tone) which was presented through headphones. Two drugs, Doriden and meprobamate, were used, in the experimental design given on page 107. A preparatory signal (a quiet tone) was always given before the signal to respond. The preparatory period, or foreperiod of reaction as it is known, was regular in the first series of stimuli and irregular in the second series, as follows:

Series (i): RTs were obtained to twenty tones which were regularly preceded by a warning tone at an interval of 3 seconds.

Series (ii): The twenty signal-to-respond tones were preceded by a warning tone at a time interval which varied from 3 seconds to 18 seconds.

In both conditions a period of about 15 seconds elapsed between the subject's response and the presentation of the next preparatory tone.

The two types of series were used since it is known that a short and uniform foreperiod permits greater readiness to react than longer, irregular, intervals. In the former case, the subject could adopt a 'set' to respond which might to some extent counteract the depressing effect of the drug, but when the time interval between warning and response signals is long it is conceivably more difficult for him to maintain vigilance under a depressant drug.

Two measurements were obtained from the regular RT data for each subject. The first was the mean of twenty readings, and the second was an estimate of the slope which these readings followed, indicating either improving or deteriorating performance in time. Only the mean RT, and not the estimate of slope, was obtained from the irregular RT data, since in this series successive RTs varied more as a function of the length of the preparatory intervals than of their numerical position in the series.

(i) *Mean reaction times*

The mean reaction time in the irregular series was found to be significantly larger than that in the regular series, as would be expected (see Table 9.1). Reaction times during both regular and irregular series are lengthened by Doriden, but are apparently unaffected by meprobamate.

TABLE 9.1

Mean reaction times in seconds under Doriden, Meprobamate, and no drug during (i) regular series, and (ii) irregular series

	Doriden	Meprobamate	No drug
Regular	0·197	0·183	0·186
Irregular	0·243	0·222	0·229
Differences between means	0·046*	0·039*	0·043*

* $p < 0{\cdot}001$.

Analyses of variance were carried out on these data, and the results are given in Table 9.2. As far as the drugs are concerned there is a significant effect only during the irregular presentation under Doriden. Order effects (i.e. performance over successive days) are not significant, which suggests that there is little practice or learning effect under the conditions of this experiment. It was clear from the raw data that subjects differed greatly in their mean reaction times, a factor reflected in the significant between subject variances in both analyses.

TABLE 9.2

(i) Mean RT—regular series

	N	S. sqrs.	m.s.v.	*F*	
Between subjects	23	261,917·78	11,387·7296	4·2878*	
treatments	2	10,385·86	5,192·9300	1·9553	n.s.
order	2	253·86	126·93	0·0478	n.s.
Residual	44	116,856·95	2,655·8398		
Total	71	389,414·45			

(ii) Mean RT—irregular series

	N	S. sqrs.	m.s.v.	*F*
Between subjects	23	213,499·32	9,282·5791	3·1450*
treatment	2	21,001·20	10,500·6000	3·5577†
order	2	16,604·78	8,302·3900	2·8129
Residual	44	129,867·36	2,951·5309	
Total	71	380,972·66		

* Significant at or beyond 1% level † Significant at or beyond 5% level

(ii) *Slope of reaction times*

An estimate of the slope of the readings during the regular series was calculated to investigate the possibility of differential performance under drugs and no drug, on the expectation that performance might deteriorate more rapidly under the drugs. In fact, the mean slopes all show a downward trend with respect to time, indicating improved performance (lowered reaction times) throughout the series under both drugs and no drug. Approximately sixteen subjects in each of the three groups improve, while the remainder show a poorer performance in time; the order of the improvement from beginning to end of the twenty responses is about 0·02 second. The slopes obtained under the different treatments do not, however, differ significantly from each other.

It is always possible that greater differences would have been obtained had the series continued longer, for as Eysenck (1957a) has argued, the effects of an inhibitory drug are likely to be more pronounced later in the series, when level of inhibition is high, than early in the series, when inhibition has had little chance to develop.

Discussion

There are three clear findings from this experiment. The first, that RTs are longer in a series with irregular preparatory periods, confirms many previous observations to the effect that RT increases when it is difficult for the subject to maintain an 'expectant' attitude, as with variable preparatory intervals prior to response.

The second is that meprobamate has no deleterious effect on RT; its means are almost identical with no-drug means, and in fact are very slightly superior to them. As meprobamate is believed to reduce muscular tension it can be assumed either that its effect was negligible in this case, or that it lowered tension but to a degree where performance is not impaired.

Third, Doriden lengthens RTs, although only in the irregular series is the effect statistically significant. Thus the attitude of vigilance is apparently impaired to a greater extent by the drug than the straightforward response as such. It is interesting to note that Doriden also depresses performance on a similar task (see Fig. 7.2, page 171) where the subject also has to respond to irregularly presented signals.

Woodworth and Schlosberg (1954) have discussed in detail the time consumed by receptor, effector, and central processes in reaction time, and their conclusion is that at least half of the auditory RT is required for brain processes. It seems likely that Doriden lowers simple RT by virtue of its effect upon central mechanisms, and that its more significant effect upon the irregular series is brought about by the greater importance of the central process in this type of reaction.

Obviously such limited data do not invite firm conclusions; neither can they be interpreted in the light of the earlier, unintegrated, findings reported in the literature. As they stand they simply suggest that Doriden has a greater effect in the traditional RT experiment when the subject is less well prepared for reaction. The absolute RTs are, however, very slightly longer under the drug, and from the applied viewpoint would matter only in tasks requiring a very high degree of precision.

10

THE CLASSIFICATION OF DRUGS ACCORDING TO THEIR BEHAVIOURAL EFFECTS: A NEW METHOD

H. J. Eysenck and S. B. G. Eysenck

PSYCHOPHARMACOLOGY is a branch of science which studies the behavioural effects of drugs. It is not primarily concerned with the *chemical* properties of the drugs in question, or the *site of action* of the drugs, or the complex *physiological* and *endocrinological* consequences of their administration. No doubt in due course it will be possible to unify the knowledge gained of the effects of drugs by pharmacologists, physiologists, biochemists, and psychologists, but at the present time such a unification appears very far off indeed, and it is clear that psychopharmacology cannot expect very much help from other disciplines. To say this is not to imply that we should neglect the established facts of other sciences; it is merely to remind ourselves that behavioural effects of drugs have to be studied empirically and cannot be predicted at present from physiological or biochemical principles.

In reviewing the field of psychopharmacology, Trouton and Eysenck (1960) found very little in the way of established facts as far as the organization of this field is concerned; they also failed to discover any signs of a suitable methodology for achieving such an end. Most writers and experimenters appeared to be content with very rough and ready classifications which often hark back to hypothetical physiological consequences; there is little agreement even on the use of terms, and in view of the lack of a general theoretical framework few deductions can be made which in their turn could mediate the experimental verification or rejection of such general theories. The literature consists almost entirely of empirical accounts of the effects of a given dose of a given drug X when applied to a given population Y under a set of conditions Z; even when the minimum experimental demands are met, such as the use of a double blind procedure (both experimenter and subject ignorant of whether drug or placebo is applied on any given occasion), this paradigm does not admit of any clear-cut interpretation of the results. This is quite obvious when we consider the make-up of the score which constitutes the dependent variable in the experiment. As Trouton and Eysenck have pointed out, the score on a psychological test is not univocal, but nearly always multidimensional, i.e. it is determined not by one ability or trait, but by several. A change in the score can therefore be produced by a given drug acting on any one or any combination of these constituent abilities; a knowledge of a change in score tells us nothing in itself of the causal relationships involved.

The same is true when we consider the definition of psychological concepts in terms of psychological theory. Suppose that we were to find that a given CNS depressant drug could be demonstrated to have a deleterious effect on the number of conditioned responses produced by a subject; this empirical finding could be interpreted either in terms of a lowering of the subject's ${}_{S}H_{R}$, or in terms of an increase in the subject's I_R, or perhaps a combination of the two. It would require a specially designed and theoretically oriented experiment to decide which of these alternatives was the correct one. Other alternatives, of course, also have to be considered; thus the action of the drug might be on D (Drive) rather than on H or I. The straight-forward empirical approach so widely favoured in psychopharmacology at the moment must therefore be recognized to have very severe limitations; here, as elsewhere in science, it is necessary to remember the words of Pasteur: 'Without theory, practice is but routine born of habit. Theory alone can bring forth and develop the spirit of invention.'

The papers in this section have attempted to test a number of deductions made from a theory advanced by one of us; and it will be conceded that, for the greater part, these deductions have been verified. However, this application of the hypothetico-deductive method cannot by itself answer certain questions and certain problems which arise in the classification of drugs. The reader will have seen that a so-called hypnotic drug (Doriden), and a so-called tranquillizing drug (meprobamate), have both been shown experimentally to have effects which could be expected from *depressant* drugs. Does this mean that there are three groups of drugs, i.e. hypnotics, tranquillizers, and depressants, or does it mean that there is one group of drugs, namely depressants, members of which may on occasion be given other names for a variety of practical and psychologically irrelevant reasons? If we were to postulate that both Doriden and meprobamate are in fact depressant drugs, how would we go about verifying or disproving such an hypothesis in as rigorous a manner as modern experimental and statistical method allows us? It is this type of question which the present chapter seeks to answer.

The method suggested here derives fundamentally from Fisher's 'discriminant function analysis', particularly that generalized form of it which goes by the name of 'canonical variate analysis'. A detailed discussion of this is given in the last part of this book (see Vol. 2), and consequently only a brief verbal description will here be given.

The first users of this method in psychology have all been concerned with a problem which, in some ways, is rather similar to the one posed here. If we have groups of normals, neurotics, and psychotics, and if all these have been submitted to a battery of personality tests which discriminate adequately between them, can we use these scores to answer a very important psychiatric question, namely that of the relative position of these three groups? In other words, do normals, neurotics, and psychotics lie along one single dimension, with neurotics, as it were, less ill psychotics, and psychotics more seriously ill neurotics, or do we require two dimensions, i.e. one of neuroticism and one of psychoticism, to deal with the test performance of these subjects? What canonical variate analysis does in this situation is essentially this. It first of all combines all the scores obtained from our subjects in such a manner as to maximize the differences between the groups; in this way we obtain our first latent vector and its associated latent root. The method then goes on to extract another combination of scores *uncorrelated* with the first, and giving us the (residual) optimum differentiation between the three groups; this gives us the second latent vector and its associated latent root. If the three groups lie along one dimension, then a test of significance applied to the second latent root would show it to be insignificant; in other words, all the differentiating power of the tests is accounted for in terms of the first vector. If, however, two dimensions are involved, then this is shown by the fact that the significance test reveals the second latent root to have a p-value smaller than 0·05 (Eysenck, 1957a).

Precisely similar reasoning can be brought to bear on the effects of drugs. Let us propose formally the hypothesis that both meprobamate and Doriden are CNS depressant drugs, i.e. that they differ from each other *only* in the strength of the effect produced, and not in the direction. We can test this hypothesis by experimentally creating three groups of subjects, i.e. those tested under Doriden, those tested under meprobamate and those tested under placebo or no-drug conditions. It would be possible to have different people in these three groups, and if tests were used scores on which changed considerably due to practice or learning, this would be the only experimental design open to us. However, in view of the great individual differences on test scores even under no-drug conditions, this design would be extremely wasteful and would require very large numbers of subjects; consequently a design seems preferable in which the three groups are made up of the same people tested under the three conditions in question. This, of course, is the design used throughout this chapter, and we can make use of the data reported to carry out our analysis.

This analysis is exactly analogous to that described in the case of our psychiatric classification problem. We have three groups (no drug, Doriden, meprobamate), and five tests, which have been applied under all three conditions; we can now calculate the latent vectors and the latent roots and assess their significance. Our hypothesis would be verified if the first root, but not the second, were to be significant at an acceptable level; our hypothesis would be infirmed if neither or both roots happened to be significant at the selected level.

Five tests were chosen from the total battery, the choice depending upon the total effectiveness of the test separating the groups, and on the necessity of maintaining experimental independence between the tests. Details of these tests have already been given on the previous pages, which also contain sufficient information about methods of scoring and direction of scoring to make repetition unnecessary. The results of the canonical variate analysis are shown in Table 10.1. It will be seen that

TABLE 10.1

Latent vectors

	X_1	X_2
1. Nonsense syllable learning	−0·040971	−0·014399
2. Reaction times	−0·013625	−0·161517
3. Level of skin resistance	−0·080835	−0·013827
4. Flicker fusion	1·000000	1·000000
5. Perimeter threshold difference	−0·475330	0·147773

Latent roots

$\lambda_1 = 0{\cdot}453220 = 90{\cdot}03\%$ $\qquad$ $\lambda_2 = 0{\cdot}050205 = 9{\cdot}97\%$

Diagonal entries of matrix $G^{-1}B = 0{\cdot}503425$

Significance of roots

$$R_1^2 = \lambda_1 : X^2 = 40{\cdot}446 : P < 0{\cdot}001$$
$$R_2^2 = \lambda_2 : X^2 = 3{\cdot}450 : \text{n.s.}$$

the first of the latent roots is significant at the 0·001 level, whereas the second latent root fails to be significant even at the 5% level. The results therefore bear out the hypothesis and show that both meprobamate and Doriden are depressant drugs, and do not differ from each other in mode of action. (The term 'mode of action' does not, of course, refer to the biochemical and physiological type of action, but simply signifies the behavioural effects of these drugs.)

Scores were computed for each subject on both canonical variates in the following manner. The latent vectors gave two sets of weights to apply to the scores obtained from the tests, so that two measures could be calculated for each subject, one for each canonical variate. These scores, Y_1 and Y_2, were obtained by multiplying the score of the subject on the tests by the appropriate weights, and summing them over the five tests. The means of these scores are given in Table 10.2. These

TABLE 10.2

Mean group scores $\left(\bar{Y} = \frac{\Sigma W_1 Y}{N}\right)$

C	$\bar{Y}_1 = 6{\cdot}030$ $\bar{Y}_2 = 8{\cdot}622$
M	$\bar{Y}_1 = 3{\cdot}873$ $\bar{Y}_2 = 9{\cdot}047$
D	$\bar{Y}_1 = 2{\cdot}989$ $\bar{Y}_2 = 8{\cdot}485$

scores enable us to calculate what, by analogy with the psychiatric classifications problems, we may perhaps call the percentile of correct classification, i.e. given that we only knew the canonical variate scores of a person, could we correctly identify him as a person who had been tested under no-drug condition, under meprobamate or under Doriden? The method used is one originally suggested by Maxwell, and the results are shown in Table 10.3; it will be seen that over 70% of accurate

TABLE 10.3

	C	M	D
C	**20**	6	1
M	1	**14**	6
D	3	4	**17**
T	24	24	24

70·8% correct classification

classifications could be made under these conditions, which is a remarkable achievement considering (*a*) the very slight amount of drug administered, and (*b*) the fact that both drugs had the same effect, and were only differentiated from the point of view of the strength of the effect. (Nearly all the discrimination is of course contributed by Y_1; Y_2 might have been omitted without much change in the number of misclassifications.)

Before turning to some further experimental results, it may be useful to discuss briefly the consequences of the statistical results reported so far. In the first place, it is suggested that we have here the beginnings of a truly scientific system of classification of drugs. The experiment reported, of course, is but a very small beginning; only two drugs, five tests, and twenty-four subjects were employed in it. This, however, does not detract from the general value of the method itself, which could easily be applied to much larger groups of drugs, subjects, and tests. In particular, it would be extremely interesting to include so-called stimulant as well as so-called depressant drugs to determine whether the unidimensionality of results could still be maintained. Furthermore, many other tests suggest themselves as being worthy of inclusion, and just as we can assess classificatory properties of the drug in terms of the test results, so we would then be able to *assess the psychological significance of each test in terms of the displacement of scores on the test by sets of drugs found to be homogeneous in their action.* In the particular case of stimulant and depressant drugs, we would also be able to test the classification of drugs in terms of tests by comparing the results with those of testing typically extraverted and introverted groups. In this way we would treat change in test score as the dependent variable, and drugs on the one hand, and selection of extraverted or introverted subjects on the other, as the independent variable.

It is necessary, however, to insert one word of caution at this point. If a latent root derived from the analysis of a given set of test scores is significant, then it is clear that the dimensionality of the universe in question cannot be less than that indicated by the number of significant roots, although it may be greater. (Thus in the psychiatric example mentioned earlier, another dimension additional to that of neuroticism and psychoticism, e.g. extraversion-introversion, might be involved, but could not be discovered by statistical analysis unless the groups were further subdivided, e.g. into hysterics and anxiety states, etc. In this way the canonical variate analysis is inferior to factor analysis by only enabling us to test the significance of specific hypotheses which are embodied in the choice of groups and tests; factor analysis, although it has other shortcomings, is not so restricted.)

When, however, one or more of the latent roots are found to be insignificant, it does not necessarily follow that no significant differences exist between groups. A faulty choice of tests may give the impression of lack of difference, when a suitable choice of tests might have given quite different results. There is no possibility of guarding against this, and particularly at the beginning of the study of such a vast field as this it is almost certain that choice of tests will be relatively haphazard, and erroneous conclusions may easily be drawn. In the present case, for instance, it is possible that if reports of subjective feelings had been included as one of the tests, then a significant second root might have been established. (It will be remembered that subjects taking meprobamate reported no after-effects, while those taking Doriden reported feelings of sleepiness, etc.)

The solution to this problem is twofold. In the first place, growth of knowledge and increase in the number of properly conceived and executed studies in this field will undoubtedly soon help us to cut down drastically the number of errors of this kind, and will help us to design batteries of tests which will cover the whole field more completely than is possible at present.

The second solution to the problem harks back to the words of Pasteur, quoted previously. What is required more than anything, in our opinion, is the creation of a firm set of theories and hypotheses linking psychopharmacology with general and experimental psychology. It is by testing, confirming, revising and improving theories of this kind that we must hope that improvement in the present unsatisfactory situation will ultimately come. Such has been the development of most scientific subjects, and it is difficult to see why psychology should be an exception to this rule.

We may now turn to some other results from this analysis which may be of interest. One obvious question which has often been raised, although few experiments have been carried out relevant to it, is that of the existence of individual differences in susceptibility to drug-taking. Most workers in this field have found that the same amount of drug may have a much greater effect on one person than on another, and there has been a considerable amount of speculation on the specificity or generality of this effect, and on possible personality correlates. The lack of reliability of change scores on any one test makes it unlikely that information on this point could be gained easily by the usual methods (cf. however the chapter by H. C. Holland), but the canonical variate scores, calculated by the optimal summation of five different tests, may increase reliability to such an extent that a correlational analysis may become possible. In the first instance, therefore, two columns were calculated, giving respectively for each of the twenty-four subjects the change from control to meprobamate condition, and secondly the change from control to Doriden condition. The correlation between these two columns is highly significant, even for the small number of subjects, and amounts to +0·58; this indicates that those subjects whose scores are changed markedly by the administration of one drug also have their scores changed markedly by the administration of the other drug; conversely, subjects whose scores are only changed slightly by one drug also have their scores changed only slightly by the administration of the other drug.

In view of the fact that the two 'change' columns are correlated reasonably well, we may add them together to obtain an *optimum estimate* of the degree to which subjects are affected by the drugs used in our study. This new 'change' column may now be correlated with the extraversion and neuroticism scores obtained from the same subjects on the Maudsley Personality Inventory; this would indicate whether or not there was any tendency for susceptibility to drugs to be correlated with these personality factors. The correlation of the change score with extraversion was positive and almost significant ($r = +0{\cdot}32$); that with neuroticism was insignificant but also positive ($r = +0{\cdot}18$). (With twenty-four subjects, a correlation would have to be 0·396 in order to be significant at the 5% level.)

In view of the small number of cases involved, and in view of the not very high reliability of the change column, it is not surprising to find that these figures are not significant, and quite clearly speculation regarding their meaning would better be postponed until a repeat study had demonstrated that at least the first of the two correlations could be duplicated experimentally. It is, however, of interest to note that Lasagna *et al.* (1954), in their study of placebo responses, found that those subjects most given to showing psychological effects after placebo administration, tended to be of the extraverted and neurotic type of personality. This, at least, is the writer's impression of the personality description given by them of the placebo reactor; to give the reader an opportunity of judging for himself, this personality description is quoted here: 'They are individuals who seem more dependent on outside stimulation than on their own mental processes. These processes tend to be less mature than in the case of the non-reactors. The reactors are in general individuals whose instinctual needs are greater and whose control over the social expression of these needs is less strongly defined and developed than in the non-reactors. While more anxious and dependent, the fact that they are also more labile and outwardly oriented may enable them to relieve this anxiety and tension more easily than the non-reactors. Over a period of time they may appear less anxious by reason of their ability to, as it were, "drain off the tension". The finding in the interviews of more "talkers" in the reactor group is probably the expression of one such mechanism. . . . We find that the non-reactors as a group do not by contrast present a "normal" picture. While showing less deviation from the normal than the reactors, they are far more rigid and emotionally controlled than the "average" for their age and background.'

Another more recent study by Shagass and Lipowski (1958) is even more relevant in this connection. These authors studied the effect of methedrine on critical flicker fusion in groups of hysterics, mixed neurotics and dysthymics. Defining CFF as 'that rate of successive light flashes from a stationary light source at which the sensation of flicker disappears and light becomes "steady"', they measured the change in CFF 10 minutes after injection of the drug. This change in dysthymics was −0·5; in the mixed neurotics it was 2·0; and the hysterics 3·8. The maximal change in their three groups was −0·2, in the mixed neurotics it was 1·5, and in the hysterics it was 4·5. Differences were statistically significant and demonstrated that the most extraverted group (hysterics) reacted most to the drug, while the most introverted group (dysthymics) reacted least to the drug. These results are therefore in agreement with our own in suggesting greater drug effects for extraverted groups. No obvious theoretical explanation suggests itself, and of course generality of this fact still remains to be established with other types of drugs and other types of reactions.

Summary and conclusions

In this section, an attempt has been made to introduce the method of canonical variate analysis for the purpose of testing certain psycho-pharmacological hypotheses. It has been shown that the behavioural effects of meprobamate and Doriden, a tranquillizer and a hypnotic respectively, are *identical* in so far as results from five selected tests are concerned; these effects are those predicted, on the basis that both drugs are CNS depressants. Susceptibility to these drugs appeared to be a constant personality feature, and correlations of this susceptibility with Extraversion and Neuroticism were found, although not at a statistically significant level of confidence.

BIBLIOGRAPHY AND AUTHOR INDEX

Numbers in italic type at the end of each entry refer to the page on which the reference is quoted.

ABBAS, T. M. Clinical trial of Glutethimide in labour. *Brit. Med. J.*, 1957, (1), 563–5. *107, 139.*

ABNEY, W. W. The sensitiveness of the retina to light and colour. *Phil. Trans. Roy. Soc.*, 1897, 190a, 155–95. *147.*

ABRAMSON, H. A., JARVIK, D. & HIRSCH, M. W. Lysergic acid diethylamide (LSD 25): X. Effect on RT to auditory and visual stimuli. *J. Psychol.*, 1955, 40, 39–52. *221.*

ALLARD, R. W. The analysis of genetic-environmental interactions by means of diallel crosses. *Genetics*, 1956, 41, 305–18. *101.*

ALPERN, M., & SPENCER, R. W. Variations of critical flicker frequency in the nasal visual field. *A.M.A. Arch. Ophthalm.*, 1953, 50, 50–63. *147.*

AMIN, A., CHAI, C. K., & REINEKE, E. P. Differences in thyroid activity of several strains of mice and F_1 hybrids. *Amer. J. Physiol.*, 1957, 191, 34–36. *7.*

AMSEL, A. The role of frustrative nonreward in noncontinuous reward situations. *Psychol. Bull.*, 1958, 55, 102–19. *39.*

ANDERSON, E. E., & ANDERSON, SARAH F. The sex hormones and emotional behavior: II. The influence of the female sex hormone upon timidity in female rats. *J. genet. Psychol.*, 1940, 56, 159–68. *39.*

ANDERSON, O. D. The spontaneous neuro-muscular activity of various pure breeds of dog and inter breed hybrids of the first and second generation. *Amer. J. Physiol.*, 1939, 126, 422–23. *11.*

ANDERSON, O. D. The role of the glands of internal secretion in the production of behavioral types in the dog. In Stockard, C. R. *The genetic and endocrinic basis for differences in form and behavior*. Philadelphia: Wistar Inst., 1941. Pp. 647–747. *11.*

ANICHKOV, S. V. Farmakologica Uslovnjkh Reflekov (The pharmacology of conditioned reflexes). *Fiziol Zh. S.S.S.R.*, 1952, 38, 3–12.

ARMSTRONG, E. A. *The folklore of birds: An enquiry into the origin and distribution of some magico-religious traditions.* London: Collins, 1958. *37.*

BAGG, H. J. Individual differences and family resemblances in animal behavior. *Amer. Naturalist*, 1916, 50, 222–36. *5.*

BAGG, H. J. Individual differences and family resemblances in behavior: A study of habit formation in various strains of mice. *Arch. of Psychol.*, 1920, No. 43, 1–58. *5.*

BAKAN, P. Extraversion-introversion and improvement in an auditory vigilance task. *Brit. J. Psychol.*, 1959, 50, 325–32. *166, 169, 172.*

BAKER, C. H. Biasing Attention to Visual Displays. *M.R.C. Appl. Psychol. Res. Unit Report*, 1956, No. 277. *165.*

BANE, A. Studies on monozygous cattle twins: XV. Sexual functions of bulls in relation to heredity, rearing intensity and somatic conditions. *Acta agric. scand.*, 1954, 4, 95–208. *11.*

BARLOW, H. B. Intrinsic noise of cones. *Nat. Phys. Lab. Report*, 1957, No. 28. *158.*

BARNETT, S. A. Behaviour components in the feeding of wild and laboratory rats. *Behaviour*, 1956, 9, 24–43. *21*.

BARNETT, S. A. Exploratory behaviour. *Brit. J. Psychol.*, 1958, 49, 289–310. *21*.

BASOWITZ, H., KORCHIN, S. J., & OKEN, D. The evocation of anxiety and performance changes under minimal doses of adrenalin. *Amer. Psychologist*, 1955, 10, 388 (Abstract). *174*.

BASTOCK, MARGARET. A gene mutation which changes a behavior pattern. *Evolution*, 1956, 10, 421–39. *10*.

BASTOCK, MARGARET, & MANNING, A. The courtship of *Drosphila. Melanogaster. Behaviour*, 1955, 8, 85–112. *10*.

BAUER, F. J. Genetic and experiential factors affecting social reactions in male mice. *J. comp. physiol. Psychol.*, 1956, 49, 359–64. *8*.

BENDER, M. B., & TEUBER, H. L. Ring scotoma and tubular fields: their significance in cases of head injury. *A.M.A. Arch. Neurol. Psychiat.*, 1946, 56, 300–26. *140*.

BENDIG, A. W., & BRAUN, H. W. The influence of the genotype on the retention of a maze habit in the rat following electroshock convulsions. *J. comp. physiol. Psychol.*, 1951, 44, 112–17. *9*.

BERGER, F. M. Meprobamate, its pharmacological properties and clinical uses. *Int. Rec. Med. Gen. Pract. Clinics*, 1956, 169, 184–96. *107, 138, 139, 152*.

BERGER, F. M., CAMPBELL, G. L., HENDLEY, C. D., LUDWIG, B. J., & LYNES, T. E. The action of tranquilizers on brain potential and serotonin. *Annal. N.Y. Acad. Sci.*, 1957, 66, 686–94. *162*.

BERLYNE, D. E. Novelty and curiosity as determinants of exploratory behaviour. *Brit. J. Psychol.*, 1950, 41, 68–80. *41*.

BEVAN, W. Sound-precipitated convulsions: 1947–1954. *Psychol. Bull.*, 1955, 52, 473–504. *7*.

BIEL, W. C., & O'KELLY, L. I. The effect of cortical lesions on emotional and regressive behavior in the rat: I. Emotional behavior. *J. comp. Psychol.*, 1940, 30, 221–40. *41*.

BIGGERS, J. D., MCLAREN, ANNE, & MICHIE, D. Variance control in the animal house *Nature* (Lond.), 1958, 182, 77–80. *5*.

BILLINGHAM, R. E., & SILVERS, W. K. Inbred animals and tissue transplantation immunity. *Transplant. Bull.*, 1959, 6, 399–403. *5*.

BILLINGSLEA, F. Y. Intercorrelational analysis of certain behavior salients in the rat. *J. comp. Psychol.*, 1942, 34, 203–11. *38*.

BINDRA, D., & THOMPSON, W. R. An evaluation of defecation and urination as measures of fearfulness. *J. comp. physiol. Psychol.*, 1953, 46, 43–5. *38*.

BIRREN, J. E., FISHER, M. B., VOLLNER, E., & KING, B. G. Effect of anoxia on performance at several simulated altitudes. *J. exp. Psychol.*, 1946, 36, 35–49. *141*.

BLANCHARD, D. B. The white-crowned sparrows (Zonotrichia leucophrys) of the Pacific seaboard: Environment and annual cycle. *Univ. Calif. Publ. Zool.*, 1941, 46, 1–178. *10*.

BLUMBERG, N., *et al.* Evaluation of a new sedative (Doriden) in a penal institute. *Pennsyl. Med. J.*, 1956, 59, 808–9. *107, 139*.

BROADBENT, D. E. Noise, paced performance and vigilance tasks. *Brit. J. Psychol.*, 1953, 44, 295–303. *165*.

BROADBENT, D. E. *Perception and Communication*. London: Pergamon Press, 1958. *186*.

BROADHURST, P. L. *Emotionality in the rat: A study of its determinants, inheritance and relation to some aspects of motivation*. Ph.D. thesis, University of London, 1956. *31, 32*.

BROADHURST, P. L. Determinants of emotionality in the rat: I. Situational factors. *Brit. J. Psychol.*, 1957a, 48, 1–12. *23, 31, 38, 41, 51, 57, 65*.

BROADHURST, P. L. Emotionality and the Yerkes-Dodson Law. *J. exp. Psychol.*, 1957b, 54, 345–52. *39*.

BROADHURST, P. L. Determinants of emotionality in the rat: II. Antecedent factors. *Brit. J. Psychol.*, 1958a, 49, 12–20. *31, 32.*

BROADHURST, P. L. Determinants of emotionality in the rat: III. Strain differences. *J. comp. physiol. Psychol.*, 1958b, 51, 55–9. *7, 21, 31, 32, 77, 79.*

BROADHURST, P. L. A 'Crespi effect' in the analysis of emotionality as a drive in rats. *Brit. J. Psychol.*, 1958c, 49, 56–8. *39.*

BROADHURST, P. L. Studies in psychogenetics: The quantitative inheritance of behaviour in rats investigated by selective and cross-breeding. *Bull. Brit. psychol. Soc.*, 1958d, 34, 2A (Abstract). *3.*

BROADHURST, P. L. Application of biometrical genetics to behaviour in rats. 1959. *Nature* (Lond.), 1959, 184, 1517–18. *3.*

BROADHURST, P. L. Analysis of maternal effects in the inheritance of behaviour. 1960a, in press. *49, 60.*

BROADHURST, P. L. The inheritance of body weight in the rat studied by the method of diallel crosses. 1960b. In preparation. *79.*

BROADHURST, P. L., & EYSENCK, H. J. Interpretations of exploratory behaviour in the rat. 1960, in press. *41.*

BROADHURST, P. L., & JINKS, J. L. Biometrical genetics and behavior: Reanalysis of published data. 1960, in press. *70.*

BRODY, ELIZABETH G. Genetic basis of spontaneous activity in the albino rat. *Comp. Psychol. Monogr.*, 1942, 17, 1–24. *16, 18, 19.*

BRODY, ELIZABETH G. A note on the genetic basis of spontaneous activity in the albino rat. *J. comp. physiol. Psychol.*, 1950, 43, 281–8. *16, 18.*

BROWN-GRANT, K., HARRIS, G. W., & REICHLIN, S. Effect of emotional and physical stress on thyroid activity in the rabbit. *J. Physiol.*, 1954, 126, 29–40. *40.*

BUNDY, R. E. A search for some effects of the 'short-ear' gene on behavior in mice. *Amer. Naturalist*, 1950, 84, 393–9. *6.*

BURSTEIN, E., & DORFMAN, D. Effects of Meprobamate vs. Placebo on paired associate learning involving a list with high inter-item competition. *J. Psychol.*, 1959, 47, 81–6. *112, 119.*

BURT, C., & HOWARD, MARGARET. The multifactorial theory of inheritance and its application to intelligence. *Brit. J. statist. Psychol.*, 1956, 9, 95–131. *24, 26, 27.*

BURT, C., & HOWARD, MARGARET. Heredity and intelligence: A reply to criticisms. *Brit. J. statist. Psychol.*, 1957a, 10, 33–63. *26.*

BURT, C., & HOWARD, MARGARET. The relative influence of heredity and environment on assessments of intelligence. *Brit. J. statist. Psychol.*, 1957b, 10, 99–104. *26, 27.*

BUTLER, L. A study of size inheritance in the house mouse: II. Analysis of five preliminary crosses. *Canad. J. Zool.*, 1952, 30, 154–71. *73.*

BUTLER, L., & METRAKOS, J. D. A study of size inheritance in the house mouse: I. The effect of the milk source. *Canad. J. Res.*, (*D.*), 1950. 28, 16–34. *18.*

CALHOUN, J. B. Hereditary differences in social behavior and social organization between DBA and C57 black inbred strains of the house mouse (Mus musculus). *Anat. Rec.*, 1950, 108, 548 (Abstract). *8.*

CANNON, W. B. *Bodily changes in pain, hunger, fear, and rage.* New York: Appleton-Century, 1929. *39.*

CARPENTER, J. R., GRÜNEBERG, H., & RUSSELL, ELIZABETH S. Genetical differentiation involving morphological characters in an inbred strain of mice: II. American branches of the C57BL and C57BR strains. *J. Morph.*, 1957, 100, 377–88. *5.*

CARR, R. M., & WILLIAMS, C. D. Exploratory behavior of three strains of rats. *J. comp. physiol. Psychol.*, 1957, 50, 621–3. *8.*

CARRIÈRE, RITA, & ISLER, H. Effect of frequent housing changes and of muscular exercise on the thyroid gland of mice. *Endocrinology*, 1959, 64, 414–18. *40.*

CARTER, T. C., *et al. mult.* Standardized nomenclature for inbred strains of mice. *Cancer Res.*, 1952, 12, 602–13. 7.

CASPARI, E. Genetic basis of behavior. In Roe, Anne, & Simpson, G. G. *Behavior and Evolution*. New Haven: Yale University Press, 1958. Pp. 103–127. *10.*

CASTLE, W. E. *Genetics and Eugenics* (4th edition). Cambridge, Mass.: Harvard University Press, 1930. *79.*

CASTLE, W. E. The domestication of the rat. *Proc. nat. Acad. Sci.* (*Wash.*), 1947, 33, 109–117. *22, 79.*

CATTELL, R. B. Research designs in psychological genetics with special reference to the multiple variance method. *Amer. J. hum. Genet.*, 1953, 5, 76–93. *4.*

CATTELL, R. B. Theory and method in psychological genetics: I. The chief multiple variance analysis equations. 1959a, in press. *4, 26.*

CATTELL, R. B. Theory and method in psychological genetics: II. Solutions, adaptations and statistical needs of the multiple variance method. 1959b, in press. *4.*

CATTELL, R. B., BLEWETT, D. B., & BELOFF, J. R. The inheritance of personality. *Amer. J. hum. Genet.* 1955, 7, 122–46. *4.*

CATTELL, R. B., STICE, G. F., & KRISTY, N. F. A first approximation to nature-nurture ratios for eleven primary personality factors in objective tests. *J. abnorm. soc. Psychol.*, 1957, 54, 143–59. *4.*

CAVALLI, L. L. An analysis of linkage in quantitative inheritance. In Reeve, E. C. R., & Waddington, C. H. (Eds.) *Quantitative Inheritance*. London: H.M.S.O., 1952. Pp. 135–44. *73.*

CHAI, C. K. Endocrine variation: Thyroid function in inbred and F_1 hybrid mice. *J. Hered.*, 1958, 49, 143–8. *40.*

CHAI, C. K., AMIN, A., & REINEKE, E. P. Thyroidal iodine metabolism in inbred and F_1 mice. *Amer. J. Physiol.*, 1957, 188, 499–502. *40.*

CHAPMAN, A. B. Effectiveness of selection in laboratory animals. *J. anim. Sci.*, 1951, 10, 3–8. *66.*

CHENEY, R. H. Reaction time behavior after caffeine and coffee consumption. *J. exp. Psychol.*, 1936, 19, 357–69. *221.*

CLARK, EUGENIE, ARONSON, L. R., & GORDON, M. Mating behavior patterns in two sympatric species of Xiphophorin fishes: Their inheritance and significance in sexual isolation. *Bull. Amer. Mus. nat. Hist.*, 1954, 103, 135–226. *9.*

COBURN, C. A. Heredity of wildness and savageness in mice. *Behav. Monogr.*, 1922, 4, No. 5, 1–71. *13.*

COOK, R. C. 'Domestication genes'. *J. Hered.*, 1941, 32, 400–1. *21.*

COOMBS, C. H. Adaptation of the galvanic response to auditory stimuli. *J. exp. Psychol.*, 1938, 22, 244–68. *198, 204, 211.*

COOPER, R. M., & ZUBEK, J. P. Effects of enriched and restricted early environments on the learning ability of bright and dull rats. *Canad. J. Psychol.*, 1958, 12, 159–164. *16.*

CRONBACH, L. J. & MEEHL, P. E. Construct validity in psychological tests. *Psychol. Bull.*, 1955, 52, 281–302. *36.*

CROZIER, W. J., & PINCUS, G. Analysis of the geotropic orientation of young rats: III. Parts 1 and 2. *J. gen. Physiol.*, 1931–2a, 15, 201–42. *6.*

CROZIER, W. J., & PINCUS, G. Analysis of the geotropic orientation of young rats: IV. *J. gen. Physiol.*, 1931–2b, 15, 243–56. *6.*

CROZIER, W. J., & PINCUS, G. Analysis of the geotropic orientation of young rats: VI. *J. gen. Physiol.*, 1931–2c, 15, 437–62. *6.*

CROZIER, W. J., & PINCUS, G. Analysis of the geotropic orientation of young rats: IX. *J. gen. Physiol.*, 1935, 19, 211–21. *6.*

CROZIER, W. J., & PINCUS, G. Analysis of the geotropic orientation of young rats: X. *J. gen. Physiol.*, 1936, 20, 111–44. *6.*

DARLINGTON, C. D., & MATHER, K. *The elements of genetics*. London: Allen & Unwin, 1949. *24, 27.*

DARROW, C. W., & SOLOMON, A. P. Galvanic skin reflex and blood pressure reactions in psychotic states. *Arch. Neurol. Psychiat.* (*Chicago*), 1934, 32, 273–99. *207.*

DAS, GITA, & BROADHURST, P. L. The effect of inherited differences in emotional reactivity on a measure of intelligence in the rat. *J. comp. physiol. Psychol.*, 1959, 52, 300–3. *39, 65.*

DAVID, P. R., & SNYDER, L. H. Genetic variability and human behavior. In Rohrer, J. H., & SHERIF, M. (Eds.) *Social Psychology at the Crossroads.* New York: Harper & Bros., 1951, pp. 53–82. *20.*

DAVIS, R. C. Factors affecting the galvanic reflex. *Arch. Psychol.*, 1930, No. 115, 5–64. *198, 220.*

DAVIS, R. C. Electrical skin resistance before, during and after a period of noise stimulation. *J. exp. Psychol.*, 1932, 15, 108–17. *198.*

DAVIS, R. C. Modification of the galvanic reflex by daily repetition of a stimulus. *J. exp. Psychol.*, 1934, 17, 504–35. *198, 205.*

DAVIS, R. C., BUCHWALD, A. M., & FRANKMAN, R. W. Autonomic and muscular responses and their relation to simple stimuli. *Psychol. Monogr.*, 1955, 69, No. 20. *198, 204.*

DAWSON, W. M. Inheritance of wildness and tameness in mice. *Genetics*, 1932, 17, 296–326. *5, 6, 14.*

DEESE, J. Some problems in the theory of vigilance. *Psychol. Rev.*, 1955, 62, 359–68. *165.*

DENENBERG, V. H. Learning differences in two separated strains of mice. *Science*, 1959, 130, 451–2. *8.*

DENENBERG, V. H., PETROPOLUS, S. F., SAWIN, P. B., & ROSS, S. Genetic, physiological, and behavioral background of reproduction in the rabbit: VI. Maternal behavior with reference to scattered and cannibalized newborn and mortality. *Behaviour*, 1959, 15, 71–6. *9.*

DENENBERG, V. H., SAWIN, P. B., FROMMER, G. P., & ROSS, S. Genetic, physiological and behavioral background of reproduction in the rabbit: IV. An analysis of maternal behavior at successive parturitions. *Behaviour*, 1958, 13, 131–42. *9.*

DICKEL, H. A., WOOD, J. A., & DIXON, H. H. Electromyographic studies on Meprobamate and the working anxious patient. *Ann. N.Y. Acad. Sci.*, 1957, 67, 780–7. *107, 138, 152.*

DICKINSON, A. G. *The effect of environment and heredity in cattle.* Ph.D. thesis: University of Birmingham, 1954. *101.*

DICKINSON, A. G., & JINKS, J. L. A generalised analysis of diallel crosses. *Genetics*, 1956, 41, 65–78. *76, 77.*

DILGER, W. C. Nest material carrying behavior of F_1 hybrids between *Agapornis fisheri* and *A. roseicollis*. *Anat. Rec.*, 1959, 134, 554 (Abstract). *10.*

DOMINO, E. F., FOX, K. E., & BRODY, T. M. Pharmacological actions of a convulsant barbiturate: I. Stimulant and depressant effects. *J. Pharm. exp. Therap.*, 1955, 114, 473–83. *160.*

DONER, R. D., INMAN, C., & DAVIS, R. T. Competitive behavior between inbred strains of mice. *Proc. S. Dak. Acad. Sci.*, 1952, 31, 172–6. *8.*

DUFFY, ELIZABETH. The concept of energy mobilisation. *Psychol. Rev.*, 1951, 58, 30–40. *197.*

DUFFY, ELIZABETH. The psychological significance of the concept of 'arousal' or 'activation'. *Psych. Rev.*, 1957, 64, 265–75. *197.*

DUFFY, ELIZABETH, & LACEY, O. L. Adaptation in energy mobilisation: changes in general level of palmar skin conductance. *J. exp. Psychol.*, 1946, 36, 437–52. *198.*

DWORKEN, S., BOURNE, W., & RAGINSKY, B. B. Change in conditioned responses brought about by anaesthetics and sedatives. *Canad. Med. Ass. J.*, 1937, 37, 136–39. *111.*

EDWARDS, A. S. The measurement of static ataxia. *Amer. J. Psychol.*, 1942, 55, 171–88. *153.*

EDWARDS, A. S. Body sway and vision. *J. exp. Psychol.*, 1946, 36, 526–35. *153.*

ENGLAND, G. J. Observations on the grazing behaviour of different breeds of sheep at Pantyrhuad Farm, Carmarthenshire. *Brit. J. anim. Behav.*, 1954, 2, 56–60. *11.*

ESTES, BETSY W. A study of the relationship between temperament of thoroughbred brood mares and performance of offspring. *J. genet. Psychol.*, 1952, 81, 273–88. *11.*

ESTES, W. K. Spontaneous recovery from extinction in maze-bright and maze-dull rats. *J. comp. Psychol.*, 1942, 34, 349–51. *16.*

EVANS, C., & MCCONNELL, T. R. A new measure of extraversion-introversion. *J. Psychol.*, 1941, 12, 111–24. *186.*

EVANS, J. T., & HUNT, J. MCV. The 'emotionality' of rats. *Amer. J. Psychol.*, 1942, 55, 528–45. *37, 38.*

EYSENCK, H. J. *Dimensions of Personality*. London: Routledge & Kegan Paul, 1947. *186, 153, 206.*

EYSENCK, H. J. *The Scientific Study of Personality*. London: Routledge & Kegan Paul, 1952. *106.*

EYSENCK, H. J. Dynamic theory of anxiety and hysteria. *J. ment. Sci.*, 1955a, 101, 28–51. *106.*

EYSENCK, H. J. Cortical inhibition, figural after-effect and theory of personality. *J. abnorm. soc. Psychol.*, 1955b, 51, 94–106. *106.*

EYSENCK, H. J. Warm-up in pursuit rotor learning as a function of the extinction of conditioned inhibition. *Acta Psychol. (Hague)*, 1956a, 12, 349–70. *183.*

EYSENCK, H. J. Reminiscence, drive and personality theory. *J. abnorm. soc. Psychol.*, 1956b, 53, 328–33. *186.*

EYSENCK, H. J. The questionnaire measurement of neuroticism and extraversion. *Rev. Psicol.*, 1956c, 50, 113–40. *109, 186.*

EYSENCK, H. J. *The Dynamics of Anxiety and Hysteria*. London: Routledge and Kegan Paul, 1957a. *105, 106, 155, 162, 163, 183, 189, 197, 210, 218, 220, 223, 227.*

EYSENCK, H. J. Drugs and personality: I. Theory and methodology. *J. ment. Sci.*, 1957b, 103, 119–31. *105, 106, 161, 162, 183.*

EYSENCK, H. J. *Manual of the Maudsley Personality Inventory*. Univ. of London Press, 1959. *109.*

EYSENCK, H. J., CASEY, S., & TROUTON, D. S. Drugs and personality. II. The effect of stimulant and depressant drugs on continuous work. *J. ment. Sci.*, 1957a, 103, 645–9. *106, 183, 186.*

EYSENCK, H. J., HOLLAND, H., & TROUTON, D. S. Drugs and personality: III. The effects of stimulant and depressant drugs on visual after-effects. *J. ment. Sci.*, 1957b, 103, 650–5. 106.

EYSENCK, H. J., HOLLAND, H., & TROUTON, D. S. Drugs and personality: IV. The effects of a stimulant and depressant drug on the rate of fluctuation of a reversible perspective figure. *J. ment. Sci.*, 1957c, 103, 656–60. *106.*

EYSENCK, H. J., & AIBA, T. Drugs and personality: V. The effects of stimulant and depressant drugs on the suppression of the primary visual stimulus. *J. ment. Sci.*, 1957d, 103, 661–5. *106.*

EYSENCK, S. B. G. An experimental study of psychogalvanic reflex responses of normal, neurotic and psychotic subjects. *J. psychosom. Res.*, 1956, 1, 258–72 *198, 202.*

FALCONER, D. S. The problem of environment and selection. *Amer. Naturalist*, 1952, 86, 293–8. *101.*

FALCONER, D. S. Selection for large and small size in mice. *J. Genet.*, 1953, 51, 470–501. *14, 66.*

FALCONER, D. S. Validity of the theory of genetic correlation. An experimental test with mice. *J. Hered.*, 1954, 45, 42–4. *54.*

FALCONER, D. S. Patterns of response in selection experiments with mice. In *Population genetics: the nature and causes of genetic variability in populations. Cold Spring Harbor Symposia on Quantitative Biology*, 1955, 20, 178–96. *13, 66.*

FALCONER, D. S. Breeding methods: I. Genetic considerations. In Worden, A. N., & Lane-Petter, W. (Eds.) *The UFAW Handbook on the Care and Management of Laboratory Animals.* London: Universities Federation for Animal Welfare, 1957. Pp. 85–107. *13, 20.*

FALCONER, D. S., & LATYSZEWSKI, M. Selection for size in mice on high and low planes of nutrition. In Reeve, E. C. R., & Waddington, C. H. (Eds.) *Quantitative inheritance.* London: H.M.S.O., 1952. Pp. 145–51. *101.*

FALCONER, D. S., & LATYSZEWSKI, M. The environment in relation to selection for size in mice. *J. Genet.*, 1952–3, 51, 67–80. *101.*

FARBER, I. E., & SPENCE, K. W. Complex learning and conditioning as a function of anxiety. *J. exp. Psychol.*, 1953, 45, 120–5. *112.*

FARRIS, E. J., & GRIFFITH, J. Q., JNR. (Eds.) *The rat in laboratory investigation* (2nd edition). Philadelphia: Lippincott, 1949. *48.*

FELSINGER, J. N. VON, LASAGNA, L., & BEECHER, H. K. The persistence of mental impairment following a hypnotic dose of a barbiturate. *J. Pharmacol. Therapeut.*, 1953, 109, 284–91 *112, 170.*

FEUER, G., & BROADHURST, P. L. Differences in thyroid hormones in rats selectively bred for emotional reactivity. 1960, in press. *40.*

FINGER, F. W. Convulsive behavior in the rat. *Psychol. Bull.*, 1947, 44, 201–48. *7.*

FISHER, J., & HINDE, R. A. The opening of milk bottles by birds. *Brit. Birds*, 1949, 42, 347–57. *10.*

FISHER, R. A. The correlation between relatives on the supposition of Mendelian inheritance. *Trans. Roy. Soc. Edin.*, 1918, 52, 399–433. *24.*

FLEISHMAN, E. A. Predicting advanced levels of proficiency in psychomotor skills. In Finch, G., & Cameron, F. (Eds.) *Symposium on Air Force Human Engineering, Personnel and Training Research.* Baltimore: A.R.D.C. Technical Report, 1956, 56–8. *161.*

FLEISHMAN, E. A., & HEMPEL, W. E. Changes in factor structure of a complex psycho-motor test as a function of practice. *Psychometrika*, 1954, 19, 239–52. *160.*

FRANKS, C. M. A conditioning laboratory for the investigation of personality and cortical functioning. *Nature* (Lond.), 1955, 175, 984. *111, 113.*

FRANKS, C. M. Conditioning and personality: a study of normal and neurotic subjects. *J. abnorm. soc. Psychol.*, 1956, 52, 143–50. *111, 113.*

FRANKS, C. M., & LAVERTY, S. G. Sodium amytal and eyelid conditioning. *J. ment. Sci.*, 101, 1955, 654–63. *106, 108, 111, 113,*

FRANKS, C. M., & TROUTON, D. Effects of amobarbital sodium and dexamphetamine sulphate on the conditioning of the eyeblink response. *J. comp. physiol. Psychol.*, 1958, 51, 220–2. *111, 113.*

FRANKS, C. M., & WITHERS, W. C. R. Photoelectric recording of eyelid movements. *Amer. J. Psychol.*, 1955, 68, 467–71. *113.*

FRAZER, D. C. The relation of an environmental variable to performance in a prolonged visual task. *Quart. J. exp. Psychol.*, 1953, 5, 31–2. *165.*

FREDERICSON, E. Reciprocal fostering of two inbred mouse strains and its effect on the modification of inherited aggressive behavior. *Amer. Psychologist*, 1952, 7, 241–2 (Abstract). *18.*

FREDERICSON, E. The wall-seeking tendency in three inbred mouse strains (Mus musculus). *J. genet. Psychol.*, 1953, 82, 143–6. *8.*

FREDERICSON, E., STORY, A. W., GURNEY, N. L., & BUTTERWORTH, K. The relationship between heredity, sex, and aggression in two inbred mouse strains. *J. genet. Psychol.*, 1955, 87, 121–30. *8.*

FREEDMAN, D. G. Constitutional and environmental interactions in rearing of four breeds of dogs. *Science*, 1958, 127, 585–6. *12.*

FREEMAN, G. L., & GEISE, W. J. The relationship between task difficulty and palmar skin resistance. *J. gen. Psychol.*, 1940, 23, 217–30. *176.*

FRIEDMAN, A. P. The treatment of chronic headache with Meprobamate. *Ann. N.Y. Acad. Sci.*, 1957, 67, 822–6. *107.*

FRINGS, H., & FRINGS, MABLE. The production of stocks of albino mice with predictable susceptibilities to audiogenic seizures. *Behaviour*, 1953, 5, 305–19. *14.*

FRINGS, H., FRINGS, MABLE, & HAMILTON, MABEL. Experiments with albino mice from stocks selected for predictable susceptibilities to audiogenic seizures. *Behaviour*, 1956, 9, 44–52. *14.*

FULLER, J. L. Individual differences in the reactivity of dogs. *J. comp. physiol. Psychol.*, 1948, 41, 339–47. *12.*

FULLER, J. L. Genetic variability in some physiological constants of dogs. *Amer. J. Physiol.*, 1951, 166, 20–4. *12.*

FULLER, J. L. *Nature and Nurture: A Modern Synthesis.* New York: Doubleday, 1954. *12.*

FULLER, J. L. Hereditary differences in trainability of purebred dogs. *J. genet. Psychol.*, 1955, 87, 229–38. *12.*

FULLER, J. L. The genetic base: Pathways between genes and behavioral characteristics. In *The nature and transmission of the genetic and cultural characteristics of human populations.* Proc. Millbank Mem. Fund., 1956. Pp. 101–11. *26.*

FULLER, J. L., & SCOTT, J. P. Genetic factors affecting intelligence: Heredity and learning ability in infra-human mammals. *Eugen. Quart.*, 1954, 1, 28–43. *11.*

FUSTER, J. M. Tachistoscopic perception in monkeys. *Fed. Proc.*, 1957, 16, 43. *188.*

GASTAUT, H., JUS, C. & A., MORRELL, F., VAN LEEUWEN, W. S., DONGIER, S., NAQUET, R., REGIS, H., ROGER, A., BEKKERING, D., KAMP, A., & WERRE, J. Étude topographique des réactions éléctro-encephalographiques conditionnées chez l'homme. *E.E.G. Clin. Neurophysiol.*, 1957, 9, 1–34. *217, 218.*

GEIER, F. M., LEVIN, M., & TOLMAN, E. C. Individual differences in emotionality, hypothesis formation, vicarious trial and error, and visual discrimination learning in rats. *Comp. Psychol. Monogr.*, 1941, 17, No. 3, 1–20. *38.*

GINSBURG, B., & ALLEE, W. C. Some effects of conditioning on social dominance and subordination in inbred strains of mice. *Physiol. Zool.*, 1942, 15, 485–506. *8.*

GLICKMAN, S. E. Effects of peripheral blindness on exploratory behaviour in the hooded rat. *Canad. J. Psychol.*, 1958, 12, 45–51. *41.*

GODFREY, J. The origin of sexual isolation between bank voles (*Clethrionomys*). *Proc. XV int. Congr. Zool. (London)*, 1959, 203–4 (Abstract). *11.*

GOLDSTONE, S. Flicker fusion measurements and anxiety level. *J. exp. Psychol.*, 1955, 49, 200–2. *152.*

GOODALE, H. D. Can artificial selection produce unlimited change? *Amer. Naturalist*, 1937, 71, 433–59. *13.*

GOODALE, H. D. A study of the inheritance of body weight in the albino mouse by selection. *J. Hered.*, 1938, 29, 101–12. *14.*

GOODALE, H. D., SANBORN, R., & WHITE, D. Broodiness in domestic fowl: data concerning its inheritance in the Rhode Island Red breed. *Mass. Agric. exp. Sta. Bull.*, 1920, 199, 99–116. *11.*

GÖSSWALD, K., & SCHMIDT, G. Zur morphologischen und biochemischen Differenzierung der Waldmeisen (Hym. Form., Gen. Formica) und ihrer waldhygienischen Bedeutung. *Waldhygiene*, 1959, 3, 37–46. *10.*

GOTTLIEB, J. S. Anti-depressive action of 5-(1,3-dimethylbutyl)-5-ethyl barbituric acid. *A.M.A. Arch. Neurol. Psychiat.*, 1951, 66, 318–28. *160.*

GOY, R. W., & JAKWAY, JACQUELINE S. The inheritance of patterns of sexual behaviour in female guinea pigs. *Anim. Behav.*, 1959, 7, 142–9. *9.*

GOY, R. W., & YOUNG, W. C. Somatic basis of sexual behaviour patterns in guinea pigs: Factors involved in the determination of the character of the soma in the female. *Psychosom. Med.*, 1957a, 19, 144–51. *9.*

GOY, R. W., & YOUNG, W. C. Strain differences in the behavioral responses of female guinea pigs to alpha-estradiol benzoate and progesterone. *Behaviour*, 1957b, 10, 340–54. *9.*

GRANGER, G. W. Psychophysiology of vision. In *Int. Rev. of Neurobiol.* Acad. Press, New York, 1959. *158.*

GRANGER, G. W. Abnormalities of Sensory Perception. In Eysenck, H. J. (Ed.) *Handbook of Abnormal Psychology*. London: Pitman, 1960. *158.*

GRAVES, ELIZABETH A. Interrelationships in performances in the albino rat. *J. comp. Psychol.*, 1936, 22, 179–86. *16.*

GRIFFING, B. A generalised treatment of the use of diallel crosses in quantitative inheritance. *Heredity*, 1956, 10, 31–50. *82.*

GRIFFITHS, W. J. Transmission of convulsions in the white rat. *J. comp. Psychol.*, 1942, 34, 263–77. *14.*

GROSS, F., TRIPOD, J., & MEIER, R. (Pharmacological characterization of the hypnotic Doriden.) *Schweiz. med. Wschr.*, 1955, 85, 305–9. *107, 139, 174.*

GRÜNEBERG, H. *The Genetics of the Mouse* (2nd edition.) The Hague: Martinus Nijhoff, 1952. *6.*

HAIZLIP, T. A., & EWING, J. A. Meprobamate Habituation. *New Eng. J. Med.*, 1958, 258, 1181–6. *138, 153.*

HALDANE, J. B. S. The interaction of nature and nurture. *Ann. Eugen.* (Camb.), 1946, 13, 197–205. *101.*

HALL, C. S. Emotional behavior in the rat: I. Defecation and urination as measures of individual differences in emotionality. *J. comp. Psychol.*, 1934, 18, 385–403. *32, 37.*

HALL, C. S. Emotional behavior in the rat: III. The relationship between emotionality and ambulatory activity. *J. comp. Psychol.*, 1936, 22, 345–52. *41, 58.*

HALL, C. S. Emotional behavior in the rat: IV. Emotionality and stereotyping of behavior. *J. comp. Psychol.*, 1937, 24, 369–75. *17.*

HALL, C. S. The inheritance of emotionality. *Sigma Xi Quart.*, 1938, 26, 17–27, 37, *17, 37, 39.*

HALL, C. S. The inheritance of emotionality in the rat. *Psychol. Bull.*, 1940, 37, 432 (Abstract). *17, 39.*

HALL, C. S. Temperament: a survey of animal studies. *Psychol. Bull.*, 1941, 38, 909–43. *17, 37, 39.*

HALL, C. S. Genetic differences in fatal audiogenic seizures between inbred strains of house mice. *J. Hered.*, 1947, 38, 3–6. *49.*

HALL, C. S. The genetics of behavior. In Stevens, S. S. (Ed.) *Handbook of Experimental Psychology*. New York: Wiley, 1951. Pp. 304–29. *5, 17, 18, 19, 20, 21, 24, 26, 30, 39, 48, 65.*

HALL, C. S., & KLEIN, L. L. Emotional behavior in the rat: VI. The relationship between persistence and emotionality. *J. comp. Psychol.*, 1941, 32, 503–6. *17.*

HALL, C. S., & KLEIN, L. L. Individual differences in aggressiveness in rats. *J. comp. Psychol.*, 1942, 33, 371–83. *17.*

HALSTEAD, W. C. *Brain and Intelligence: A Quantitative Study of the Frontal Lobes.* Chicago: Univ. of Chicago Press, 1947. *162.*

HARRIS, H. *Human Biochemical Genetics*. Cambridge: Cambridge University Press, 1959. *10.*

HARRIS, R. E. An analysis of the maze-learning scores of bright and dull rats with reference to motivational factors. *Psychol. Rec.*, 1940, 4, 130–6. *16.*

HARRISON, B. J. Reversal of a secondary sex character by selection. *Heredity*, 1953, 7, 153–64. *60.*

HAUTY, G. T. The effects of drugs upon the components of hand steadiness. *Air. Univ. USAF Sch. Avia. Med.*, 1954, Rep. No. 5, Proj. No. 21-1601-0004. *176.*

HAYMAN, B. I. The theory and analysis of diallel crosses. *Genetics*, 1954a, 39, 789–809. *75, 76, 82, 87, 92.*

HAYMAN, B. I. The analysis of variance of diallel crosses. *Biometrics*, 1954b, 10, 235–44. *82, 89, 91.*

HAYMAN, B. I. Interaction, heterosis and diallel crosses. *Genetics*, 1957, 42, 336–55. *76.*

HAYMAN, B. I. The theory and analysis of diallel crosses: II. *Genetics*, 1958, 43, 63–85. *76.*

HAYMAN, B. I., & MATHER, K. The description of genic interactions in continuous variation. *Biometrics*, 1955, 11, 69–82. *67.*

HERON, W. T. The inheritance of maze learning ability in rats. *J. comp. Psychol.*, 1935, 19, 77–89. *15.*

HERON, W. T. The behavior of active and inactive rats in experimental extinction and discrimination problems. *Psychol. Rec.*, 1940, 4, 23–31. *16.*

HERON, W. T. The inheritance of brightness and dullness in maze learning ability in the rat. *J. genet. Psychol.*, 1941, 59, 41–9. *15.*

HERON, W. T., & SKINNER, B. F. The rate of extinction of maze-bright and maze-dull rats. *Psychol. Rec.*, 1940, 4, 11–18. *16.*

HERON, W. T., & YUGEND, S. Basal metabolism and maze learning in rats. *J. genet. Psychol.*, 1936, 48, 471–4. *16.*

HERTER, K. Das thermotaktische Optimum bei Nagetieren, ein mendelendes Art und Rassenmerkel. *Z. vergl. Physiol.*, 1936, 23, 605–50. *6.*

HERTER, K. Die Beziehungen zwischen Vorzugstemperatur und Hautbeschaffenheit bei Mäusen. *Zool. Anz.* (*Suppl.*), 1938, 11, 48–55. *6.*

HERTER, K., & SGONINA, K. Vorzugstemperatur und Hautbeschaffenheit bei Mäusen. *Z. vergl. Physiol.*, 1938, 26, 366–415. *6.*

HESS, E. H. Comparative psychology. *Annu. Rev. Psychol.*, 1956, 7, 305–22. *12.*

HESS, W. R. *Diencephalon: autonomic and extra-pyramidal functions.* London: Heinemann, 1954. *39.*

HIMMELWEIT, HILDE T. Speed and accuracy of work as related to temperament. *Brit. J. Psychol.*, 1946, 36, 132–44. *134.*

HIMWICH, H. E. (Ed.). *Tranquilising drugs.* Amer. Assoc. Adv. Sci., 1957, No. 46. *107, 139.*

HINDE, R. A. The behaviour of certain cardueline F_1 interspecies hybrids. *Behaviour*, 1956a, 9, 202–13. *10.*

HINDE, R. A. Breeding success in cardueline interspecies pairs, and an examination of the hybrids' plumage. *J. Genet.*, 1956b, 54, 304–310. *10.*

HINDE, R. A. Behaviour and speciation in birds and lower vertebrates. *Biol. Rev.*, 1959, 34, 85–128. *10.*

HINDE, R. A., & TINBERGEN, N. The comparative study of species-specific behaviour. In Roe, Anne, & Simpson, G. G., *Behavior and Evolution.* New Haven: Yale University Press, 1958. Pp. 251–68. *10.*

HIRSCH, J. Recent developments in behavior genetics and differential psychology. *Dis. nerv. Sys., Monogr. Suppl.*, 1958, 19, 17–24. *17.*

HIRSCH, J. Studies in experimental behavior genetics: II. Individual differences in geotaxis as a function of chromosome variations in synthesized *Drosophila* populations. *J. comp. physiol. Psychol.*, 1959, 52, 304–8. *10.*

HIRSCH, J., & BOUDREAU, J. C. Studies in experimental behavior genetics: I. The heritability of phototaxis in a population of *Drosophila melanogaster. J. comp. physiol. Psychol.*, 1958, 51, 647–51. *17.*

HIRSCH, J., & TRYON, R. C. Mass screening and reliable individual measurement in the experimental behavior genetics of lower organisms. *Psychol. Bull.*, 1956, 53, 402–10. *17.*

HOCH, P., KUBIS, J. F., & ROUKE, F. L. Psychogalvanometric investigations in psychoses and other abnormal mental states. *Psychosom. Med.*, 1944, 6, 237–43. *207.*

HOLLISTER, L. E., ELKINS, H., HILER, E. G., & ST. PIERRE, R. Meprobamate in chronic psychiatric patients. *Ann. N.Y. Acad. Sci.*, 1957, 67, 789–98. *107.*

HONEYMAN, M. S. A quantitative genetic study of a nutritional strain difference in mice. *J. Hered.*, 1957, 48, 84–7. *29, 73,*

HOVENER, W. H. Comparison of flicker perimetry with standard perimetric methods. *A.M.A. Arch. Ophthalm.*, 1954, 52, 91–105. *147.*

HOVLAND, C. J. Experimental studies in rote learning theory: II. Reminiscence following learning by massed and by distributed practice. *J. exp. Psychol.*, 1938, 22, 201–24. *121, 135.*

HOWELL, C. A. A. 'Doriden'. Letter to *Brit. Med. Journal.*, 1956. *107, 139.*

HOWELL, T. R. Racial and sexual differences in migration in *Sphyrapicus varius*. *Auk*, 1953, 70, 118–26. *10.*

HUGHES, K. R., COOPER, R. M., & ZUBEK, J. P. Effect of glutamic acid on the learning ability of bright and dull rats: III. Effect of varying dosages. *Canad. J. Psychol.*, 1957, 11, 253–5. *16.*

HUGHES, K. R., & ZUBEK, J. P. Effects of glutamic acid on the learning ability of bright and dull rats: I. Administration during infancy. *Canad. J. Psychol.*, 1956, 10, 132–8. *16.*

HUGHES, K. R., & ZUBEK, J. P. Effect of glutamic acid on the learning ability of bright and dull rats: II. Duration of the effect. *Canad. J. Psychol.*, 1957, 11, 182–4. *16.*

HULL, C. L. The influence of caffeine and other factors on certain phenomena of rote learning. *J. gen. Psychol.*, 1935, 13, 255–67. *111.*

HULL, C. L. *Mathematico-deductive theory of rote learning—a study in scientific methodology.* New Haven: Yale University Press, 1940. *110, 121, 130, 131.*

HULL, C. L. *Principles of Behavior.* New York: Appleton-Century-Crofts, 1943. *130, 131, 188.*

HULL, C. L. *A Behavior System.* New Haven: Yale University Press, 1952. *130.*

HUNT, H. F. Some effects of drugs on classical (Type S) conditioning. *Ann. N.Y. Acad. Sci.*, 1955, 65, 258–67. *111, 119.*

HUNT, H. F. Some effects of Meprobamate on conditioned fear and emotional behavior. *Ann. N.Y. Acad. Sci.*, 1957, 67, 712–22. *111, 119, 138.*

HUNT, H. F., & OTIS, L. S. Conditioned and unconditioned emotional defecation in the rat. *J. comp. physiol. Psychol.*, 1953, 46, 378–82. *38.*

HURST, C. C. *Experiments in genetics.* Cambridge (Engl.): Univ. Press, 1925. *11.*

HUTT, F. B. *Genetics of the Fowl.* New York: McGraw-Hill, 1949. *11.*

IDESTROM, C. Flicker fusion in chronic barbiturate usage: a quantitative study in the pathophysiology of drug addiction. *Acta psychiat.* (*Kbh.*), 1954, Supp. 91, 93. *148.*

IKUI, H., NAKANA, K., & OSHIO, S. The influence of oxygen deficiency on vision: I. The changes of the field of vision by oxygen deficiency. *Jap. J. Clin. Exp. Med.*, 1947, 24, 250–1. *141.*

INGHAM, J. G. Body sway suggestibility and neurosis. *J. ment. Sci.*, 1954, 100, 432–41. *153.*

JAKWAY, JACQUELINE S. The inheritance of patterns of mating behaviour in the male guinea pig. *Anim. Behav.*, 1959, 7, 150–62. *9.*

JENSEN, A. R. The Maudsley Personality Inventory. *Acta Psychol.* (*Hague*), 1958, 14, 314–25. *155.*

JINKS, J. L. The analysis of continuous variation in a diallel cross of *Nicotiana rustica* varieties: I. The analysis of F_1 data. *Genetics*, 1954, 39, 767–88. *76.*

JINKS, J. L. A survey of the genetical basis of heterosis in a variety of diallel crosses. *Heredity*, 1955, *9*, 223–38. *76, 85, 86.*

JINKS, J. L. The F_2 and backcross generation from a set of diallel crosses. *Heredity*, 1956, 10, 1–30. *76.*

JINKS, J. L., & JONES, R. M. Estimation of the components of heterosis. *Genetics*, 1958, 43, 223–34. *67, 72, 73.*

JONES, H. G. The status of inhibition in Hull's system: A theoretical revision. *Psychol. Rev.*, 1958, 65, 179–82. *182, 187.*

JONES, H. G. Learning and abnormal behavior. In Eysenck, H. J. (Ed.) *Handbook of Abnormal Psychology*. London: Pitman, 1960.

JONES, R. M., & MATHER, K. Interaction of genotype and environment in continuous variation: II. Analysis. *Biometrics*, 1958, 14, 489–98. *101.*

JOST, H., RUILMAN, G. J., HILL, T. S., & GULO, M. J. Studies in hypertension: I. Technics and control data. Central & ANS reactions of normal adults to sensory and ideational (frustration) stimulation. *J. Nerv. Ment Dis.*, 1952, 115, 35–48. *207.*

KALMUS, H. The genetic and genetical aspects of behaviour. *Brit.J. anim. Behav.*, 1955, 3, 38 (Abstract). *3.*

KAUFMAN, LAURA. On the mode of inheritance of broodiness. *Proc. VIII. World Poult. Congr. (Copenhagen)*, 1948, 301–4. *11.*

KEELER, C. E. The association of the black (non-Agouti) gene with behavior in the Norway rat. *J. Hered.*, 1942, 33, 371–84. *21.*

KEELER, C. E. Gene determined physical modifications affecting the sociometry of rats. *Sociometry*, 1945a, 8, 30–41. *21.*

KEELER, C. E. Les effets de variation du poil sur la morphologie, la physiologie, et la conduite du rat Norvégien. *Bull. Soc. Zool. France*, 1945b, 70, 123–44. *21.*

KEELER, C. E. Modification of brain and endocrine glands as an explanation of altered behavior trends in coat character mutant strains of the Norway rat. *J. Tenn. Acad. Sci.*, 1947, 22, 202–9. *21.*

KEELER, C. E. Materials for the synthesis of hereditary behavior trends in mammals. *J. comp. physiol. Psychol.*, 1948, 41, 75–81. *21.*

KEELER, C. E., & KING, HELEN D. Multiple effects of coat-color genes in the rat with special reference to the 'marks of domestication'. *Anat. Rec. (Suppl.)*, 1941, 81, 48–9 (Abstract). *21.*

KEELER, C. E., & KING, HELEN D. Multiple effects of coat color genes in the Norway rat with special reference to temperament and domestication. *J. comp. Psychol.*, 1942, 34, 241–50. *21.*

KEELER, C. E., & TRIMBLE, H. C. Inheritance of position preference in coach dogs. *J. Hered.* 1940, 31, 51–4. *11.*

KELLEY, R. B., & SHAW, H. E. B. Fertility in sheep: An experimental study of periodicity of oestrus and non-breeding seasons in Australia. *Austral. Council sci. indust. Res. Bull.*, 1943, 166, 1–28. *11.*

KEMPTHORNE, O. The theory of the diallel cross. *Genetics*, 1956, 41, 451–9. *76.*

KEMPTHORNE, O. *An Introduction to Genetic Statistics*. New York: Wiley, 1957. *27, 76.*

KILLAM, EVA K. The effects of psychotherapeutic compounds on the central afferent and limbic pathways. *Ann. N.Y. Acad. Sci.*, 1957, 66, 784–805. *153.*

KIMBLE, G. A., & HORENSTEIN, B. R. Reminiscence in motor learning as a function of the length of interpolated rest. *J. exp. Psychol.*, 1948, 38, 239–44. *185.*

KING, HELEN D. Selective fertilization in the rat. *Arch. Entw. mechan. Org.*, 1929, 116, 202–19. *9.*

KING, J. A. Maternal behavior and behavioral development in two subspecies of *Peromyscus maniculatus*. *J. Mammol.*, 1958, 39, 177–190. *8.*

KING, J. A., & DESHAIES, J. C. A comparison of two subspecies of *Peromyscus maniculatus* at weaning. *Anat. Rec.*, 1959, 134, 595 (Abstract). *8.*

KING, J. A., & ELEFTHERIOU, B. E. Effects of early handling upon adult behavior in two subspecies of deermice, *Peromyscus maniculatus*. *J. comp. physiol. Psychol.*, 1959, 52, 82–8. *8.*

KING, J. A., & MAVROMATIS, A. The effect of a conflict situation on learning ability in two strains of inbred mice. *J. comp. physiol. Psychol.*, 1956, 49, 465–86. *8.*

KORKMAN, N. Selection with regard to the sex difference of body weight in mice. *Hereditas*, 1957, 43, 665–78. *14.*

KRECH, D., ROSENZWEIG, M. R., & BENNETT, E. L. Dimensions of discrimination and level of cholinesterase activity in the cerebral cortex of the rat. *J. comp. physiol. Psychol.*, 1956, 49, 261–8. *15.*

KRECH, D., ROSENZWEIG, M. R., BENNETT, E. L., & KRUECKEL, B. Enzyme concentrations in the brain and adjustive behavior-patterns. *Science*, 1954, 120, 994–6. *15.*

KRECHEVSKY, I. Hereditary nature of 'hypotheses'. *J. comp. Psychol.*, 1933, 16, 99–116. *15.*

KRUSE, MARIAN. Food satiation curves for maze-bright and maze-dull rats. *J. comp. Psychol.*, 1941, 31, 13–21. *16.*

KRUSHINSKI, L. V. (Hereditary 'fixation' of individually acquired forms of behaviour of animals and the origin of instincts.) *Zh. obshch. Biol.*, 1944, 5, 261–83. (*Biol. Abstr.*, 1947, 21, No. 24055 (Abstract)). *11.*

KRUSHINSKI, L. V. (The inheritance of passive defence behavior (cowardice) in relation to types of nervous system in dogs.) *Akad. Meditsinskitch Nauk S.S.S.R.*, 1947, 1, 61. (*Biol. Abstr.*, 1951, 25, No. 26381. (Title only.)) *11.*

KUBIS, J. F. Adaptation of the psychogalvanic response (PGR) to a visual, auditory and ideational stimulus. *Amer. Psychologist*, 1948, 3, 256. *207.*

KUDRJAWZEW, P. N. Polyallele Kreuzung als Prüfungsimethode für die Leistungfähigkeit von Zuchtebern. *Zuchtungskunde*, 1934, 9, 444–452. *76.*

KUPPASAWNY, B. Laws of heredity in relation to general mental ability. *J. gen. Psychol.*, 1947, 36, 29–43. *14.*

Laboratory Animals Centre. *Catalogue of uniform strains of Laboratory animals maintained in Great Britain* (2nd edition). London: Laboratory Animals Centre, 1958. *78.*

LACEY, J. L. The evaluation of autonomic responses: toward a general solution. *Ann. N.Y. Acad. Sci.*, 1956, 67, 123–64. *202, 205, 212, 216.*

LANDIS, C. An annotated bibliography of flicker fusion phenomena. *The Armed Forces National Research Council*, Michigan, 1953. *147.*

LANDIS, C. Determinants of the critical flicker-fusion threshold. *Physiol. Rev.*, 1954, 34, 259–86. *147.*

LANSING, R. W. The relationship of brain and tremor rhythms to visual reaction time. *E.E.G. clin. Neurophysiol.*, 1957, 9, 497–504. *188.*

LANSING, R. W., SCHWARTZ, E., & LINDSLEY, D. B. Reaction time and EEG activation. *Amer. Psychologist*, 1956, 11, 433 (Abstract). *188.*

LASAGNA, L., MUSTELLER, F., FELSINGER, J. M., & BEECHER, H. K. A study of placebo responses. *Amer. J. Med.*, 1954, 16, 770–9. *232.*

LATIES, V. G. Effects of meprobamate on fear and palmar sweating. *Fed. Proc.*, 1957, 16, 315 (Abstract). *176, 197.*

LAWLOR, MONICA M. Hereditary determinants of social dominance in the golden hamster. *Brit. J. anim. Behav.*, 1956, 4, 75–6 (Abstract). *11.*

LEOPOLD, A. S. The nature of heritable wildness in turkeys. *Condor*, 1944, 46, 133–97. *10.*

LERNER, I. M. *Population genetics and animal improvement: As illustrated by the inheritance of egg production.* Cambridge (Eng.): Cambridge University Press, 1950. *20.*

LERNER, I. M. *Genetic basis of selection.* New York: Wiley, 1958. *27, 66.*

LEVINE, L. Studies on sexual selection in mice: I. Reproductive competition between albino and black-agouti males. *Amer. Naturalist*, 1958, 92, 21–6. *9.*

LEWIS, W. L., & WARWICK, E. J. Effectiveness of selection for body weight in mice: from inbred and outbred populations derived from common parent stocks. *J. Hered.*, 1953, 44, 233–8. *14.*

LINDEMANN, E. Psychological changes in normal and abnormal individuals under the influence of sodium amytal. *Amer. J. Psychiat.*, 1932, 1083–91. 106.

LINDQUIST, E. F. *Design and analysis of experiments in psychology and education.* Cambridge, Mass.: Houghton Mifflin Co., 1953. *71.*

LINDQUIST, T. Finger tremor and the a-waves of the electroencephalogram. *Acta. med. scand.*, 1941, 108, 580–5. *174.*

LINDSLEY, D. B. Psychophysiology and motivation. In Jones, M. R. (Ed.) *Nebraska*

Symposium on Motivation, 1957. Lincoln: Univ. of Nebraska Press, 1957. *188, 189.*

LINDZEY, G. Emotionality and audiogenic seizure susceptibility in five inbred strains of mice. *J. comp. physiol. Psychol.*, 1951, 44, 389–93. *7.*

LITCHFIELD, H. R. Clinical evaluation of Meprobamate in disturbed and pre-psychotic children. *Ann. N.Y. Acad. Sci.*, 1957, 67, 828–31. *138, 139.*

LITTLE, C. C. Coat colour genes in rodents and carnivores. *Quart. Rev. Biol.*, 1958, 33, 103–37. *79.*

LLOYD, V. V. A comparison of critical fusion frequencies for different areas in the fovea and periphery. *Amer. J. Psychol.*, 1952, 65, 346–57. *147.*

LORENZ, K. The evolution of behaviour. *Sci. Amer.*, 1958, 199 (Dec.), 67–78. *10.*

LUSH, J. L. *Animal breeding plans.* (2nd edition.) Ames: Iowa State College Press, 1943. *20.*

MACARTHUR, J. W. Genetics of body size and related characters: I. Selecting small and large races of the laboratory mouse. *Amer. Naturalist*, 1944a, 78, 142–57. *14.*

MACARTHUR, J. W. Genetics of body size and related characters: II. Satellite characters associated with body size in mice. *Amer. Naturalist*, 1944b, 78, 224–37, *14.*

MACARTHUR, J. W. Selection for small and large body size in the house mouse. *Genetics*, 1949, 34, 194–209. *14.*

MACKWORTH, N. H. Researches on the measurement of human performance. *M.R.C. Spec. Rep. Ser. No. 268.* London: H.M.S.O., 1950. *165, 170.*

MACKWORTH, N. H. Some factors affecting vigilance. *The Advancement of Science*, 1957, 53, 393–398. *165.*

MAHUT, HELEN. Breed differences in the dog's emotional behaviour. *Canad. J. Psychol.*, 1958, 12, 35–44. *11.*

MALMO, ROBERT B. Measurement of drive: an unsolved problem in psychology. In Nebraska Symposium on Motivation. (Ed. M. R. Jones) 1958, 6, 229–65. *219.*

MALTZMAN, I., SMITH, W. H., & BROOKS, W. D. Some effects of different training conditions and manifest anxiety upon target tracking. *Psychol. Abstr.*, 1956, 30, 5642 (Abstract). *176.*

MANN, IDA, & SHARPLES, F. W. The normal visual (rod) field of the dark adapted eye. *J. Physiol.*, 1946, 104, 384–91. *140.*

MARBLE, D. R. Genetics of egg shape. *Poultry, Sci.*, 1943, 22, 61–71. *13.*

MARDONES, R. J., SEGOVIA, M. N., & HEDERRA, D. A. Herencia del alcoholismo en ratas: I. Comportamiento de la primera generación de ratas bebedoras, colocadas en dieta carenciada en factor N_1. *Bol. Soc. Biol. Santiago.*, 1950, 7, 61–2. *8.*

MARDONES, R. J., SEGOVIA, M. N., & HEDERRA, D. A. Heredity of experimental alcohol preference in rats: II. Coefficient of heredity. *Quart. J. Stud. Alc.*, 1953, 14, 1–2. *8.*

MARGOLIS, L. H. Pharmacotherapy in psychiatry: A review. *Ann. N.Y. Acad. Sci.*, 1957, 66, 698–718. *138.*

MARQUIS, D. G., KELLY, E. L., MILLER, J. G., GERARD, R. W., & RAPAPORT, A. Experimental studies of behavioral effects of meprobamate on normal subjects. *Ann. N.Y. Acad. Sci.*, 1957, 67, 701–10. *119, 138, 139, 176, 197.*

MARSHALL, W. H. Recent evidence for neural mechanisms in vision leading to a general theory of sensory acuity. In H. Kluver (Ed.) Visual Mechanisms. *Biol. Sympos.*, 1942, 7, 117–64. *140.*

MARSHALL, W. H., & TALBOT, S. A. Recovery cycle of the lateral geniculate of the nembutalized cat. *Amer. J. Physiol.*, 1940, 129, 417–18. *140.*

MARTIN, R. F., & HALL, C. S. Emotional behaviour in the rat: V. The incidence of behavior derangements resulting from air-blast stimulation in emotional and non-emotional strains of rats. *J. comp. Psychol.*, 1941, 32, 191–204. *17, 40.*

MATHER, K. *Biometrical Genetics: The Study of Continuous Variation.* London: Methuen, 1949. *24, 26, 27, 67, 70, 72, 73, 76, 92.*

MATHER, K., & HARRISON, B. J. The manifold effect of selection. *Heredity*, 1949, 3, 1–52, and 131–62. *40, 44, 66.*

MATHER, K., & JONES, M. R. Interaction of genotype and environment in continuous variation: I. Descriptions. *Biometrics*, 1958, 14, 343–59. *101.*

MATHER, K., & VINES, A. The inheritance of height and flowering time in a cross of *Nicotiana rustica.* In Reeve, E. C. R., & Waddington, C. H. (Eds.) *Quantitative Inheritance.* London: H.M.S.O., 1952. Pp. 49–79. *73.*

MCCLEARN, G. E. Performance differences among mouse strains in a learning situation. *Amer. Psychologist*, 1958, 13, 405 (Abstract). *8.*

MCCLEARN, G. E. The genetics of mouse behavior in novel situations. *J. comp. physiol. Psychol.*, 1959, 52, 62–7. *7, 41.*

MCCLEARN, G. E., & RODGERS, D. A. Differences in alcohol preferences among inbred strains of mice. *Quart. J. Stud. Alc.*, 1959, 20, 691–5. *8.*

MCFARLAND, R. A., & HALPERIN, M. H. The relation between foveal visual acuity and illumination under reduced oxygen tension. *J. gen. Physiol.* 1940, 23, 613–30. *141.*

MCFARLAND, R. A., *et al.* The effect of oxygen deficiency on the relation between stimulus intensity and the latency of visual after-images. *Amer. J. Physiol.*, 1943, 140, 354–66. *141.*

MCGEOCH, J. A., & IRION, A. L. *The Psychology of Human Learning.* (2nd edition.) New York: Longmans Green, 1952. *183.*

MCNEMAR, Q. *Psychological Statistics.* (2nd edition.) New York: Wiley, 1955. *55.*

METFESSEL, M. The relationships of heredity and environment in behavior. *J. Psychol.*, 1940, 10, 177–98. *10.*

MILES, W. R. Static equilibrium as a useful test of motor control. *J. Indust. Hygiene.* 1922, 3, 316–61. *153.*

MILLER, N. E. Experimental studies of conflict. In Hunt, J. McV. (Ed.) *Personality and the Behavior Disorders.* New York: Ronald Press Co., 1944. Pp. 431–65. *39.*

MONTAGUE, E. K. The role of anxiety in serial rote learning. *J. exp. Psychol.*, 1953, 45, 91–6. *112.*

MORUZZI, G., & MAGOUN, H. W. Brain stem reticular formation and activation of the E.E.G. *E.E.G. clin. Neurophysiol.*, 1949, 1, 455–73. *168.*

MUNDY-CASTLE, A. C., & MCKIEVER, B. L. The psychophysiological significance of the galvanic skin response. *J. exp. Psychol.*, 1953, 46, 15–24. *198.*

MUNN, N. L. *Handbook of Psychological Research on the Rat.* London: Harrap, 1950. *6.*

MYERS, A. K. Avoidance learning as a function of several training conditions and strain differences in rats. *J. comp. physiol. Psychol.*, 1959, 52, 381–6. *6.*

NACHMAN, M. The inheritance of saccharin preference. *J. comp. physiol. Psychol.*, 1959, 52, 451–7. *8, 14.*

NACHTSHEIM, H. Untersuchungen über Variation und Vererbung des Gesäuges beim Schwein. *Z. Tierzuchtg.*, 1925, 2, 113–61. *76.*

NACHTSHEIM, H. Das Porto-Santo-Kaninchen. Ein beitrag zum Rasse und Artproblem. *Umshau*, 1941, 45, 151–4. *9.*

NELDER, J. A. Statistical models in biometrical genetics. *Heredity*, 1953, 7, 111–19. *29.*

NIELSON, H. C., DOTY, R. W., & RUTLEDGE, L. T. Motivational and perceptual aspects of subcortical stimulation in cats. *Amer. J. Physiol.*, 1958, 194, 427–32. *188.*

NISSEN, H. W. 'Freezing' behavior in rats. *Science*, 1946, 103, 27. *41.*

OAKLEY, S. R. *Extraversion and Neuroticism as Factors in Pursuit Rotor Learning and Reminiscence.* Unpubl. Thesis. Univ. of Pittsburgh. 1958. *189.*

O'KELLY, L. I. The validity of defecation as a measure of emotionality in the rat. *J. gen. Psychol.*, 1940, 23, 75–87. *38.*

OLSON, H. H., & PETERSEN, W. E. Uniformity of semen production and behaviour in monozygous triplet bulls. *J. dairy Sci.*, 1951, 34, 489–90 (Abstract). *11.*

OSGOOD, C. E., & HEYER, A. W. A new interpretation of figural after-effects. *Psychol. Rev.*, 1952, 59, 98–118. *140.*

OSINSKI, W. A. Treatment of anxiety states with Meprobamate (Miltown). *Inter. Rec. med. gen. prac. Clinics*, 1956, 169, 589–95. *107.*

PAINTAL, A. S. A comparison of the galvanic skin responses of normals and psychotics. *J. exp. Psychol.*, 1951, 41, 425–8. *207.*

PARKER, M. M. The interrelationship of six different situations in the measurement of emotionality in the adult albino rat. *Psychol. Bull.*, 1939, 36, 564–5 (Abstract). *37, 38.*

PAVLOV, I. P. *Conditioned Reflexes* (Trans. G. V. Anrep). London: Oxford Univ. Press, 1927. *110.*

PAWLOWSKI, A. A., & SCOTT, J. P. Hereditary differences in the development of dominance in litters of puppies. *J. comp. physiol. Psychol.*, 1956, 49, 353–8. *12.*

PEARSON, E. S., & HARTLEY, H. O. *Biometrika Tables for Statisticians*. Vol. I. Cambridge (Eng.): University Press, 1958. *55, 97.*

PEIRCE, J. T. Cerebral cholinesterase activity and 'hypotheses' behavior in a problemless maze. *J. comp. physiol. Psychol.*, 1959, 52, 168–71. *15.*

PETRIE, A. *The Study of Experimental Methods of Assessing Personality*. Unpubl. Thesis. Univ. of London, 1946. *173.*

PETTERSSON, M. Diffusion of a new habit among greenfinches. *Nature*, 1956, 177, 709–10. *10.*

PETTERSSON, M. Diffusion of a new habit among Greenfinches. *Nature*, 1959, 184, 649–50. *10.*

PHILLIPS, J. C. Note on wildness in ducklings. *J. anim. Behav.*, 1912, 2, 363–4. *10.*

PIRENNE, M. H., MARRIOT, F. H. C., & O'DOHERTY, E. F. Individual differences in night vision efficiency. *Med. Res. Council, Special Report No. 294*, London: H.M.S.O., 1957. *147, 158.*

PORTER, J. M., JNR. Adaptation of the galvanic skin response. *J. exp. Psychol.*, 1938, 23, 553–7. *195.*

RABINOVITCH, M. S., & ROSVOLD, H. E. A closed-field intelligence test for rats. *Canad. J. Psychol.*, 1951, 5, 122–8. *16, 65.*

RASMUSSEN, E. W. Wildness in rats: Heredity or environment? *Acta Psychol. (Hague)*, 1939, 4, 295–304. *18.*

RASMUSSEN, E. W. The relation between strength of sexual drive and fertility as evident from experimental investigations. *Proc. II int. Congr. anim. Reprod. (Copenhagen)*, 1952, 1, 188–91. *14.*

REED, JANET G. A study of the alcoholic consumption and amino acid excretion patterns of rats of different inbred strains. *Univer. Texas Publ.*, 1951, 5109, 144–9. *8.*

REITMAN, R. The comparative effects of placebo, Ultran and Meprobamate on psychological test performance. *Antibiot. Med. Clin. Therap.*, 1957, 4, 158–64. *162.*

RICHTER, C. P. Domestication of the Norway rat and its implications for the problem of stress. In Wolff, H. G., Wolf, S. G., & Hare, C. C. (Eds.) *Life Stress and Bodily Disease* (Res. Publ. Assoc. Res. nerv. ment. Dis., 29). Baltimore: Williams and Wilkins Co., 1950. Pp. 19–47. *21.*

RICHTER, C. P. Domestication of the Norway rat and its implication for the study of genetics in man. *Amer. J. hum. Genet.*, 1952, 4, 273–85. *21.*

RICHTER, C. P. Rats, man, and the welfare state. *Amer. Psychologist*, 1959, 14, 18–28. *21.*

RIDDELL, L. A. The use of the flicker phenomenon in the investigation of the field of vision. *Brit. J. Ophthalm.*, 1936, 20, 385–410. *147.*

RIESS, B. F. A possible explanation of 'freezing' behavior in rats. *Science*, 1945, 102, 570. *41.*

RIESS, B. F. A correction. *Science*, 1946a, 103, 27. *41.*

RIESS, B. F. 'Freezing' behavior in rats and its social causation. *J. soc. Psychol.*, 1946b, 24, 249–51. *41.*

ROBACK, G. S., KRASNO, L. R., & IVY, A. C. Effect of analeptic drugs on the somnifacient effect of Seconal and antihistaminics as measured by the flicker fusion threshold.

ROBINSON, R. Genetic studies of the rabbit. *Bibliograph. Genet.*, 1958, 17, 229–558. *9.*

RODGERS, D. A., & MCCLEARN, G. E. Genetic factors in alcohol preference in laboratory mice. *Amer. Psychologist*, 1959, 14, 396 (Abstract). *8.*

ROSENZWEIG, M. R., KRECH, D., & BENNETT, E. L. Brain chemistry and adaptive behavior. In Harlow, H. F., & Woolsey, C. N. (Eds.) *Biological and Biochemical Bases of Behavior.* Madison: University of Wisconsin Press, 1958a. Pp. 367–400. *15.*

ROSENZWEIG, M. R. KRECH, D., & BENNETT, E. L. Brain enzymes and adaptive behaviour. In Wolstenholme, G. E. W., & O'Connor, Cecilia M. (Eds.) *The Neurological Basis of Behaviour.* (Ciba Foundation symposium.) Churchill: London, 1958b. Pp. 337–58. *15, 20, 63.*

ROSENZWEIG, M. R., KRECH, D., & BENNETT, E. L. Individual differences in behavior and their correlates in brain chemistry. *Proc. XV int. Congr. Psychol. (Brussels)*, 1957, 182–3. Amsterdam: North-Holland Publishing Co., 1959 (Abstract). *15.*

ROSENZWEIG, M. R., KRECH, D., BENNETT, E. L., & LONGUEIL, C. L. Strain differences in rats in behavior and brain chemistry. *Amer. Psychologist*, 1958, 13, 405 (Abstract). *15.*

ROSS, R. T. Foveal fusion frequency as a function of effective cone population. *Psychol. Bull.*, 1935, 32, 712. *147.*

ROSS, R. T. A comparison of the regional gradient of fusion frequency and visual acuity. *Psychol. Monogr.*, 1936, 47, 306–10. *147.*

ROSS, R. T. The fusion frequency in different areas of the visual field: I. The foveal fusion frequency. *J. gen. Psychol.*, 1936, 15, 133–47. *147.*

ROSS, R. T. The fusion frequency in different areas of the visual field: II. The regional gradient of fusion frequency. *J. gen. Psychol.*, 1936, 15, 161–70. *147.*

ROSS, R. T. The fusion frequency in different areas of the visual field: III. Foveal fusion frequency as a function of the light dark ratio for constant retinal illumination at fusion. *J. gen. Psychol.*, 1938, 18, 111–22. *147.*

ROYCE, J. R. The factorial analysis of animal behavior. *Psychol. Bull.*, 1950, 47, 235–59. *38.*

RUNDQUIST, E. A. Inheritance of spontaneous activity in rats. *J. comp. Psychol.*, 1933, 16, 415–38. *16.*

RUNDQUIST, E. A., & BELLIS, C. J. Respiratory metabolism of active and inactive rats. *Amer. J. Physiol.*, 1933, 106, 670–5. *16.*

RUNDQUIST, E. A., & HERON, W. T. Spontaneous activity and maze learning. *J. comp. Psychol.*, 1935, 19, 297–311. *16.*

RUSSELL, R. W. Experimental studies of hereditary influences on behaviour. *Eugen. Rev.*, 1953a, 45, 19–30. *5, 19, 48.*

RUSSELL, R. W. Behaviour under stress. *Int. J. Psychoanal.*, 1953b, 34, Suppl., 1–12. *76.*

SADOVNIKOVA-KOLTZOVA, MARY P. Genetic analysis of temperament in rats. *J. exp. Zool.*, 1926, 45, 301–18. *5.*

SADOVNIKOVA-KOLTZOVA, MARY P. (Genetical analysis of mental faculties of rats: II). *Zh. eksp. Biol. (A)*, 1928, 4, 65–76 (*Biol. Abstr.*, 1929, 3, No. 17450 (Abstract)). *5.*

SADOVNIKOVA-KOLTZOVA, MARY P. Genetische Analyse des Temperamentes der Ratten. *Z. ind. Abst. Vererblehre.*, 1929, 49, 131–45. *5.*

SADOVNIKOVA-KOLTZOVA, MARY P. (Genetical analysis of mental faculties of rats: III). *Zh. eksp. Biol.*, 1931, 7, 265–83. *5.*

SADOVNIKOVA-KOLTZOVA, MARY P. (Genetical analysis of mental faculties in rats: IV). *Biol. Zh. Mosk.*, 1933, 2, 184–95. *5.*

SARGANT, W., & SLATER, E. *An Introduction to Physical Methods of Treatment in Psychiatry*. Edinburgh & London: E. & S. Livingstone, Ltd., 1954. *106.*

SAVAGE, R. D. *Constitutional Determinants of Emotionality in the Rat: An experimental study of Fear, Frustration and Conflict*. Ph.D. Thesis, University of London, 1960. *39.*

SAWIN, P. B., & CRARY, D. D. Genetic and physiological background of reproduction in the rabbit: II. Some racial differences in the pattern of maternal behavior. *Behaviour*, 1953, 6, 126–46. *9.*

SAWIN, P. B., & CURRAN, R. H. Genetic and physiological background of reproduction in the rabbit: I. The problem and its biological significance. *J. exp. Zool.*, 1952, 128, 165–201. *9.*

SCHAEFER, V. H. Differences between strains of rats in avoidance conditioning without an explicit warning stimulus. *J. comp. physiol. Psychol.*, 1959, 52, 120–2. *6.*

SCHMIDT, J. La valeur de l'individu à titre de générateur appreciée suivant la méthode du croisement diallèle. *C. R. Lab. Carlsberg*, 1919, 14, No. 6, 1–33. *75, 76.*

SCOTT, J. P. Hereditary differences in social behavior (fighting of males) between two inbred strains of mice. *Anat. Rec.*, 1940, 78, Suppl., 103 (Abstract). *8.*

SCOTT, J. P. Genetic differences in the social behavior of inbred strains of mice. *J. Hered.*, 1942, 33, 11–15. *8.*

SCOTT, J. P. Effects of single genes on the behavior of drosophila. *Amer. Naturalist*, 1943, 77, 184–90. *9, 17.*

SCOTT, J. P. The genetic determination of a social relationship. *Anat. Rec.*, 1952, 113, 543 (Abstract). *12.*

SCOTT, J. P. Biomathematical problems in animal behavior. In Kempthorne, O., (Ed.) *Statistics and Mathematics in Biology*. Ames: Iowa State College Press, 1954a. *11, 12.*

SCOTT, J. P. The effects of selection and domestication upon the behavior of the dog. *J. nat. Cancer Res. Inst.*, 1954b, 15, 739–58. *11, 12, 21.*

SCOTT, J. P. Analysis of hereditary factors affecting a threshold of stimulation for playful fighting behavior in puppies. *Anat. Rec.*, 1955, 122, 423 (Abstract). *12.*

SCOTT, J. P. Critical periods in the development of social behavior in puppies. *Psychosom. Med.*, 1958a, 20, 24–54. *12.*

SCOTT, J. P. *Animal Behavior*. Chicago: Chicago Univer. Press, 1958b. *12.*

SCOTT, J. P. *Aggression*. Chicago: Chicago Univer. Press, 1958c. *12.*

SCOTT, J. P., & CHARLES, MARGARET S. Some problems of heredity and social behavior. *J. gen. Psychol.*, 1953, 48, 209–30. *12.*

SCOTT, J. P., & CHARLES, MARGARET S. A case of genetic differences modified by thresholds and habit formation. *J. genet. Psychol.*, 1954, 84, 175–88. *12.*

SCOTT, J. P., & FREDERICSON, E. The causes of fighting in mice and rats. *Physiol. Zool.*, 1951, 24, 273–309 *8, 30.*

SCOTT, J. P., & FULLER, J. L. Research on genetics and social behavior. *J. Hered.*, 1951, 42, 191–7. *11, 48.*

SCOTT, J. P., & FULLER, J. L. Heredity and the development of social behavior traits in dogs. *Proc. XV int. Congr. Psychol. (Brussels)*, *1957*, 554–5. Amsterdam: North-Holland Publishing Co., 1959a (Abstract). *11.*

SCOTT, J. P., & FULLER, J. L. Inheritance of seasonal breeding behavior in the basenji (African barkless) dog. *Anat. Rec.*, 1959b, 134, 636 (Abstract). *12.*

SCOTT, J. P., & GAULT, MONA M. Genetic differences in the reactions of dogs to a barrier problem. *Anat. Rec.*, 1953, 117, 565 (Abstract). *12.*

SEARLE, L. V. The organization of hereditary maze-brightness and maze-dullness. *Genet. Psychol. Monogr.*, 1949, 39, 279–325. *15, 63.*

SEASHORE, R. H., DUDEK, F. J., & HOLTZMAN, W. A factorial analysis of arm-hand precision tests. *J. appl. Psychol.*, 1949, 33, 579–84. *174.*

SETTLAGE, P. The effects of sodium amytal on the formation and elicitation of conditioned reflexes. *J. comp. Psychol.*, 1936, 22, 339–43. *111.*

SEWARD, J. P., & SEWARD, G. H. The relation of galvanic skin reactions to preceding resistance. *J. exp. Psychol.*, 1935, 18, 64–79. *198.*

SHAGASS, C. Sedation threshold. A neurophysiological tool of psychosomatic research. *Psychosom. Med.*, 1956, 18, 410–19. *119.*

SHAGASS, C. A measurable neurophysiological factor of psychiatric significance. *J. E.E.G. clin. Neurophysiol.*, 1957, 9, 101–8. *119.*

SHAGASS, C., & LIPOVSKI, F. J. Effects of methedrine on critical flicker fusion and its relation to personality and affect. *J. nerv. ment. Dis.*, 1958, 127, 407–16 *232.*

SHAGASS, C., & NAIMAN, J. The sedation threshold, manifest anxiety and some aspects of ego function. *A.M.A. Arch. Neurol. Psychiat.*, 1955, 74, 397–406. *119.*

SHARPLES, F. W. Relation between illumination and the extent of the visual field. *J. Physiol.*, 1946, 105, 215–22. *140.*

SHARPLESS, S., & JASPER, H. Habituation of the arousal reaction. *Brain*, 1956, 79, 655–680. *217.*

SIGG, E. B., SCHNEIDER, J. A., & HOLLAND, R. Non-barbiturate depressants: Effect on EEG and central polysynaptic mechanisms. *Fed. Proc.*, 1957, 16, No. 1. *168.*

SILVERMAN, W., SHAPIRO, F., & HERON, W. T. Brain weight and maze learning in the rat. *J. comp. Psychol.*, 1940, 30, 279–82. *16.*

SIMONSON, E., & BROZEK, J. Flicker fusion frequency: background and application. *Physiol. Rev.*, 1952, 32, 349–78. *148, 152.*

SINES, J. O. Selective breeding for development of stomach lesions following stress in the rat. *J. comp. physiol. Psychol.*, 1959, 52, 615–17. *14.*

SINGH, S. D. Conditioned emotional response in the rat: I. Constitutional and situational determinants. *J. comp. physiol. Psychol.*, 1959, 52, 574–8. *39.*

SINGH, S. D. Conditioned emotional response in the rat: II. Effect of stimulant and depressant drugs. *Acta Psychol. (Hague)*, 1960, in press. *39.*

SINGH, S. D., & EYSENCK, H. J. Conditioned emotional response in the rat: III. Drug antagonism. *J. gen. Psychol.*, 1960, in press. *39.*

SINHA, S. N., FRANKS, C. M., & BROADHURST, P. L. The effect of a stimulant and a depressant drug on a measure of reactive inhibition. *J. exp. Psychol.*, 1958, 56, 349–54. *39.*

SKILLICORN, S. A. Presenile cerebellar ataxia in chronic alcoholics. *Neurology*, 1955, 5, 527–34. *153.*

SMITH, R. P., WAGMAN, ALTHEA I., & RIOPELLE, A. J. Effects of reserpine on conditioned monkeys. *J. Pharmacol.*, 1956, 117, 136–41. *111.*

SMITH, W. I., & POWELL, E. K. The role of emotionality in hoarding. *Behaviour*, 1955, 8, 57-62. *7.*

SNEDECOR, G. W. *Statistical Methods applied to Experiments in Agriculture and Biology*. (5th edition.) Ames: Iowa State College Press, 1956. *23, 58, 63, 80.*

SPENCE, K. W., & FARBER, J. C. Conditioning and extinction as a function of anxiety. *J. exp. Psychol.*, 1953, 45, 116–19. *111.*

SPENCE, K. W., FARBER, I. E., & MCFANN, H. H. The relation of anxiety (drive) level to performance in competitional and noncompetitional paired-associate learning. *J. exp. Psychol.*, 1956, 52, 296–305. *112.*

SPENCE, K. W., & TAYLOR, JANET A. Anxiety and the strength of the UCS as determiners of the amount of eyelid conditioning. *J. exp. Psychol.*, 1951, 42, 183–8. *111.*

SPENCE, K. W., & TAYLOR, JANET A. The relation of conditioned response strength to anxiety in normal, neurotic and psychotic subjects. *J. exp. Psychol.*, 1952, 45, 265–72. *111.*

SPENCE, K. W., TAYLOR, J., & KETCHEL, R. Anxiety (drive) level and degree of competition in paired associate learning. *J. exp. Psychol.*, 1956, 52, 306–10. *112.*

STAATS, JOAN. Behaviour studies on inbred mice: A selected bibliography. *Anim. Behav.*, 1958, 6, 77–84. *6.*

STAMM, J. S. Genetics of hoarding: I. Differences between homozygous strains of rats. *J. comp. physiol. Psychol.*, 1954, 47, 157–61. *7.*

STAMM, J. S. Hoarding and aggressive behavior in rats. *J. comp. physiol. Psychol.*, 1955, 48, 324–6. *7.*

STAMM, J. S. Genetics of hoarding: II. Hoarding behavior of hybrid and backcrossed strains of rats. *J. comp. physiol. Psychol.*, 1956, 49, 349–52. *7.*

STEINBERG, HANNAH, & SUMMERFIELD, A. Environmental conditions and behavior. Effects of drugs: effects of nitrous oxide on learning and retention. *Bull. Brit. psychol. Soc.*, 1955, 26, Inset 6–7 (Abstract). *112.*

STEINBERG, HANNAH, & SUMMERFIELD, A. Influence of a depressant drug on acquisition in rote learning. *Quart. J. Psychol.*, 1957, 9, 138–45. *112.*

STEPHENSON, W. Some observations on Q technique. *Psychol. Bull.*, 1952, 49, 483–98. *105.*

STEVENS, S. S. (Ed.) *Handbook of Experimental Psychology*. New York: Wiley & Sons, 1951. Pp, 1–55. *121.*

STEVENS, S. S. On the psychophysical law. *Psychol. Rev.*, 1957, 64, 513–81. *155.*

STONE, C. P. Wildness and savageness in rats of different strains. In Lashley, K. S. (Ed.) *Studies in the Dynamics of Behavior*. Chicago: University of Chicago Press, 1932. Pp. 1–55. *21.*

STONE, C. P. Methodological resources for the experimental study of innate behavior as related to environmental factors. *Psychol. Rev.*, 1947, 54, 342–7. *4, 5.*

STONE, C. P., & BARKER, R. G. Change of the age of puberty in albino rats by selective mating. *Proc. Soc. exp. Biol. Med.*, 1940, 44, 48–50. *14.*

STOUFFER, S. A., GUTTMAN, L., SUCHMAN, E. A., LAZARSFELD, P. F., STAR, SHIRLEY A., & CLAUSEN, J. A. *Studies in Social Psychology in World War II:* Vol. 4. *Measurement and Prediction*. Princeton: Princeton Univer. Press, 1950. *37.*

STOUFFER, S. A., LUMSDAINE, A. A., LUMSDAINE, MARION H., WILLIAMS, R. M., JNR., SMITH, M. B., JANIS, I. L., STAR, SHIRLEY A., & COTTRELL, L. S., JNR. *Studies in Social Psychology in World War II:* Vol. 2. *The American Soldier: Combat and its Aftermath*. Princeton: Princeton Univer. Press, 1949. *37.*

SUMMERFIELD, A., & STEINBERG, HANNAH. Reducing interference in forgetting. *Quart. J. Psychol.*, 1957, 9, 146–54. *112, 135.*

TALBOT, S. A., & MARSHALL, W. H. Physiological studies on neural mechanisms of visual localization and discrimination. *Amer. J. Ophthalm.*, 1941, 24, 1255–64. *140.*

TAYLOR, J. G., & REICHLIN, B. A contribution to the theory of the inheritance of behavior tendencies in the white rat. *J. soc. Res. (Pretoria)*, 1950, 1, 159–71. *14.*

TEICHNER, W. H. Recent studies of simple reaction time. *Psychol. Bull.*, 1954, 51, 128–149. *221.*

THOMPSON, W. D., JNR., & SONTAG, L. W. Behavioral effects in the offspring of rats subjected to audiogenic seizure during the gestational period. *J. comp. physiol. Psychol.*, 1956, 49, 454–6. *18.*

THOMPSON, W. R. Exploratory behavior as a function of hunger in 'bright' and 'dull' rats. *J. comp. physiol. Psychol.*, 1953a, 46, 323–6. *16, 37.*

THOMPSON, W. R. The inheritance of behaviour: Behavioural differences in fifteen mouse strains. *Canad. J. Psychol.*, 1953b, 7, 145–55. *7, 19, 21.*

THOMPSON, W. R. The inheritance and development of intelligence. In *Genetics and the Inheritance of Integrated Neurological and Psychiatric Patterns*. (Proc. Ass. Res. nerv. ment. Dis., 23.) Baltimore: Williams & Wilkins, 1954. Pp. 209-31. *7, 16, 19.*

THOMPSON, W. R. The inheritance of behavior: Activity differences in five inbred mouse strains. *J. Hered.*, 1956, 47, 147–8. *7.*

THOMPSON, W. R. Influence of prenatal maternal anxiety on emotionality in young rats. *Science*, 1957, 125, 698–9. *18.*

THOMPSON, W. R., & BINDRA, D. Motivational and emotional characteristics of 'bright' and 'dull' rats. *Canad. J. Psychol.*, 1952, 6, 116–22. *16, 65.*

THOMPSON, W. R., & FULLER, J. L. The inheritance of activity in the mouse. *Amer. Psychologist*, 1957, 12, 433 (Abstract). *7.*

THOMPSON, W. R., & FULLER, J. L. The genetics of activity in the mouse. 1960, in press. *7, 12.*

THOMPSON, W. R., & KAHN, A. Retroaction effects in the exploratory activity of 'bright' and 'dull' rats. *Canad. J. Psychol.*, 1955, 9, 173–82. *16.*

THOMPSON, W. R., & SOLOMON, L. M. Spontaneous pattern discrimination in the rat. *J. comp. physiol. Psychol.*, 1954, 47, 104–7. *16.*

THORNE, F. C. The inheritance of shyness in dogs. *J. genet. Psychol.*, 1944, *65*, 275–9. *11.*

TOBACH, ETHEL, & BLOCH, H. A study of the relationship between behavior and susceptibility to tuberculosis in rats and mice. *Adv. Tuberc. Res.*, 1955, 6, 62–89. *8.*

TOLMAN, E. C. The inheritance of maze learning in rats. *J. comp. Psychol.*, 1924, 4, 1–18. *15.*

TOLMAN, E. C., & JEFFRESS, L. A. A self-recording maze. *J. comp. Psychol.*, 1925, 5, 455–463. *15.*

TOLMAN, E. C., TRYON, R. C., & JEFFRESS, L. A. A self-recording maze with an automatic delivery table. *Univer. Calif. Publ. Psychol.*, 1929, 4, 99–112. *15.*

TOMAN, J. E. P., EVERETT, G. M., & JEANS, R. F. Seizure latency method and other procedures for antipsychotic drugs. In Himwich, H. E. (Ed.) *Tranquilizing Drugs*. American Association for the Advancement of Science. No. 46. 1957. *174.*

TRAQUAIR, H. M. *An Introduction to Clinical Perimetry*. 5th edition. London: Henry Kimpton, 1948. *139, 140.*

TRAVIS, L. E. The relation of voluntary movement to tremors. *J. exp. Psychol.*, 1929, 12, 515–24. *174.*

TRAVIS, L. E., & HUNTER, T. A. Tremor frequencies. *J. gen. Psychol.*, 1931, 5, 225–60. *174.*

TREADWELL, E. *Motor Reminiscence and Individual Personality Differences*. Unpubl. Thesis: Univ. of Belfast, 1956. *186.*

TROUTON, D. S., & EYSENCK, H. J. The effects of drugs on behaviour. In H. J. Eysenck (Ed.) *Handbook of Abnormal Psychology*. London: Pitman, 1960. *138, 160, 161, 163, 225.*

TRYON, R. C. Genetics of learning ability in rats: Preliminary report. *Univer. Calif. Publ. Psychol.*, 1929, 4, 71–89. *15, 26.*

TRYON, R. C. The inheritance of mental ability. *Psychol. Bull.*, 1932, 29, 663–4 (Abstract). *15.*

TRYON, R. C. Genetic differences in maze-learning ability in rats. *Yearb. nat. Soc. Stud. Educ.*, 1940, 39, 111–19. *15, 18, 26.*

TRYON, R. C. Individual differences. In Moss, F. A. (Ed.). *Comparative Psychology*. (2nd edition.) New York: Prentice Hall, 1942. Pp. 330–65. *15, 26.*

UTSURIKAWA, N. Temperamental differences between outbred and inbred strains of the albino rat. *J. anim. Behav.*, 1917, 7, 111–29. *5.*

VALENSTEIN, E. S., RISS, W., & YOUNG, W. C. Sex drive in genetically homogeneous and highly inbred strains of male guinea pigs. *J. comp. physiol. Psychol.*, 1954, 47, 162–5. *9.*

VALENSTEIN, E. S., RISS, W., & YOUNG, W. C. Experiential and genetic factors in the organisation of sexual behavior in male guinea pigs. *J. comp. physiol. Psychol.*, 1955, 48, 397–403. *9.*

VAN DER VEEN, J. H. The 2 × 2 genotype-environment table. *Heredity*, 1959, 13, 123–6. *101.*

VENABLES, P. H. The relationships between PGR scores and temperature and humidity. *Quart. J. exp. Psychol.*, 1955, 7, 12–18. *199, 200.*

VENABLES, P. H. Car driving consistency and measures of personality. *J. appl. Psychol.*, 1956, 40, 21–4. *134.*

VICARI, EMELIA M. Mode of inheritance of reaction time and degrees of learning in mice. *J. exp. Zool.*, 1929, 54, 31–88. *5.*

VON HÖRMANN-HECK, SYBILLE. Untersuchungen über der Erbgang einiger Verhaltensweisen bei Crillen-bastarden (Cryllus compestris L. ~ cryllus bimaculatus de Cear). *Z. Tierpsychol.*, 1957, 14, 137–83. *10.*

WARREN, E. P., & BOGART, R. Effect of selection of age at time of puberty on reproductive performance in the rat. *Tech. Bull. Ore. agric. Sta.*, 1952, No. 25, 1–27. *14.*

WATERMAN, A. J., & MOORE, W. M. Thyroid activity in inbred and selected mice in relation to behavior. *Anat. Rec.*, 1958, 131, 607 (Abstract). *14.*

WATSON, R. H. J. The investigation of a psycho-pharmacological and genetic problem. *Bull. Brit. psychol. Soc.*, 1958, 35, A23 (Abstract). *39, 40.*

WATSON, R. H. J. Constitutional differences between two strains of rats with different behavioural characteristics. *Psychosom. Adv. Med.*, 1960, 1, 160–5. *39, 40.*

WESTON, D. T. Treating insomnia with Doriden, a new non-barbiturate sedative. *Lancet*, 1956, 3477. *107, 139.*

WHALEN, R. E. Sexual behavior of descendants of Tryon's maze-bright and maze-dull rats. *Amer. Psychologist*, 1959, 14, 396–7 (Abstract). *15.*

WHERRY, R. J. Determination of the specific components of maze ability for Tryon's bright and dull rats by means of factorial analysis. *J. comp. Psychol.*, 1941, 32, 237–52. *15.*

WHITNEY, L. F. Inheritance of the trail-barking propensity in dogs. *J. Hered.*, 1929, 20, 561–2. *11.*

WIESNER, B. P., & SHEARD, N. M. *Maternal Behaviour in the Rat.* Edinburgh: Ol ver & Boyd, 1933. *48.*

WILLETT, R. A. Drugs and Personality: The effect of a stimulant and a depressant drug on the serial rate learning of nonsense syllables (unpublished paper). *112, 113.*

WILLIAMS, R. J., BERRY, L. J., & BEERSTECHER, E., JNR. Biochemical individuality: III. Genetotrophic factors in the etiology of alcoholism. *Arch. Biochem.*, N.Y., 1949, 23, 275–90. *8.*

WILLINGHAM, W. W. The organization of emotional behavior in mice. *J. comp. physiol. Psychol.*, 1956, 49, 345–8. *38, 41.*

WILSON, W. K. A tame-wild rabbit cross. *J. Hered.*, 1936, 27, 127–31. *9.*

WOLFSON, A. Regulation of spring migration in Juncos. *Condor*, 1942, 44, 237–63. *10.*

WOOD-GUSH, D. G. M. The behaviour of the domestic chicken: A review of the literature. *Brit. J. anim. Behav.*, 1955, 3, 81–110. *11.*

WOOD-GUSH, D. G. M. Genetic differences in the reproductive behavior of domestic cockerels. *Anat. Rec.*, 1959, 134, 658–9 (Abstract). *10.*

WOOD-GUSH, D. C. M., & OSBORNE, R. A study of differences in the sex drive of cockerels. *Brit. J. anim. Behav.*, 1956, 4, 102–10. *10.*

WOODWORTH, R. S. *Experimental Psychology.* London: Methuen, 1939. *149.*

WOODWORTH, R. S., & SCHLOSBERG, H. *Experimental psychology.* New York: Henry Holt, 1954. *147, 221, 224.*

WRIGHT, S. Systems of mating: II. The effects of inbreeding on the genetic composition of a population. *Genetics*, 1921, 6, 124–43. *67.*

WRIGHT, S. The genetics of quantitative variability. In Reeve, E. C. R., & Waddington, C. H. (Eds.) *Quantitative inheritance.* London: H.M.S.O., 1952. Pp. 5–41. *24.*

YATES, F. Analysis of data from all possible reciprocal crosses between a set of parental lines. *Heredity*, 1947, 1, 287–301. *89.*

YEAKEL, ELEANOR H., & RHOADES, RUTH P. A comparison of the body and endocrine gland (Adrenal, thyroid and pituitary) weights of emotional and non-emotional rats. *Endocrinology*, 1941, 28, 337–40. *17, 39, 40.*

YERKES, ADA W. Comparison of the behavior of stock and inbred albino rats. *J. anim. Behav.*, 1916, 6, 267–96. *5.*

YERKES, R. M. The heredity of savageness and wildness in rats. *J. anim. Behav.*, 1913, 3, 286–96. *5.*

YOSHIOKA, J. G. Learning versus skill in rats. *J. genet. Psychol.*, 1932, 41, 406–16. 37.

YOUNG, W. C. Genetic and psychological determinants of sexual behavior patterns. In Hoagland, H. (Ed.) *Hormones, Brain Function and Behavior*. New York: Academic Press, 1957. Pp. 75–98. *9.*

ZIMMERMAN, R. Kreuzungs versuche zwischen Wild-kaninchen und zahmen Pelzkaninchen. *Berl. tierarztl. Wschr.*, 1916, 32, 213. *9.*

SUBJECT INDEX

For Product Safety Concerns and Information please contact our EU representative GPSR@taylorandfrancis.com Taylor & Francis Verlag GmbH, Kaufingerstraße 24, 80331 München, Germany